PREFACE AND CAUTION

DO NOT BUY THIS BOOK BEFORE YOU READ THIS WARNING!

It is not like any other medical book you may have read. It is informal and does not obey generally accepted publishers' conventions.
BUT:

1) It contains a unique and plentiful collection of representative ECGs--more than 450!

2) The unusual "horizontal" presentation was chosen in order to present the majority of tracings with a full-size format.

3) It manifests a healthy scorn for the expensive prevalence of computerized Misinterpretations.

4) Many EKGs with rhythm abnormalities are provided with ladder-diagram analysis to foster logical stepwise interpretation.

5) It does not offer pages and pages of References seldom if ever to be consulted.

If you can tolerate such academic heresy, this book is for you. Enjoy--and hopefully learn!

WN
HM
DS

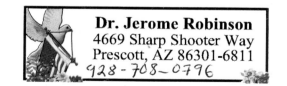

Dr. Jerome Robinson
4669 Sharp Shooter Way
Prescott, AZ 86301-6811
928-708-0796

Concepts
and Cautions in Electrocardiography

First Edition

William P. Nelson, M.D.
Director of Cardiology Education
Saint Joseph Hospital
Denver, Colorado

Henry J.L. Marriott, M.D.
Professor of Clinical Medicine
University of South Florida College of Medicine
Tampa, Florida

Douglas D. Schocken, M.D.
Professor of Medicine
University of South Florida College of Medicine
Tampa, Florida

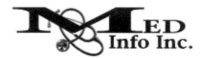

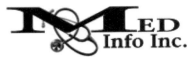

Cover photograph is used with permission and is courtesy of:

Einthoven Foundation
Department of Cardiology
Leiden University Medical Center
P.O. Box 9600, 2300 RC Leiden
The Netherlands
Email: info@einthoven.nl

Library of Congress Control Number: 2006935435

Care has been taken to confirm the accuracy of the information presented and to describe generally accepted practices. However, the authors, editors, and publisher are not responsible for errors or omissions or for any consequences from application of the information in this book and make no warranty, expressed or implied, with respect to the currency, completeness, or accuracy of the contents of the publication. Application of this information in a particular situation remains the professional responsibility of the practitioner.

To purchase additional copies of this book, fax orders to (866) 779-5922, or order online at www.MDpocket.com.

MedInfo Inc.
1650 Irma Drive, Suite 17D
Northglenn, Colorado 80233

Printed in the United States of America
ISBN: 0-9765440-3-2
ISBN-13: 978-0-9765440-3-6

Contents

DEDICATION

With gratitude to the many "students" from whom we have learned.

AN INTRODUCTION

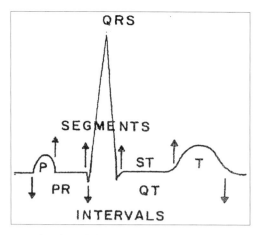

The heart is an electrically activated mechanical pump, and the interpretation of its electrical activity provides important information. The recording of the amplitude of the electrical signal on a time axis constitutes the electrocardiogram (EKG--some prefer the abbreviation ECG). Components of the EKG waveform are familiar to all and will not be discussed at this time. In the illustration, note the *intervals* and *segments* of the typical EKG recording.

Several generalizations regarding the EKG should be made before proceeding further.

1. Once a few basic concepts are grasped, there is little mystique in the EKG; most concepts make sense, and only minimal "memorization" is required.

2. In some circumstances, there is considerable precision in the EKG (e.g. arrhythmias), but in others there is not. The range of normal is wide, and there is overlap between normal and abnormal. The EKG should be regarded as an imprecise tool and too much should not be expected of it. Thus, the patient may have serious heart disease, with little abnormality in the tracing or no detectable heart disease but an abnormal tracing.

3. The EKG must be interpreted in relation to other aspects of the patient's evaluation and always compared to previous tracings, when available.

4. The limb and precordial leads represent differing vantage points of the same event, and do not "look at" particular areas of the heart.

5. The computer is a poor substitute for the human intellect. Computer errors are common and sometimes disastrous!

P-QRS-T analysis is made from three variables:
Amplitude (millivolts)
Duration (milliseconds)
Direction (electrical axis)

Amplitude of Deflections:
The EKG components must be compared to a known electrical signal. By convention, the normal standardization is that 10 mm of stylus excursion is equal to 1 mV of electrical discharge. In the current electrocardiograph, the reference standardization impulse is automatically inserted at the beginning or end of the recording.

Duration of Deflections and Intervals:
At normal recording speed (25 mm/sec.) each small box on the paper represents 0.04 sec. (40 millisec.) and the five boxes between darker vertical lines, thus, define a time of 0.20 sec. (200 millisec.).

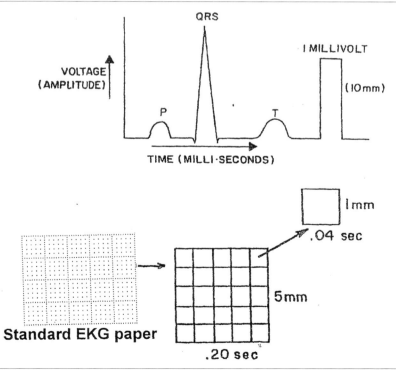

Standard EKG paper

Although the duration of some of events varies with the heart rate, the upper limits of normal, for practical purposes (and for the time being), may be considered to be the following:

P wave - 0.12 sec. (120 msec.)
PR interval - 0.20 sec. (200 msec.)
QRS duration - 0.10 sec. (100 msec.)
Q to the end of T interval - 0.40 sec. (400 msec.) at a heart rate of 60/min.

Determination of the heart rate at a glance: if P-P (or R-R) intervals are separated from each other by one major division (0.20 sec.), the rate is 300/min.; if by two such intervals, the rate is 150/min. This leads to an easy rule: divide the number of divisions separating events into 300 and an approximate rate is obtained. Thus, in the example shown: 300 divided by five= 60/min. For a more accurate assessment of heart rate, the illustration below may be used, however, there is little merit in spending time to determine the *exact* heart rate, and an approximate rate is usually adequate.

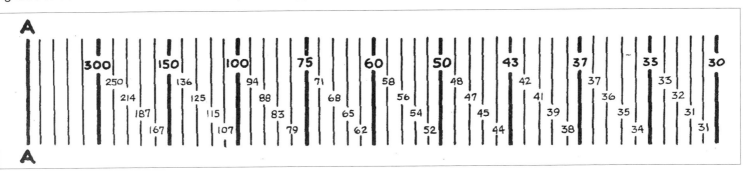

Direction of Deflections:

Essential in electrocardiography is an understanding of the direction (electrical axis) that can be defined for each of the EKG deflections. The easiest way to do this is by envisioning each deflection as a <u>vector</u>, recalling that a vector has a magnitude, direction, and sense (positive or negative). Thus, for example, the QRS deflection on any given lead can be easily measured for amplitude (magnitude) and a composite of leads allows us to define its direction.

As illustrated in the figure below, the projection of the QRS vector on any given lead can be considered as though a light source cast a shadow of the vector on that lead. When the lead is given an arbitrarily polarity, a vector pointing toward the positive pole will be represented as an upright (positive) deflection and one directed toward the negative pole will be represented as a downward (negative) deflection.

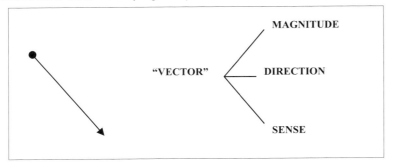

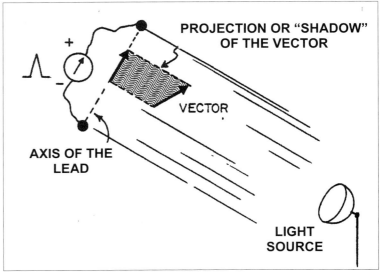

With a moment's reflection on the illustration, it is obvious that if the vector lies *parallel* to the axis of the lead, the shadow cast will be identical to the original vector. Similarly when the vector is *perpendicular* to the axis of the lead, it will cast no shadow, and its representation on that lead will therefore be none (isoelectric). Using a simple concept we can formulate two easy rules for determination of the electrical axis of any deflection:

1. The vector is parallel to the lead with the largest deflection.
2. The vector is perpendicular to the lead with the smallest deflection.

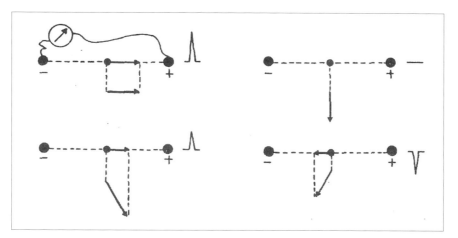

In deciding on the polarity of any given EKG complex it must be realized that in most cases this consists of a biphasic deflection (i.e. one that is partly positive and partly negative). To establish the <u>mean</u> vector, the algebraic sum of positive and negative deflection must be assessed.

The Limb Leads, The Einthoven Triangle, The Triaxial and Hexaxial Reference Figures

The original leads used for EKG recording were <u>bipolar</u> limb leads, connecting the right arm, left arm, and left leg.
The bipolar limb leads and their polarity are depicted in the figure.
Lead I: The potential difference between the right arm and left arm (the left arm is the positive pole).
Lead II: The potential difference between right arm and left leg (the left leg is positive).
Lead III: The potential difference between left arm and left leg (the left leg is the positive pole).

When the three bipolar limb leads are depicted as being joined together, the Einthoven isosceles triangle is constructed, and the leads reflect the cardiac electrical activity as though the heart was in the center of the triangle. It is convenient to relocate the leads in the diagram as though they shared a common center point. Now the bipolar limb leads can be envisioned as constituting the diameters of a circle ("spokes of a wheel"). This transposition of leads does not alter their angular relationship, and the three leads divide a 360 degree circle into six zones of 60° each. This is the so-called <u>triaxial reference figure</u> and it is used to define the vectoral direction in degrees. By convention, 0° on the reference figure is located at the positive pole of lead I. Departures from this, in a clockwise direction, are positive degrees; in a counterclockwise direction they are negative degrees. Thus, the perpendicular to lead I, pointing inferiorly, is (+) 90°.

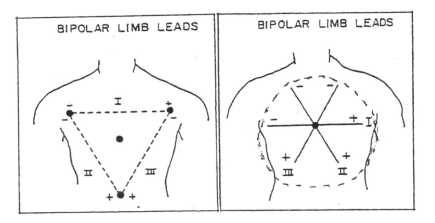

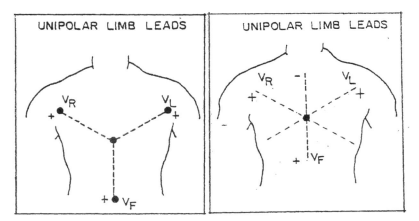

The <u>unipolar limb leads</u> are constructed with a positive pole and an indifferent electrode of zero potential. Thus, as shown in the figure: **1**. In lead aVR, the right arm is positive.
           2. In lead aVL, the left arm is positive.
           3. In lead aVF, the left foot is positive.

The unipolar limb leads can be visualized as additional diameters of the circle (as additional spokes in the wheel) and their lead axes bisect the 60 degree angles established by the bipolar leads.

Using all six leads, known as the "frontal plane leads," we have the <u>hexaxial reference figure</u> with which it is possible to define the axis of the vector more accurately, since the angular separation between the leads is now 30°. Note that the unipolar limb leads do not add new information, but merely adds some precision in electrical axis determination. Note also the relationship of the unipolar to the bipolar leads. Lead aVF is the perpendicular of lead I; aVL is the perpendicular of lead II; and aVR the perpendicular of lead three. With a little practice you can quickly draw a reference figure. If the lead designations are placed as shown in the illustration, the <u>positive pole</u> of each is indicated. Little practices is required, using the two rules already defined, to become proficient in defining the electrical axis. At first it is a rewarding exercise to actually plot the vector of the EKG component under consideration; later the reference figure can be visualized and the axis determined at a glance.

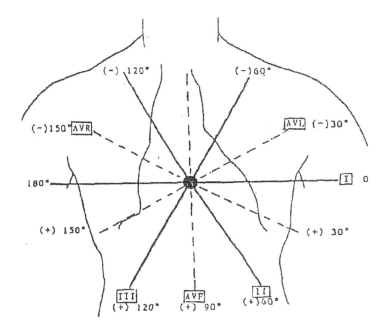

4

To start, it is valuable to assign the vector a *general direction* in a quadrant, using the "I and aVF rule." Since leads I and aVF are perpendicular to each other, they identify four quadrants which can be designated as follows:

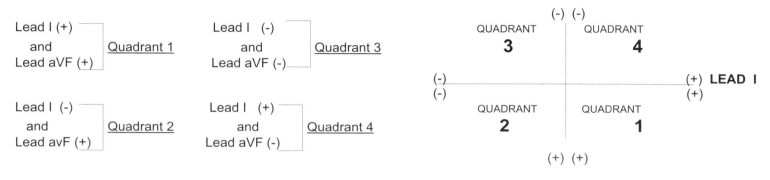

Lead I (+)
and   Quadrant 1
Lead aVF (+)

Lead I (-)
and   Quadrant 3
Lead aVF (-)

Lead I (-)
and   Quadrant 2
Lead avF (+)

Lead I (+)
and   Quadrant 4
Lead aVF (-)

(-) (-)

QUADRANT 3	QUADRANT 4

(-)   (+) **LEAD I**
(-)   (+)

QUADRANT 2	QUADRANT 1

(+) (+)

LEAD aVF

Using this rule, you can, at a glance, determine the general orientation of the electrical event.

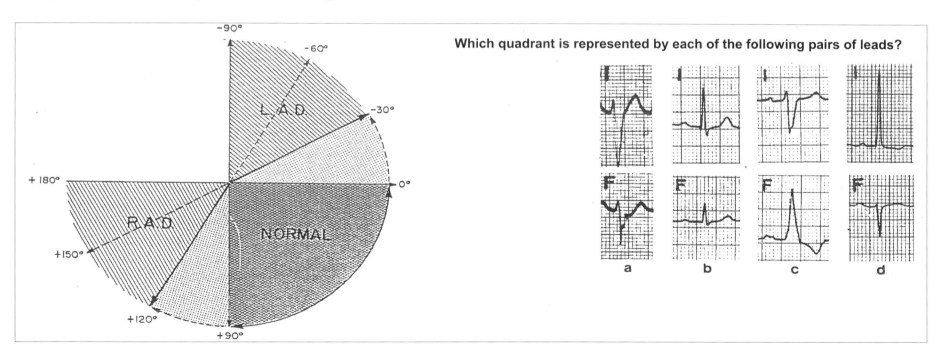

Which quadrant is represented by each of the following pairs of leads?

a   b   c   d

5

P Wave Axis

In the normal individual, the mean axis of the P wave has a limited range of approximately (+) 30° to (+) 70°. If the P wave is directed more leftward and superiorly (inverted in leads III and aVF), it may be inferred that the pacemaker has been displaced in the low atrium. In chronic obstructive lung disease, the P wave axis is commonly (+) 90°.

QRS Axis

The electrical axis of the mean QRS vector has a normal range that depends on age. In infancy, we all show "right ventricular preponderance", and in childhood, the QRS axis may normally be located in quadrant 2. In the normal young adult, it is situated in quadrant 1--between 0° and 90°. In the older adult, it may shift leftward in quadrant 4 to (-) 30 degrees. After childhood, an electrical axis beyond (+) 90° constitutes right axis deviation; an axis shift beyond (-) 30° constitutes left axis deviation. There is disagreement about the zone between 0° and (-) 30°. Some regard it as left axis deviation, others think of it is within the normal range. The computer begs the issue with the term "leftward axis", but this is uninformative. We will regard a *single* tracing with a QRS axis of less than (-) 30° as normal. Of importance is the comparison of serial tracings. If an earlier EKG showed an axis of (+) 60° and the current tracing shows (-) 15°, left axis has developed. Possible causes for these abnormal electrical axes will be discussed subsequently.

T wave Axis

In general, the electrical axis of the T wave vector tends to parallel that of the QRS vector. In bygone days, this observation led to the rule: "the T-wave is upright in leads in which the QRS vector is upright". When both are plotted, the angular separation between the two vectors is called the QRS-T angle. It does not normally exceed 60°. Causes of "wide QRS-T angle" will be discussed later.

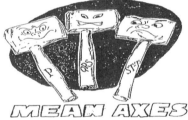

MEAN AXES

For some practice with determination of the mean electrical axis of the EKG components, cover the answers and try plotting the axis for the P wave, QRS, and T-wave in the following examples.

Example #1

The P wave is (+) in both leads I and aVF and is located in quadrant 1. It is smallest (isoelectric) in lead aVL and, thus, it is perpendicular to that lead--P axis = (+) 60°.....
The QRS complex is (+) in leads I and aVF and, thus, is also in quadrant 1. Since it is smallest in lead III, it is perpendicular to that lead--QRS axis = (+) 30°.....
The T wave is (-) in lead I and (+) in aVF and is located in quadrant 2. It is smallest in lead aVR, thus, the T vector must be perpendicular to lead aVR--T axis = (+) 120°......
The QRS-T angle is the separation between the axis of the QRS vector (+ 30°) and the T wave vector (+ 120°) = 90°--an abnormality.

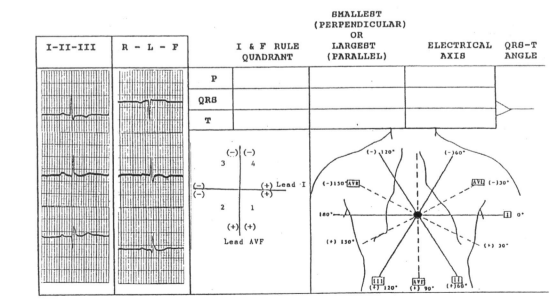

Example #2

The P wave is virtually isoelectric in lead I and is (-) in lead aVF.
Thus, it is reasonably perpendicular to lead I--axis = (-) 90°.
The QRS complex is (+) in lead I and negative in lead aVF and is
therefore in quadrant 4. It is most isoelectric in lead II. The
perpendicular to II, in quadrant four, defines an axis of (-) 30°.
The T wave is (+) in lead I and isoelectric in aVF and is located
at 0°. The angular separation between the QRS axis (- 30°) and
the T wave axis (0°) is 30°--within the normal range.

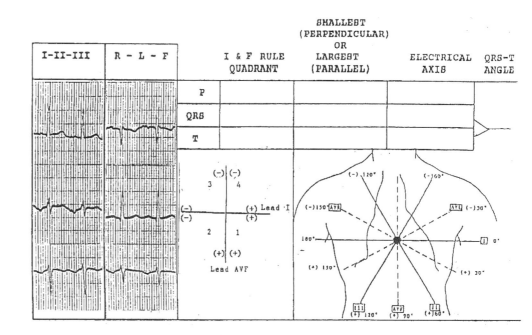

I-II-III	R - L - F	I & F RULE QUADRANT	SMALLEST (PERPENDICULAR) OR LARGEST (PARALLEL)	ELECTRICAL AXIS	QRS-T ANGLE
P					
QRS					
T					

Example #3

With fewer words, but the same concept;

P wave = (+) in lead I
= Isoelectric aVF → **Axis = 0°**

QRS complex = (-) in lead I   Quadrant 2
= (+) in aVF   Isoelectric in aVR → **Axis = (+) 120°**

T wave = (+) in lead I   Quadrant 4
= (-) in aVF   Isoelectric in aVR → **Axis = (-) 60°**

QRS-T angle = 180°--which is markedly abnormal....

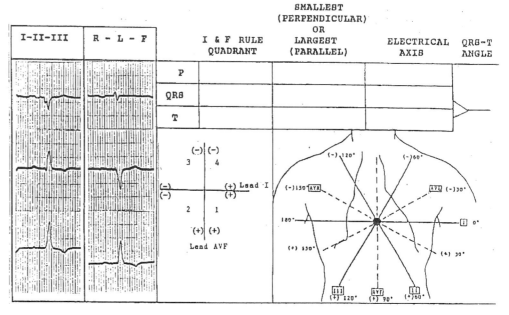

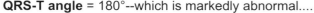

I-II-III	R - L - F	I & F RULE QUADRANT	SMALLEST (PERPENDICULAR) OR LARGEST (PARALLEL)	ELECTRICAL AXIS	QRS-T ANGLE
P					
QRS					
T					

Example #4

P wave = (+) in lead I   <u>Quadrant 4</u>
    = (−) in aVF   Isoelectric in II   → **Axis = (−) 30°**

QRS complex = (+) in lead I   <u>Quadrant 1</u>
        = (+) in aVF   Isoelectric in aVL → **Axis = (+) 60°**

T wave = (−) in lead I   <u>Quadrant 2</u>
    = (+) in aVF   Isoelectric in aVR   → **Axis = (+) 120°**

QRS-T angle = 60°

Example #5

P wave = (+) in lead I   <u>Quadrant 1</u>
    = (+) in aVF   Isoelectric in aVL   → **Axis = (+) 60°**

QRS complex = (+) in lead I   <u>Quadrant 4</u>
        = (−) in aVF   Isoelectric in aVR → **Axis = (−) 60°**

T wave = (+) in lead I   <u>Quadrant 1</u>
    = (+) in aVF   Isoelectric in aVL   → **Axis = (+) 60°**

QRS-T angle = (+) 120°--markedly abnormal

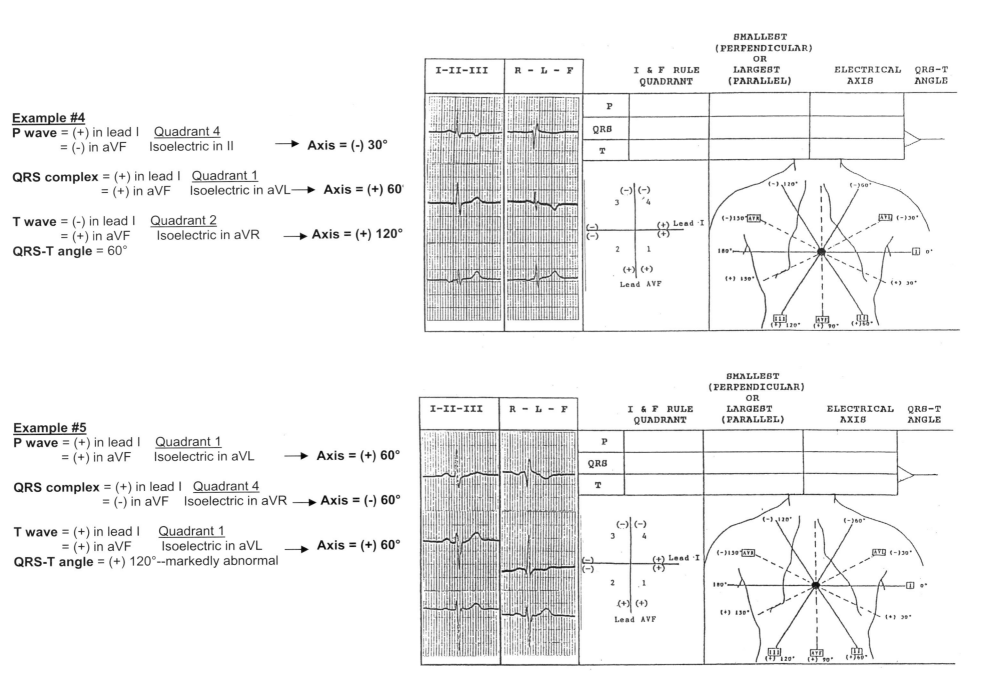

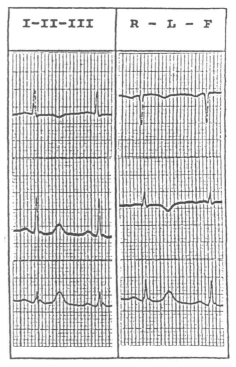

These examples were selected because the P-QRS-T components are
<u>reasonably isoelectric</u> (smallest) in a given lead (or largest in another lead).
Obviously, such is not always the case, but the principles still
apply. In the tracing shown there is no isoelectric lead for the QRS complex,
but it is (+) in both leads I and aVF, and is therefore situated in quadrant 1.
Since it is of small amplitude in leads III and aVL, it must be "almost perpendicular"
to those leads. If the QRS complex was isoelectric to lead III, the electrical axis
would be (+) 30°; and if isoelectric to aVL it would be (+) 60°. A reasonable
compromise is that the mean axis of the QRS is (+) 45°. Thus, with little practice,
it is possible to provide an assessment of direction with <u>adequate precision</u>.
Determination of the exact electrical axis is rarely necessary.

An example of an "indeterminate QRS axis". Note that
the complex is reasonably isoelectric in <u>all leads</u>, with
early and late forces oriented in opposite directions.
This pattern can be normal in youth, but is abnormal in
the older adult, and is frequently associated with serious
chronic obstructive pulmonary disease.

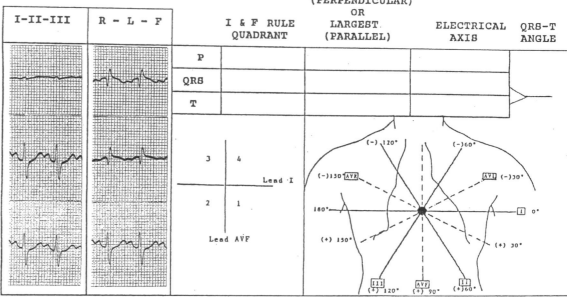

The determination of the "electrical direction" of events is the basis of most of the abnormalities in the EKG. To hone your skills with axis determination, you are invited to review the examples below. Please plot the mean QRS axis, the T wave axis, and the QRS-T angle before looking at the answer at the top of the next page.

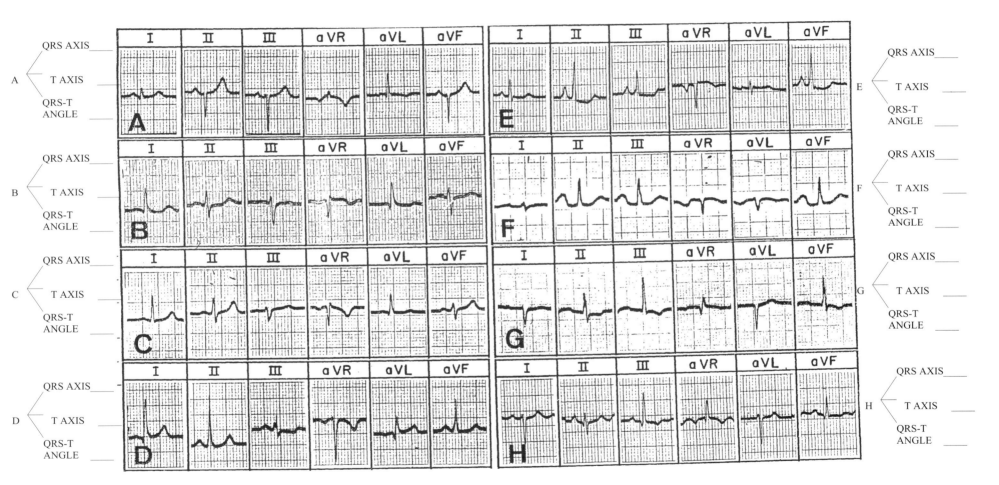

A) QRS = (-) 60° T= (+) 60° QRS-T angle= 120°	**E**) QRS = (+) 60° T = (+) 30° QRS-T angle = 30°
B) QRS = (-) 30° T= (+) 30° QRS-T angle= 60°	**F**) QRS = (+) 90° T = (+) 90° QRS-T angle = 0°
C) QRS = 0° T= (+) 60° QRS-T angle= 60°	**G**) QRS= (+) 120° T = (-) 60° QRS-T angle = 180°
D) QRS = (+) 30° T= (+) 30° QRS-T angle= 0°	**H**) QRS= (+) 150° T = 0° QRS-T angle = 150°

Precordial Leads: The Horizontal Plane

It is obvious that electrical activity exists not only in the frontal plane, but in three dimensions. The precordial leads serve to depict the spatial direction of electrical forces, i.e., their anterior or posterior direction.

Precordial lead placement has arbitrarily been located as follows:

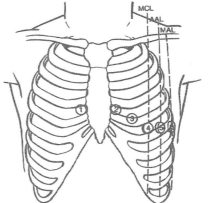

Lead V1: at the fourth intercostals space, just to the right of the sternum
Lead V2: at the fourth intercostals space, just to the left of the sternum
Lead V3: midway between leads V2 and V4
Lead V4: in the midclavicular line, in the fifth intercostals space
Lead V5: in the anterior axillary line, at the same level as lead V4
Lead V6: in the midaxillary line, at the same level as lead V4

We can depict the heart with a transverse "slice" through the chest-the horizontal plane. The precordial leads can then be envisioned as extending from the skin surface through the theoretical center of the heart. The positive pole is the point of electrode placement. Thus, if the electrical activity is directed toward an electrode, it is recorded as a positive event; if directed away, a negative deflection results. If we consider this sequence of ventricular activation, the normal "pattern" in the precordial leads can be appreciated. The first portion of the ventricular myocardium to undergo depolarization is the ventricular septum, with its activation occurring predominantly via the left bundle branch. The resulting multiple electrical wave fronts of septal activation are oriented anteriorly and to the right, and can be depicted by a single vector-vector 1.

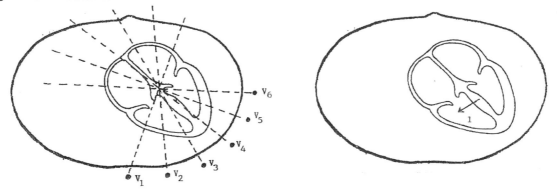

Subsequently, the free walls of the right and left ventricles are rapidly depolarized. The summation of the multiple instantaneous of the left and right ventricles can also be represented by single vector arrows-vector 2. The electrical forces of LV and RV are in opposite directions and, in the adult, those of LV origin exceed the RV forces. The electrical influence of the RV is effectively "erased" and only the dominate LV vector is seen. Thus, the latter portion of the QRS complex is normally oriented left lateral and posterior.

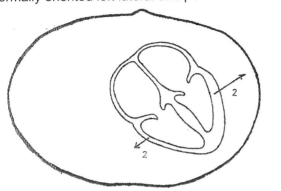 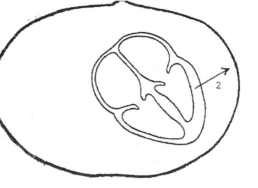 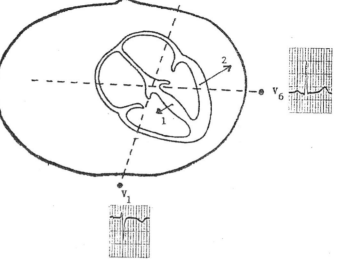

The registration of these vectors in leads V1 and V6 can be easily appreciated. The initial component, vector1, is recorded as a small positive deflection in V1 and a negative deflection in V6. The terminal portion results in a predominant S wave in V1 and R wave in V6.

The other precordial leads serve as additional "vantage points" for these electrical events. In the illustration, note that the axis of lead V3 is reasonably perpendicular to both vectors 1 and 2. Theoretically, this lead should show no deflection (i.e., "isoelectric"), but instead it records positive and negative forces of equal size. This is the so-called "transition lead" and indicates the point at which the QRS morphology changes from predominantly negative to predominantly positive. We will encounter examples of "early transition" and "late transition" and their meaning will be reviewed at that time.

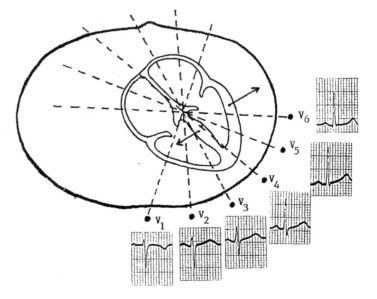

The QRS morphology warrants further dissection. The first upright deflection is an R wave. If it is preceded by a negative deflection, that deflection is a Q Wave; and any negative deflection that follows the R wave is an S wave. If a second positive wave follows the S wave, it is called R' (R prime). When the ventricular complex consists of a single negative deflection without any positive waves, it is described as a QS complex. A handy convention is the use of capital letters (Q, R, S) for the large waves and small letters (q, r, s) for smaller waves. Capitals are generally used for waves measuring 5 mm or more; small letters for waves of less than 5 mm. If the entirely positive QRS ascends haltingly - stepwise - with a notch early in the upstroke, it may be labeled rR'. Regardless of which waves it contains, even if it doesn't have a Q wave or an S wave, any ventricular complex, by convention, is referred to as the "QRS."

The figure illustrates a variety of ventricular ("QRS") complexes

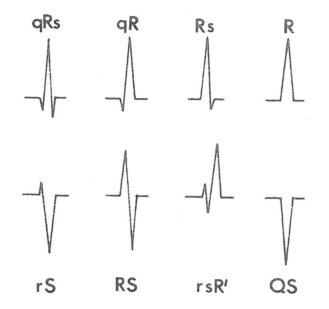

Descriptive labeling of a variety of QRS complexes

MYOCARDIAL ISCHEMIA and INFARCTION

Although all aspects of electrocardiography are informative, perhaps the most important is the recognition of myocardial ischemia and infarction. First, let's review the classical presentation of acute myocardial infarction.

The insult of myocardial infarction mainly involves the left ventricle. For now, pretend that the L.V. walls are the only ones involved in the process (We will discuss right ventricular infarction later). The left ventricle can be envisioned as a cone of muscle, with an aortic valve outlet and a mitral valve inlet. Its three-dimensional character allows separation into five area--inferior wall (**1**), lateral wall (**2**), apex (**3**), anterior (**4**), and posterior walls (**5**)--and these are the zones where infarction can be identified. Although some myocardial infarctions are localized to one of the areas, many "spill" from one to another (e.g. inferolateral, inferoposterior, anterolateral, etc.).

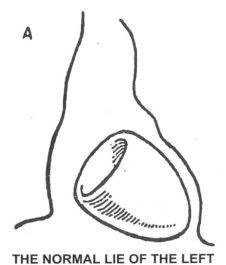

THE NORMAL LIE OF THE LEFT VENTRICLE

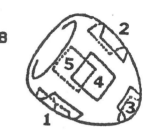

THE FIVE REGIONS OF THE HEART WHERE AN INFARCT MAY OCCUR

The illustration depicts an idealized sequence of ventricular activation.
A) Pretend that left ventricular depolarization consists of seven areas (vectors) that occur simultaneously. The influence of vector #1 "counterbalances" that of #7, vector #2 negates vector #6, and #3 partially removes the influence of vector #5.
B) The end result of these vector subtractions is the "mean QRS vector".
C) If there is a lateral wall infarction, the areas reflected by vectors #6 and 7 are no longer present.
D) Vectors #1 and 2 have no opposing vector and, thus, redirect initial forces to the right and inferior. The terminology for the new initial vector varies, but the concept is straightforward. The rule becomes, the "initial forces" (Q waves) become oriented <u>away</u> from the infarct zone--the "dead zone" <u>*depolarization*</u> effect.

14

The <u>repolarization</u> abnormalities occurring with infarction include those involving the ST segment ("injury") and T-wave ("ischemia"). The injury effect occurs as the process of myocardial infarction begins, and indicates that the process is <u>acute</u>. Since these are the cells that are active in this portion of repolarization, the ST segment ("injury vector") points <u>toward</u> the involved area. Cells that are more remote from the central dead zone can depolarize and initiate repolarization appropriately. However, they are not normal and the major portion of their repolarization (the T-wave) is either less rapid or decreased in amplitude, and opposing areas are dominant. Thus, the ischemic T vector points <u>away</u> from the area of abnormality.

The illustration depicts a myocardial infarction with a central dead area, surrounded by injured and ischemic zones. The vectoral directions of the injury vector (ST), dead zone and ischemic T vector of a lateral wall myocardial infarction are shown. The ST segment is directed toward the injured zone. It would be elevated in leads I and aVL and (reciprocally) depressed in leads III and aVF. The initial forces (IF) are oriented away from the "dead zone" and, since they are directed toward the negative pole of leads I and aVL, they register as <u>Q waves</u> in these leads (and frequently in leads with a similar vantage--leads V5 and V6). The T vector (T) becomes oriented away from the lateral wall and is inscribed negative in leads I and aVL. The generalizations about the direction of these abnormal events apply to *all* areas of myocardial infarction. The examples to follow show common locations and typical EKG's.

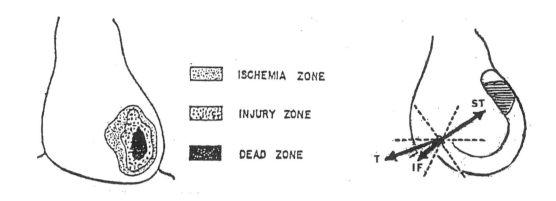

QRS–ST –T EVENTS IN ACUTE MYOCARDIAL INFARCTION

In the typical evolution of acute myocardial infarction, the direction of abnormal depolarization and repolarization vectors can be considered as <u>INDICATIVE</u> changes. Because of the orientation and polarity of the lead axes, for every indicative vectoral direction there must be a <u>RECIPROCAL</u> event. These changes may occur during the acute event or evolve in the hours and days following the initial injury. This is outlined below.

<u>**INDICATIVE**</u>   <u>**RECIPROCAL**</u>

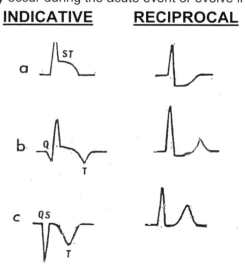

ECG CHANGES OF MYOCARDIAL INFARCTION
<u>INDICATIVE</u> – Any or all of:
    Significant Q waves ("necrosis")
    ST-T elevation ("injury")
    T-wave inversion ("ischemia")

<u>RECIPROCAL</u> – Any or all of:
    Increased height of R wave
    ST-T depression
    Tall, symmetrical T waves

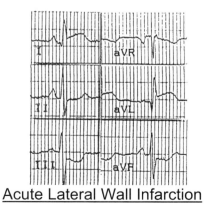

Acute Lateral Wall Infarction

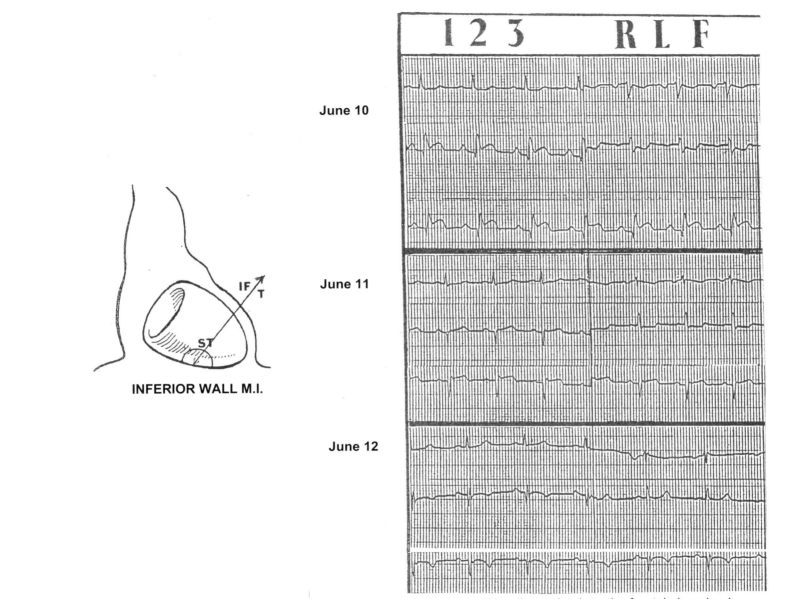

INFERIOR WALL M.I.

An example of the evolution of an acute inferior myocardial infarction. For now, attention will be directed only to the frontal plane leads.
On June 10, the mean QRS axis is (+) 60°. The ST segment is elevated in leads II, III, and aVF--*the indicative leads*--and are reciprocally depressed in leads I and aVL. The ST vector is oriented at (+) 120°, and directed toward the left ventricular inferior wall. Initial forces (IF)--Q waves--are already present in the leads with ST elevation. On June 11, the ST segment elevation is receding. The Q waves in II, III, and aVF have increased in depth and breadth, resulting in a left shift of the QRS axis to (-) 60°. On June 12, T wave inversion has developed in the indicative leads, oriented left and superior "away from" the ischemic zone surrounding the infarction.

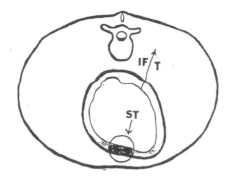

ANTERIOR WALL M.I.

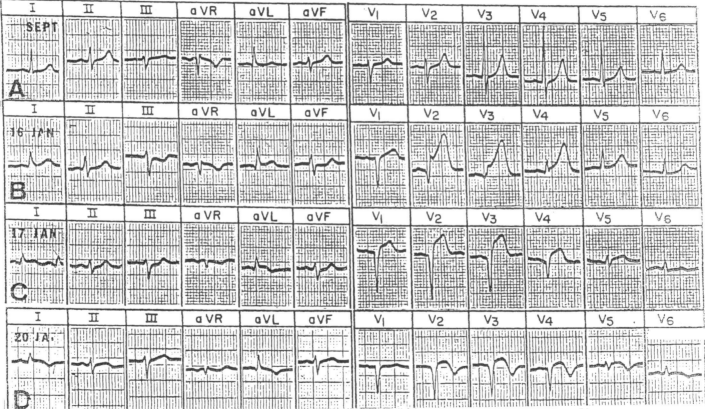

For now, let's ignore the frontal plane leads and concentrate on the horizontal plane. In September, a routine EKG shows normal precordial QRS-ST-T morphology. The large R wave in V3 is probably due to a misplaced electrode. On 16 Jan., there is ST segment elevation in V1-V4; this "injury vector" is oriented toward the anterior wall of the left ventricle, and identifies an acute process. There is already a loss of R waves in leads V1-V3. On 17 Jan., the ST segments remain elevated and there is a "QS" pattern in V1-V4--indicating that the initial forces (IF) have shifted away from the infarcted anterior wall. On 20 Jan., the elevated ST segments continued to recede and the ischemic T vector has appeared.

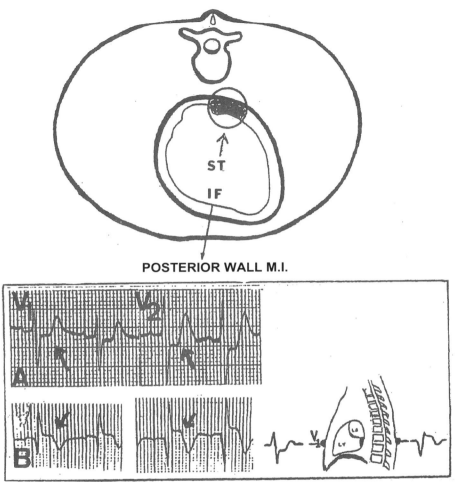

POSTERIOR WALL M.I.

Posterior wall infarctions are a potential problem. The rules regarding vectoral directions apply, but since the precordial leads are only located anteriorly, the recorded pattern is "upside down." Since the ST injury vector is directed toward the involved posterior wall, it is recorded *negative* in V1-V2- V3. Similarly, the "dead zone" effect is directed anteriorly away from the involved area. Thus, initial forces (IF) are recorded as <u>R waves</u> in these leads. With evolution of the infarction, the ischemic T-waves parallel the initial R waves and are upright in V1-V2-V3. **In segment A** - the recorded morphology of a posterior MI in V1-V2 is shown. **In segment B** - the image in A has been inverted and shows the typical "pattern" of an acute infarction--ST elevation, prominent Q waves, and T-wave inversion. This would also be the pattern if posterior chest leads were recorded.

The cases to follow are additional examples of myocardial infarction. Try your hand at interpreting them before reading the legends. See if you agree with the computer interpretation.

```
PR      152   +   Normal sinus rhythm, rate 93 [Now Present]
QRSD     80   -   [Now Absent]   Sinus Tachycardia, rate 109
QT      314   -   [Now Absent]   Multiple atrial premature complexes
QTc     390   -   [Now Absent]   Right axis deviation
              -   [Now Absent]   Right bundle branch block
--AXES--      -   [Now Absent]   Left atrial enlargement
P        69                                    - NORMAL ECG -
QRS      74
T        54
```

**66 YEAR OLD MAN
DO YOU AGREE?**

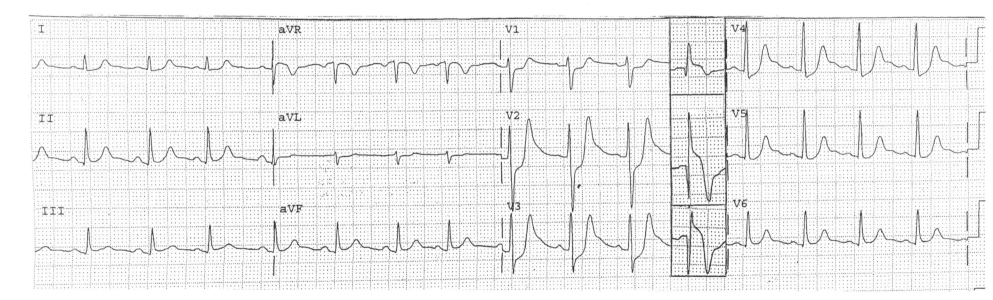

A grievous computer error! The ST segment depression in leads V1-V4 is obvious. It should not be interpreted as "nonspecific depression"--let alone as normal. The pattern is typical of an acute posterior wall MI. The injury vector is oriented toward the involved area and the "dead zone" and T wave vectors oriented away from the posterior wall. The insert has had the leads V1-V3 inverted and the resulting pattern is recognized as that of an acute infarction. Happily, the computer error was recognized and the patient admitted to the hospital.

49 YEAR OLD WOMAN- 12/2
ANY WORRIES??

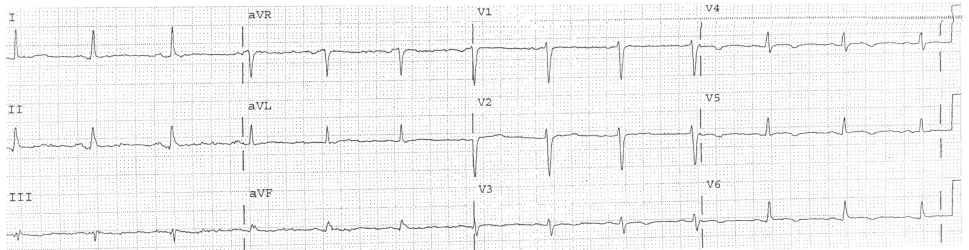

This woman presented with recurring chest discomfort and the EKG above. There are generalized, but nonspecific, T-wave abnormalities. Two days later (below) she retuned with severe chest pain and diffuse and marked T wave inversions. The rise in enzyme markers was not accompanied by ST elevation or the localizing "dead zone" effect of Q waves - but the tracing indicates acute myocardial infarction.

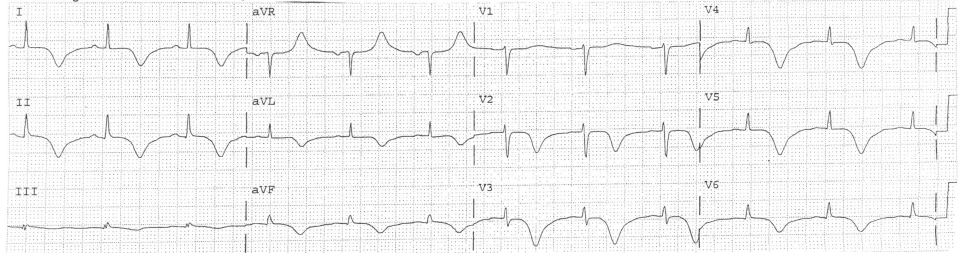

The EKG terminology regarding myocardial infarction has varied through the years. The earliest recognition emphasized the typical presentation with "ST elevation" and "Q waves." With the realization that these features were not always present, there evolved terms that (incorrectly) suggested the anatomy and prognosis of the infarction--"*subendocardial infarction*"--"*non-transmural infarction*"--"*non-Q wave infarction.*" None of these designations provided adequate correlation with clinical severity or postmortem findings. Currently there is recognition that the EKG features may show typical "ST elevation myocardial infarction" (<u>STEMI</u>) or frequently "non-ST elevation myocardial infarction," (<u>NONSTEMI</u>). These cumbersome, but perhaps more accurate, abbreviations are in common use.

73 YEAR OLD WOMAN
YOUR OBSERVATIONS INCLUDE??

RT. CHEST LEADS

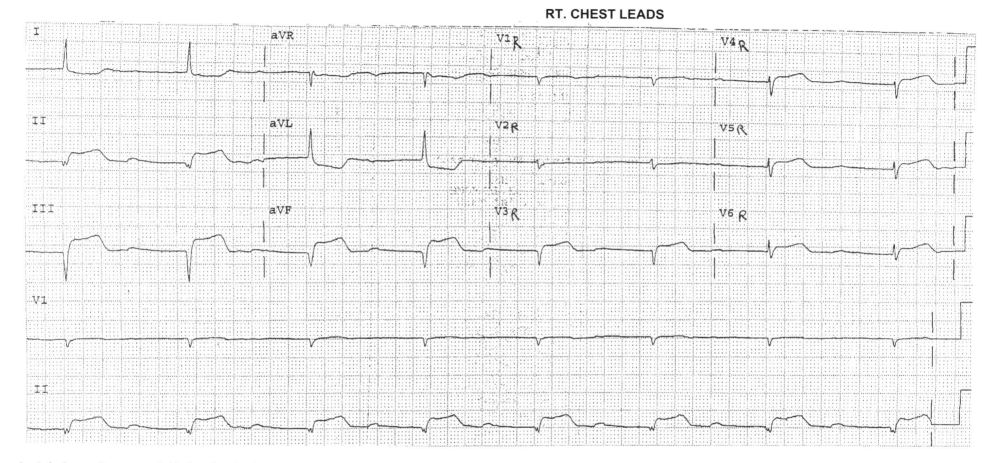

An inferior wall myocardial infarction is always due to occlusion of the posterior descending coronary artery. This vessel is commonly a continuation of the right coronary artery. If the RCA is obstructed near its origin, the branches to the right ventricle will be lost. The result will be an acute inferior M.I. accompanied by infarction of the RV. The EKG manifestation of this is typical evidence of inferior M.I. in the frontal leads, and ST segment elevation in leads recorded over the right chest (V1R to V6R) particularly V4R, V5R or V6R. Patients with RV infarction have an increased incidence of AV block, ventricular arrhythmias, and cardiogenic shock, and a poorer prognosis than those with only a localized inferior M.I. Right chest leads are inexpensive additional "vantage points" that should be recorded with <u>ALL</u> tracings showing acute inferior MI.

This woman has marked sinus bradycardia of 40/min. with a prolonged PR interval of 0.40 sec. The frontal plane leads show an acute inferior M.I. and the ST elevation in V3R to V6R indicates an associated right ventricular infarction.

49 YEAR OLD MAN
WHAT IS THE "BEZOLD-JARISCH" REFLEX??
WHAT Rx??
WHAT IS ESCAPE-CAPTURE BIGEMINI??

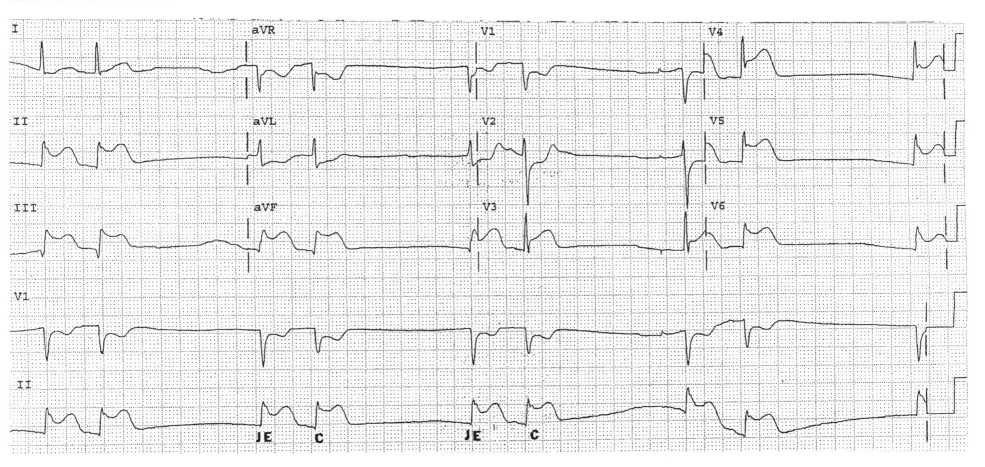

The Bezold-Jarisch reflex occurs when there is activation of ventricular stretch receptors, located (primarily) in the inferior wall of the LV. It is commonly associated with inferior wall infarctions. It causes a vagatonic depression of the sinus and/or AV node, resulting in bradycardia, or AV block, or both; and vasodilatation resulting in hypotension. It is a dangerous combination in a bad setting! If the sinus bradycardia is marked, a junctional "escape" (**JE**) can occur. If the JE is followed by the sluggish sinus node discharge, the P wave can "capture" (**C**) the ventricles, resulting in "escape--capture bigemini." Since the reflex is a vagal influence, it usually is eliminated by IV administration of atropine.

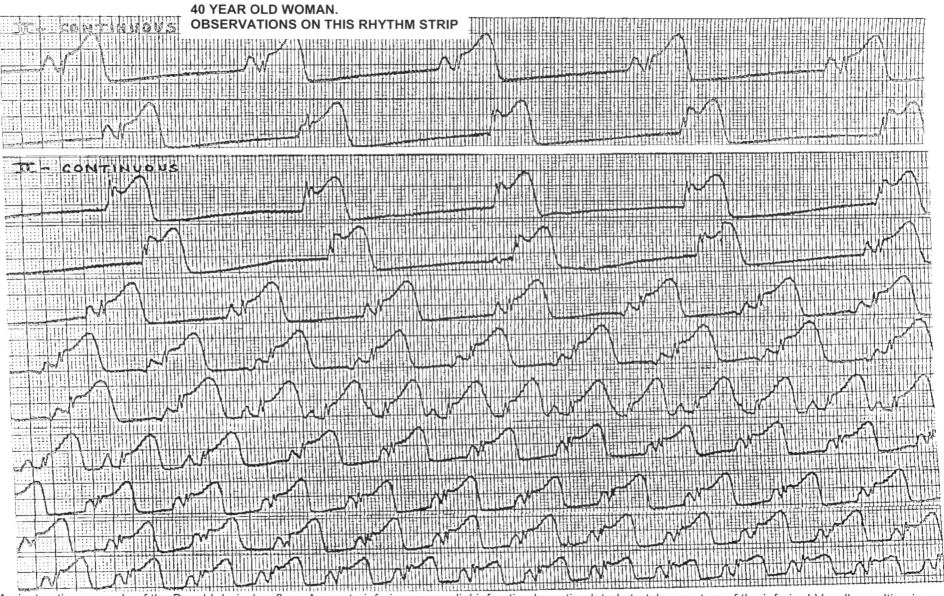

40 YEAR OLD WOMAN.
OBSERVATIONS ON THIS RHYTHM STRIP

An instructive example of the Bezold-Jarisch reflex. An acute inferior myocardial infarction has stimulated stretch receptors of the inferior LV wall, resulting in striking sinus bradycardia. In the second strip, the laggardly P waves are replaced by an escaping junctional focus at a 30/min. The lower continuous recording of lead II shows the prompt and dramatic effect of 1 mg IV atropine. P waves reappear, the rate increases, and the magnitude of the injury current decreases. Her subsequent course was uneventful.

59 YEAR OLD MAN – 3/23 "SIR, I THINK YOUR CHEST PAIN IS DUE TO _____"???

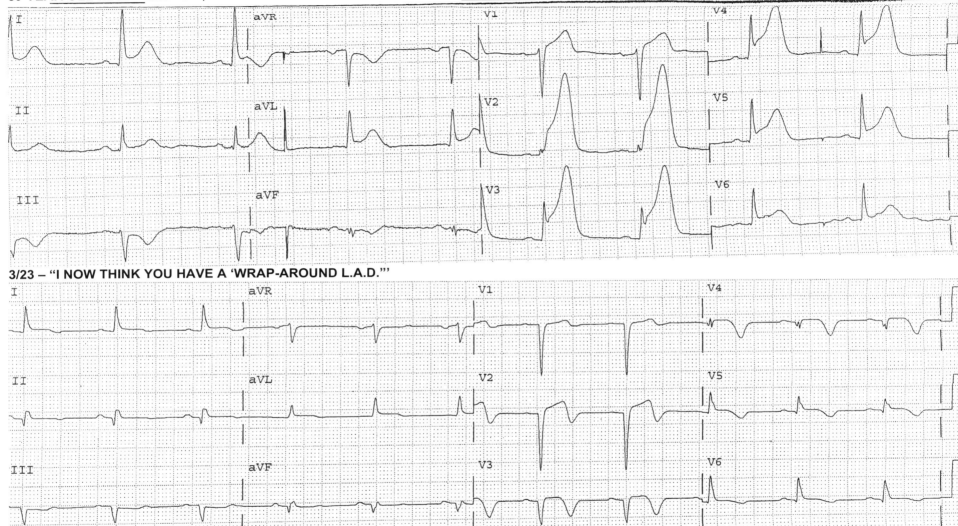

3/23 – "I NOW THINK YOU HAVE A 'WRAP-AROUND L.A.D.'"

The top tracing has ST segment elevation in leads I and aVL, and all the precordial leads, indicating an extensive and anteroseptal--lateral MI. Later in the day, the bottom tracing shows the evolution of the infarction. In addition, there are now Q waves in leads II, III, and aVF, indicating that an inferior wall infarct has joined the anterior. Why this unusual combination? Some of us are born with a left anterior descending coronary artery that "wraps around" the base of the interventricular septum, and supplies the apex and some of the inferior L.V. wall. When the LAD vessel is occluded, part of the inferior wall becomes infarcted--an additional and threatening insult.

24

```
PR      254     (SR     ) . Sinus rhythm, rate 81   - - - - -
QRSD     93     (1AVB   ) . First degree AV block - - - - - - -
QT      423     (LQT    ) . QT Interval long for rate - - -
QTc     491     (SD1AN  ) . Nonspecific Anterior ST depression -

--AXES--
P        76                              - ABNORMAL ECG -
QRS      74
T        74
```

70 YEAR OL WOMAN
MINOR COMPUTER UNDERCALL??

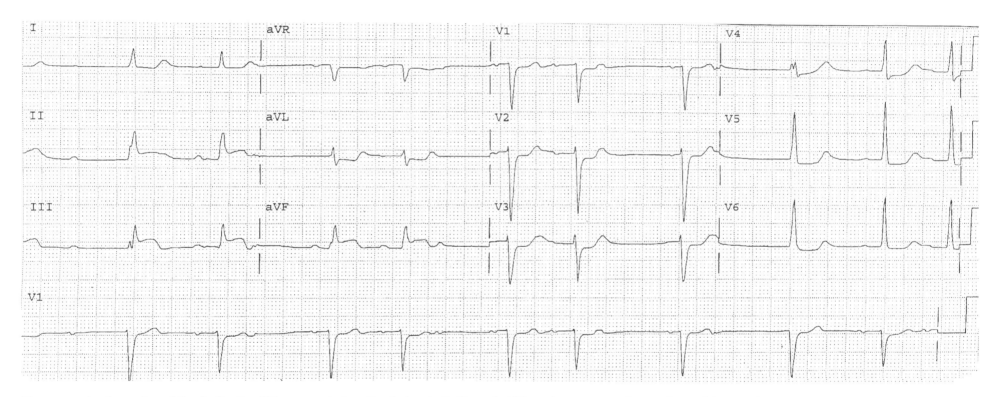

The computer has missed the *indicative* ST segment elevation in leads II, III, and aVF, and accompanying *reciprocal* depression in leads I and aVL. The ST segment depression in the precordial leads should <u>not</u> be regarded as "nonspecific," but rather as a current of injury involving the posterior LV wall. The prolonging PR intervals and "dropped beats" indicate Wenckebach (Type 1) second degree AV block. Type 1 AV block is common with inferior infarction, and if symptomatic, usually responds to atropine.

```
PR     170  . Normal sinus rhythm, rate 90
QRSD   108  . Left axis devation, consider LAFB
QT     344  . Early transition
QTc    421  . Nonspecific Inferior T abnormalities

--AXES--
P       45                          - ABNORMAL ECG -
QRS    -43
T      -10
```

47 YEAR OLD MAN
DO YOU AGREE WITH THE COMPUTER?

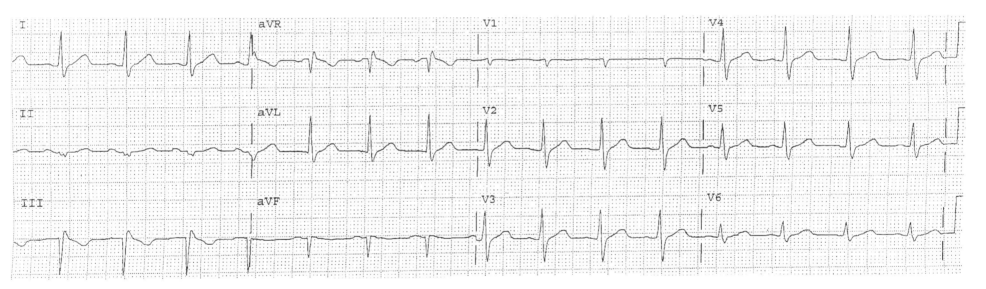

The computer has made a correct observation, but for the wrong reason! The left axis deviation results from the "Q waves" present in leads II, III, and aVF, and is due to an age undetermined inferior myocardial infarction. The "early transition" in the horizontal plane indicates an accompanying posterior infarction--often the case, and frequently ignored!

```
PR     167  . Normal sinus rhythm, rate 72
QRSD    87  - Borderline low voltage in frontal leads
QT     371  - Anterolateral region ST depression
QTc    406  - Consistent with subendocardial injury

--AXES--
P       58                                    - ABNORMAL ECG -
QRS     46
T       76
```

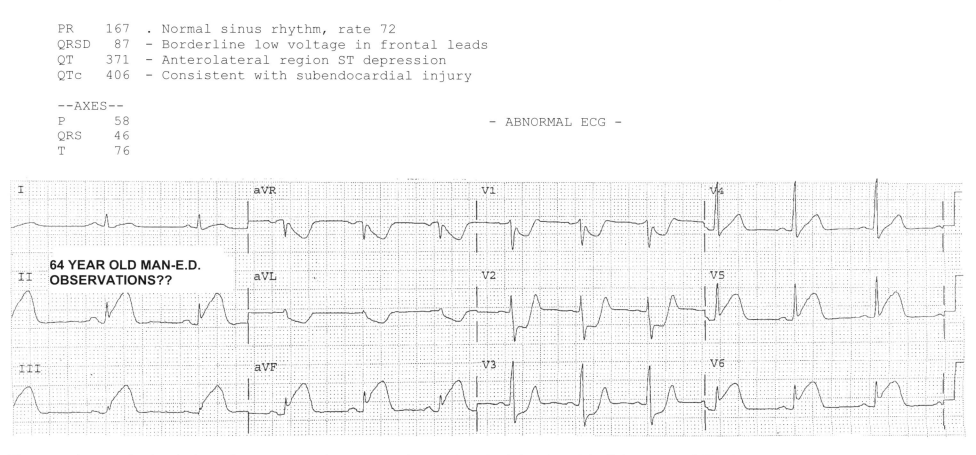

64 YEAR OLD MAN-E.D. OBSERVATIONS??

The computer uses the terminology of yesteryear, and suggests an incorrect anatomic location of the "injury current." The ST segment elevation in frontal leads II, II, and aVF indicate an acute *inferior* MI; the ST depression in V1-2-3 a *posterior* infarction; and the ST elevation in V5-6 a *lateral* MI.

69 YEAR OLD WOMAN
"OUTREACH ECG"
DO YOU AGREE WITH THE COMPUTER?

```
SINUS TACHYCARDIA WITH SHORT PR WITH FREQUENT PREMATURE ECTOPIC
COMPLEXES IN A PATTERN OF BIGEMINY
INDETERMINATE AXIS
PULMONARY DISEASE PATTERN
NONSPECIFIC T WAVE ABNORMALITIES
ABNORMAL ECG
WHEN COMPARED WITH ECG IN 14-OCT 14:09
PREMATURE ECTOPIC COMPLEXS ARE NOW PRESENT
PR INTERVAL HAS DECREASED
```

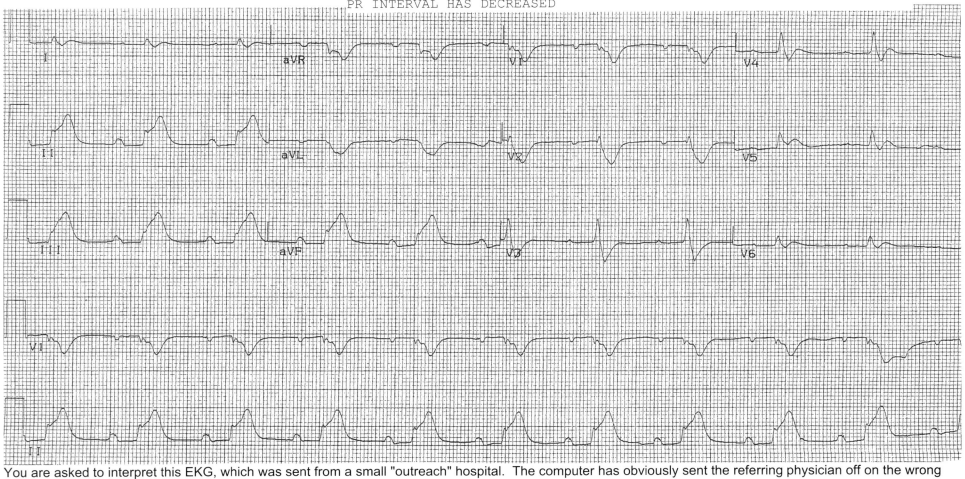

You are asked to interpret this EKG, which was sent from a small "outreach" hospital. The computer has obviously sent the referring physician off on the wrong trail! Corrections include:

1. Sinus P waves are conducted with a <u>long PR interval</u>.
2. No "ectopic complexes" are present.
3. The "nonspecific T waves" are really *specific* ST segment currents of injury, oriented toward the inferior, posterior, and lateral ventricular walls.

73 YEAR OLD MAN —4/22 -13:22 WHAT ARE HYPERACUTE T WAVES?

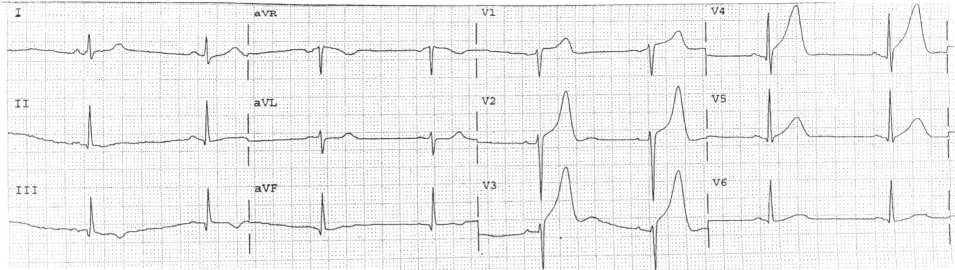

As experience with EKG manifestations of MI grew, observers came up with some interesting and picturesque descriptive terms, one of which was "hyperacute T waves." Although it has no specific meaning, the term emphasizes that the ST segment elevations and tall T waves are sending a message "loud and clear" that an acute infarction is in progress.

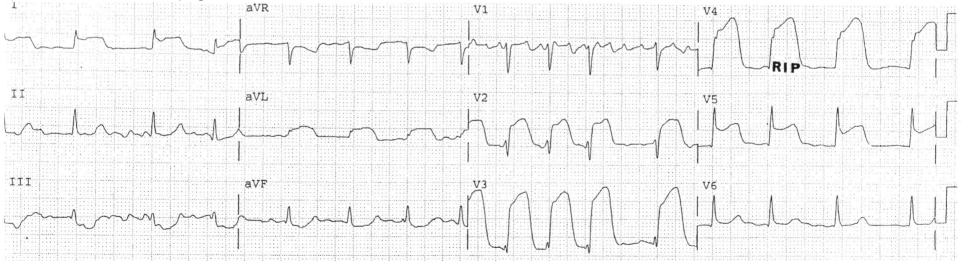

An evident acute anteroseptal-lateral infarction, accompanied by atrial fibrillation. Early interpreters were reminded of familiar objects and labeled the striking repolarization changes as "Tombstone T waves," probably reflecting the grim prognosis at the time.

29

84 YEAR OLD MAN - 8/31 - WHAT IS REPORTED TO BE EVIDENCE OF LEFT MAIN CORONARY ARTERY DISEASE?

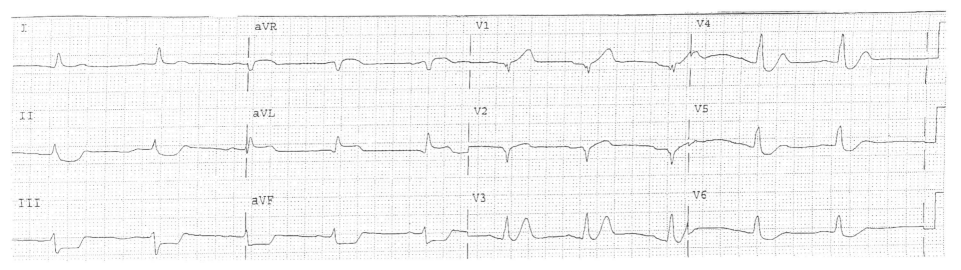

The tracing shows sinus rhythm at 60/min. with low-voltage QRS complexes and diffuse repolarization abnormality. The frontal plane leads I and aVL show ST elevation consistent with acute lateral wall "injury," and the precordial leads probable septal MI--what else? There have been several articles indicating that ST segment elevation in lead aVR, which is more than that in lead V1, provides evidence that there is _left main_ coronary artery occlusive disease. Consider this: if there is left main obstruction, both the left anterior descending and circumflex arteries are compromised. The resulting ST "injury" vector becomes the result of two wavefronts - as diagrammed. The resultant vector is oriented to the right and superior, and would be recorded (+) in aVR. Look for this possibility and for angiographic correlation.

CIRC

LAD

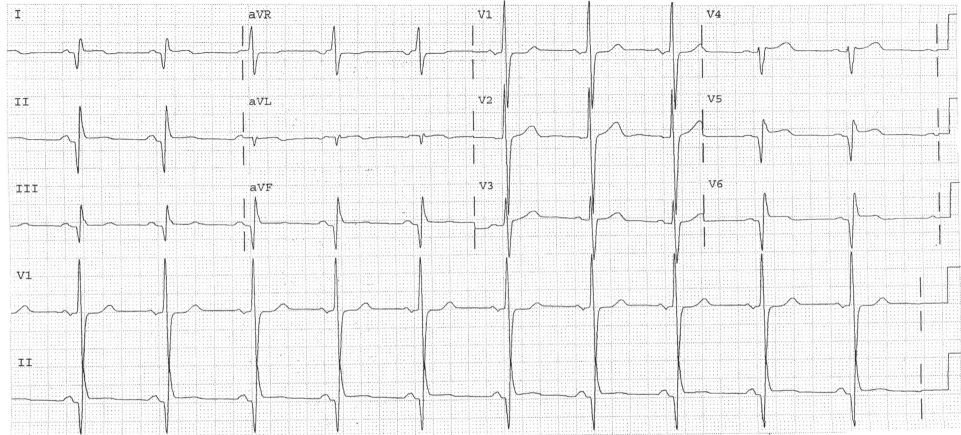

In the frontal plane leads, an inferior and lateral wall infarction both participate in altering the initial forces (Q waves). The resultant vectoral direction is a composite of these two wavefronts. Inferior MI directs the early events to the *left* and *superior*, and the forces of lateral MI become oriented *right* and *inferior*. The vectoral "addition" results in a direction right and superior, and records Q waves in all the limb leads (except for the broad R wave in aVR). The precordial leads display a prominent R wave in V1 and V2 and Q waves in V5 and V6, indicating a probable posterior MI and confirming the lateral wall contribution to the extensive infarction.

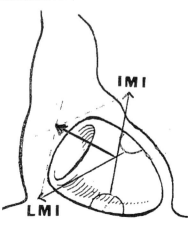

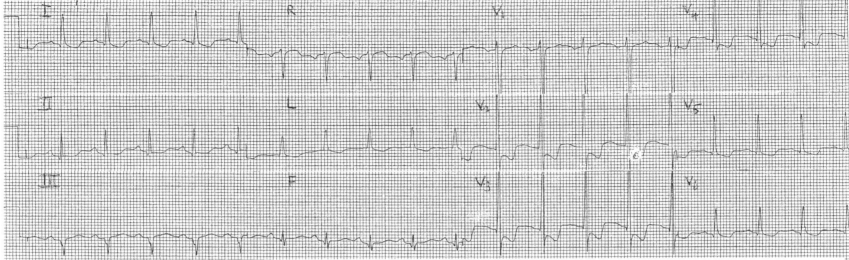

12/8-ANY EVIDENCE OF M.I. WHAT IS "NORMALIZATION BY CANCELLATION"??

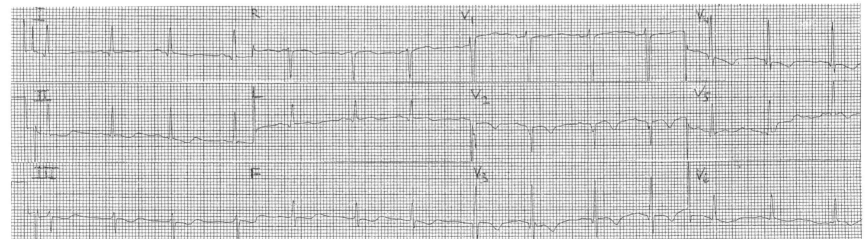

The importance of serial tracings is seen in this "Case of the Canceling Infarcts." In the top tracing, the "inferior Q waves" and tall R waves in V1-V2 indicates a recent (? acute) inferior--posterior MI. In the bottom EKG, the Q waves that had been present in leads II, III and aVF have disappeared, and have been replaced by small Q waves in leads I and aVL. Under more common circumstances, these Q waves might be regarded as insignificant; however Q waves are now present in V1-2-3. The reorientation of *initial* forces, due to an anterolateral MI, has erased the evidence of the prior inferior MI.

41 year old man – 10/3 – 14:13

10/3 – 14:16 Anything else?   **Right Chest Leads**

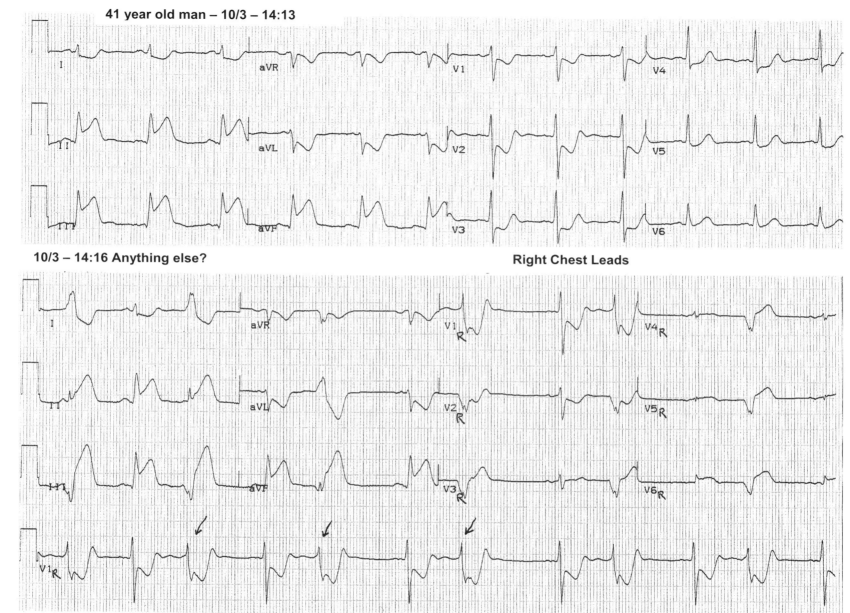

The ST segment elevation in leads II, III, and aVF, accompanied by reciprocal depression in leads I and aVL, identifies an acute inferior M.I. The ST segment depression in the precordial leads incriminates a posterior wall infarction. A tracing three minutes later, obtained with the <u>right chest leads</u>, shows ST segment elevation in lead V4R, V5R and V6R indicating that the right ventricle shares in the destructive process. The presence of VPCs (arrows) with every sinus-conducted complex is an ominous addition.

57 YEAR OLD WOMAN
DO YOU AGREE WITH THE COMPUTER?

SINUS TACHYCARDIA
OTHERWISE NORMAL ECG
WHEN COMPARED WITH ECG OF _____
VENT. RATE HAS INCREASED BY 58 BPM

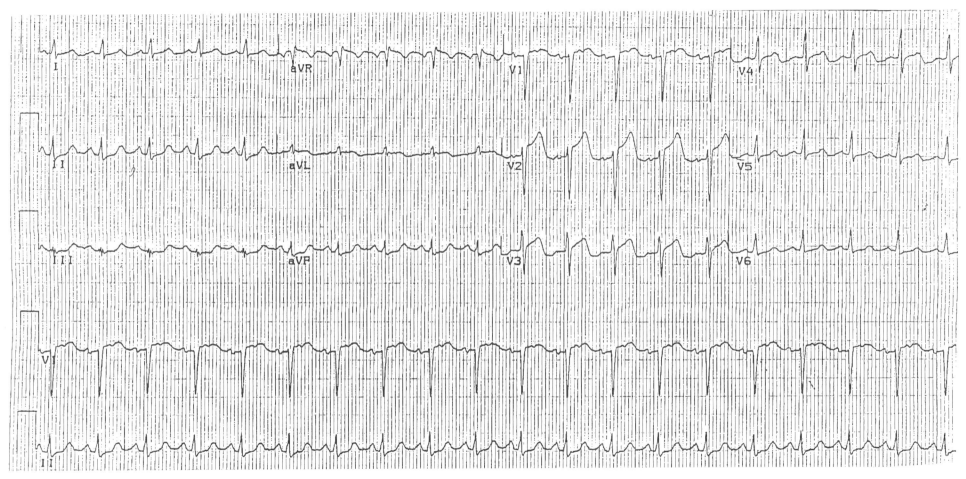

Let's be disagreeable! The slight ST segment elevation in leads I and aVL is accompanied by a reciprocal depression in leads II, III, and aVF. If there is lingering doubt, the obvious ST segment elevation in the precordial leads screams acute anterolateral MI. The P wave configuration is consistent with bi-atrial abnormality.

MYOCARDIAL INFARCTION MIMICS

Nowadays, when thrombolytics and percutaneous coronary interventions have proven their value, and when 1-2 mm. of ST segment elevation in two adjacent leads is frequently cited as adequate indication for administering them, it is doubly important to be sure that the ST elevation present is indeed secondary to coronary occlusion and to recognize the fact that such ST elevation can be seen in situations other than myocardial infarction. In some of these, e.g., pericarditis or intracranial bleeding, the administration of a thrombolytic agent may be a lethal disaster. ST segment elevation, of even gross degree, can result from numerous non-cardiac problems. Many of the well-documented causes of ST elevation are listed in the table and examples of some will be provided. In addition, an "old" infarction can be simulated by non-infarction Q waves and some of the causes of such Q waves are provided in the adjoining table. Some conditions, including acute cor pulmonale, can produce both abnormal Q waves and ST segment elevation.

SOME NON-INFARCTION CAUSES OF ST SEGMENT ELEVATION	SOME CAUSES OF NON-INFARCTION Q WAVES
Acute Pericarditis	Hypertrophic Cardiomyopathy
Early repolarization	Accessory Pathway Activation (W.P.W.)
Acute Cor Pulmonale	Chronic Obstructive Pulmonary Disease
Hyperkalemia	Pulmonary Embolization
Intracranial Hemorrhage	Incomplete L.B.B.B.
"Variant" (Prinzmetal) Angina	L.V. Hypertrophy
Acute Pancreatitis	Left Anterior Fascicular Block
Acute Cholecystitis	Cardiac Amyloidosis
Myocardial Metastases	Myocardial Infiltration
	-Cardiac Amyloidosis
	-Hemachromatosis
	-Sarcoidosis
	Misplaced Leads
	Cardiac Displacement (e.g. pneumothorax)

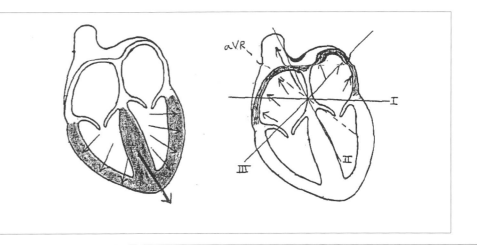

33 YEAR OLD MAN
DIFFERENTIAL DIAGNOSIS?

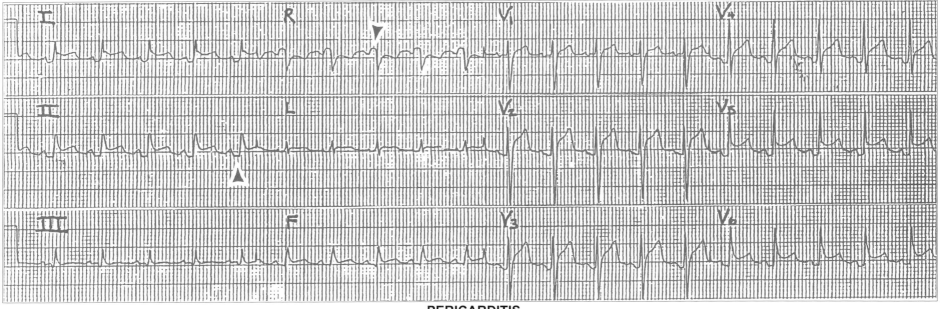

PERICARDITIS

An important fact--the pericardium itself has no electrical activity and, if there is a pericarditis with <u>EKG change</u>, there is myocarditis. The inflammatory process present involves the entire myocardium and is not zonal (as in myocardial infarction). Thus, there are multiple vectors reflecting the diffuse myocardial injury. The sum of these is indicated by one vector oriented to the left and inferiorly, resulting in ST segment elevation in the limb leads. Unlike the ST vector in myocardial infarction, there is no reciprocal depression, except in lead aVR. The injury process is also present in the horizontal plane, with ST elevation usually occurring in all the precordial leads. Supporting the diffuse nature of the myocarditis, their often is evidence of *atrial* myocardial injury, indicated by an abnormality of the *PR segment* (the ST segment of the P wave). This vector is oriented to the right and superior, and is recorded negative in many leads (P-R segment depression-**up arrow**-) and positive only in lead aVR.

78 YEAR OLD WOMAN – 2/10
CHEST PAIN

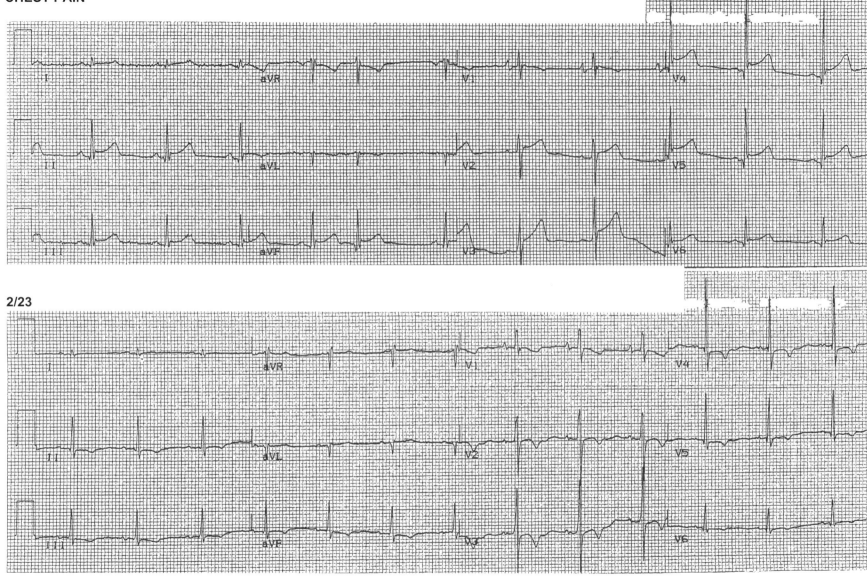

2/23

Dr. David Spodick has emphasized that the pattern of acute pericarditis recedes in stages. The initial tracing, with diffuse ST segment elevation is termed stage one. Later, the elevated segments regress (stage two) and the T waves invert (stage three). Ultimately, and hopefully, the tracing returns to normal. Given only the lower EKG, the obvious concern would be "diffuse ischemia."

EARLY REPOLARIZATION

The ST segment elevation of this normal variant can be quite dramatic and may be associated with marked T wave inversion. The example below was recorded in a healthy 19-year-old college student.

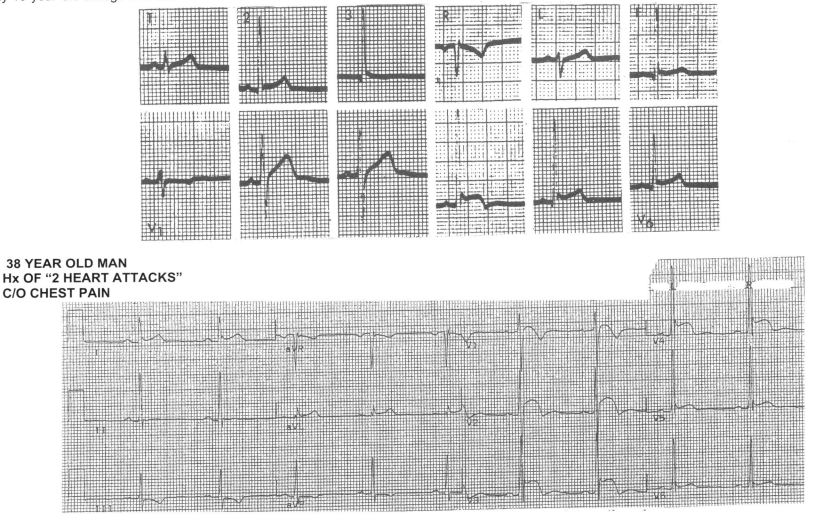

38 YEAR OLD MAN
Hx OF "2 HEART ATTACKS"
C/O CHEST PAIN

"The case of the man who cried wolf." A dramatic example of early repolarization, and an interesting story. This 38-year-old man was a prisoner and, when he was bored with jail life, he would complain of chest pain. Because of his EKG and history of "two heart attacks," he would be hospitalized and infarction "ruled out." This occurred on five occasions and, on each, his tracing consistently showed these marked changes. During the last admission, coronary arteriograms were performed and his vessels and cardiac function were normal. It was suggested that he not pull this stunt again!

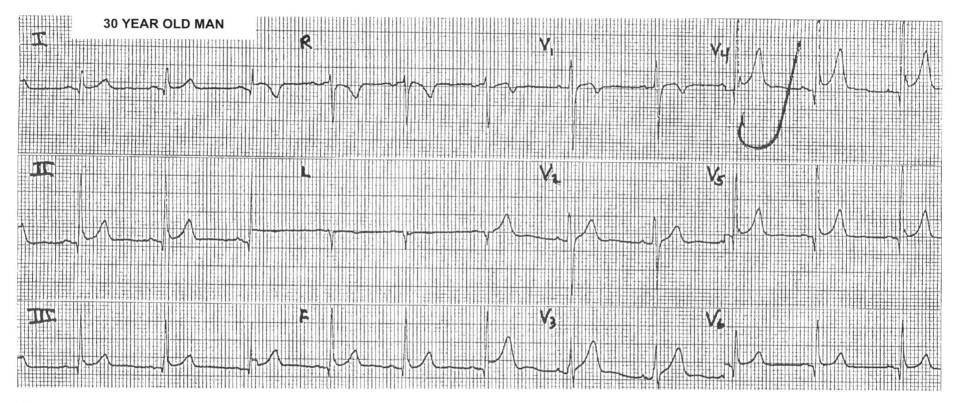

30 YEAR OLD MAN

Usually, however, the ST segment elevation is more moderate and the T wave remains upright. In the example above, from a healthy 30-year-old man, notice the little "barbs" at the beginning of repolarization in leads V4 and V5. This is a common finding in this innocent pattern; and, combined with the J-shaped ST-T, forms a "fishhook." <u>One of the most helpful features of this pattern, to exclude the diagnosis of infarction, is the absence of any sign of ST segment depression in lead aVL</u>.

```
(RAT08)   .  SINUS BRADYCARDIA, RATE 43
(STE95)   .  PROBLABLE EARLY REPOLARIZATION PATTERN
(QM102)   .  ARTIFACT IN LEAD(S): L1, L2, L3, L5,…REPEAT ECG REQUESTED
                        -OTHERWISE NORMAL ECG-
```

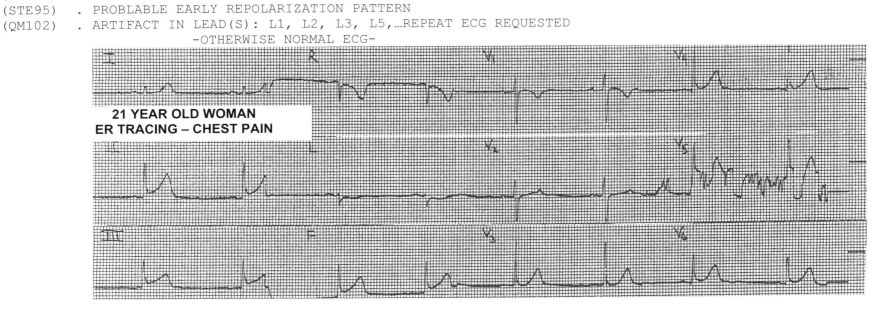

21 YEAR OLD WOMAN
ER TRACING – CHEST PAIN

This was ignored in this young woman. Note the ST depression in aVL. Based on the computer EKG interpretation, she was discharged from the emergency department, only to present dead on arrival at another hospital. At her autopsy, the acute inferior myocardial infarction was due to a coronary artery anomaly.

DIFFERENTIATION BETWEEN EARLY REPOLARIZATION AND MYOCARDIAL INFARCTION

EKG	EARLY REPOLARIZATION	MYOCARDIAL INFARCTION
ST segment elevation	Yes "fishhook" concave upward	Yes Convex upward
ST reciprocal depression	No	Yes
Q waves	No	Yes
CLINICAL		
Sex	Male	Both
Age	Usually young	Older
Symptoms	No	Yes

At times, it is difficult to distinguish pericarditis from the pattern of early repolarization. Pericarditis occurs in both sexes, whereas early repolarization is virtually a male monopoly. The T waves are generally less tall in pericarditis and, in V6, there is less difference between the level of ST elevation and the height of the T wave in pericarditis than in early repolarization. Presence of PR segment change helps to indicate that the ST changes are due to pericarditis and not early repolarization. Obviously, the patient's symptoms are a major deciding factor.

```
PR      144       . Sinus Tachycardia, rate 111
QRSD     57       - Probable early repolarization pattern [Remains]
QT      278
QTc     378

--AXES--
P        77
QRS      32
T        13
```

31 YEAR OLD WOMAN – E.R.
AGREE WITH REVIEWER?

    - OTHERWISE NORMAL ECG -

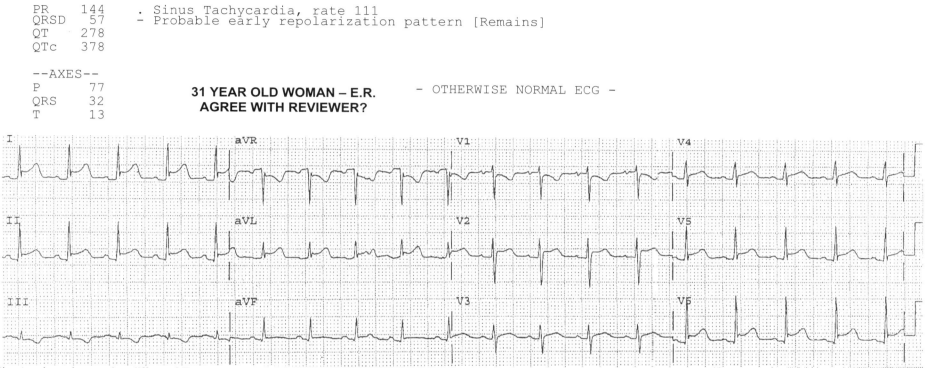

In the tracing above, the diffuse ST segment elevation without reciprocal depression (except aVR), accompanied by PR segment depression, identifies acute pericarditis. The EKG features of early repolarization (**A**) and acute pericarditis (**B**) are contrasted in the illustration below, and the clinical differences are outlined in the table.

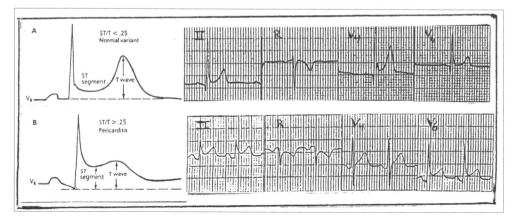

DIFFERENTIATION BETWEEN "EARLY REPOLARIZATION" AND ACUTE PERICARDITIS

Early repolarization	Pericarditis
All males	Both Sexes
Taller T waves	Less tall T waves
"fishhook" at J point	No "fishhook"
In V6, ST < 25% of T	In V6, ST > 25% of T
Bradycardia	Tachycardia

ACUTE COR PULMONALE

The most common cause of this is, of course, pulmonary embolism. Several different patterns in the EKG have been described as characteristic. Included are: the "S1-Q3-T3 pattern" (the classic Mcginn-White pattern), prominent S waves in the majority of leads, new RBBB, and atrial tachycardias. While any or all of these may be seen, the most helpful pattern is the *simultaneous development of abnormalities in both the inferior and anteroseptal leads*. This can be summed up as follows: when you look at the limb leads and suspect *inferior* ischemia, injury, or infarction, and then look at the precordial leads and think of *anteroseptal* ischemia, injury, or infarction - suspect pulmonary embolization. For example in the figure below, the QRS-T configuration in lead III is suggestive of acute inferior infarction, but lead V1 looks like acute anteroseptal MI.

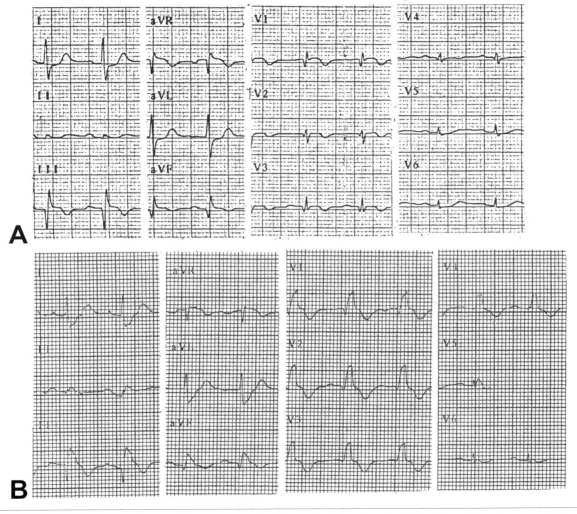

Acute cor pulmonale from pulmonary embolism. A. The classical S1-Q3 pattern is present, but note the Q waves, ST elevation and T-wave inversion, suggesting acute myocardial infarction, in both leads 3 and V1. **B.** Twenty minutes later, slight increase in rate and RBBB has developed.

```
PR      133   (AT  ).  Atrial tachycardia, rate 111
QRSD    150   (RBBB ).  Right bundle branch block
QT      380   (CLAE ).  Consider left atrial enlargement
QTc     516   STE31T).  Probable Anterior Subepicardial injury
--AXES--
P       234                            - ABNORMAL ECG -
QRS     253
T        59
```

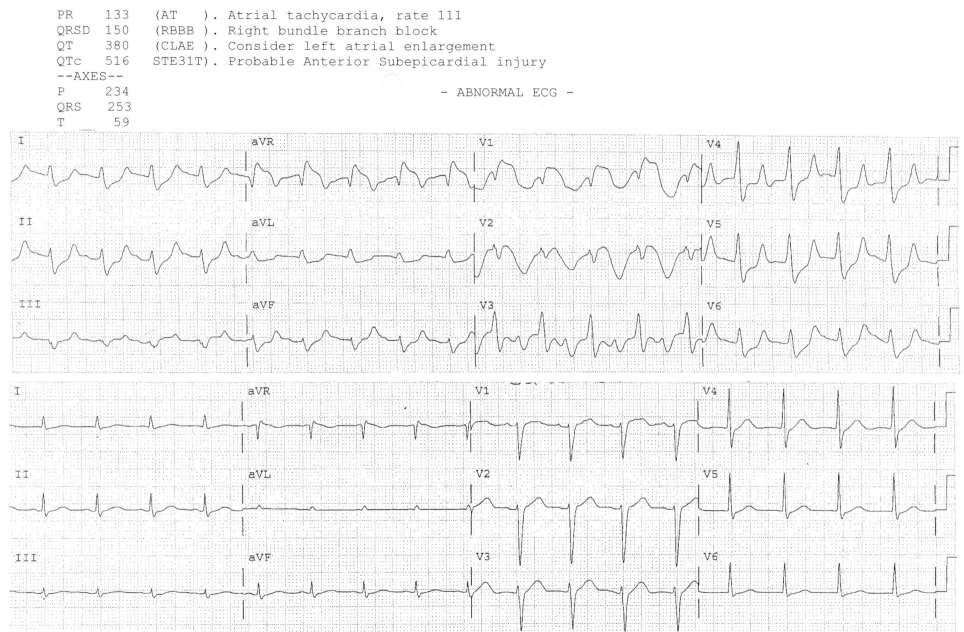

This diabetic man, with chronic renal failure, has a serum potassium of 8.9meq, and the pattern shown in the upper tracing. The marked depolarization and repolarization abnormalities that occur with advanced hyperkalemia can simulate acute myocardial infarction. With treatment, the next day the changes have regressed and the evidence of infarction has disappeared.

VARIANT ANGINA

Dr. Myron Prinzmetal championed the concept that angina could be due to coronary artery "spasm." It was atypical in that it did not occur with exercise but at rest, often in the early morning hours. When EKGs were obtained during episodes, striking, but transient, ST segment elevation was recorded. This continuous Holter monitoring was performed on a 40-year-old woman with recurrent nocturnal episodes of "chest pressure." Her initial diagnosis was "esophageal reflux and spasm". The demonstrated ST segment change obtained during one attack clarified her problem. Coronary arteriograms were normal, but spasm could be provoked.

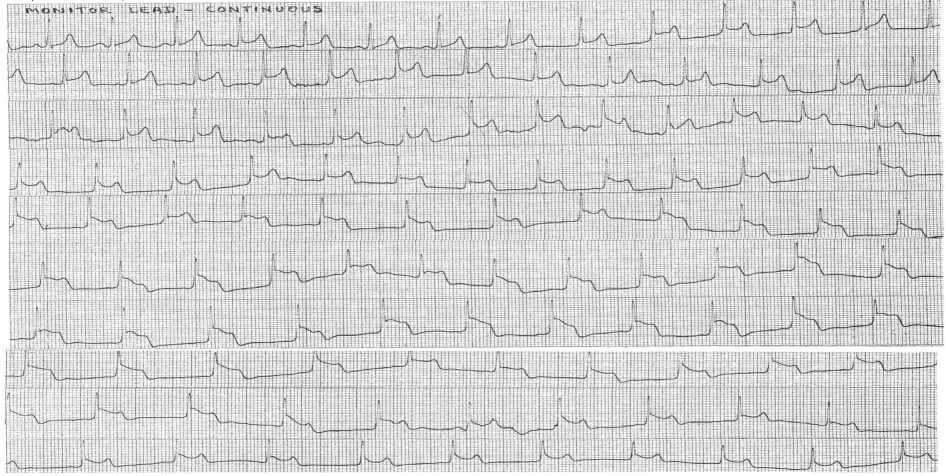

INTRACRANIAL HEMMORHAGE

Subdural, subarachnoid, and cerebral hemorrhages can be accompanied by marked ST segment elevation or by major T wave abnormalities (elevation or inversion), either of which may strongly suggest acute or recent myocardial infarction.

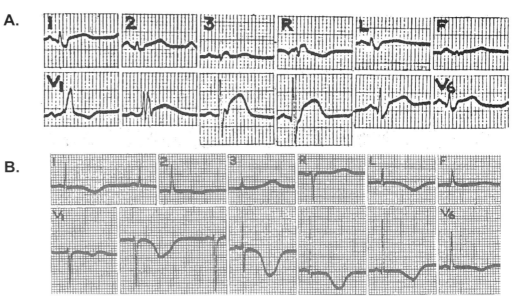

A. Subdural hematoma in a 72-year old man. **B. Cerebral hemorrhage.**

THE ACUTE ABDOMEN

Documented cases of acute cholecystitis and acute pancreatitis producing significant ST-T elevation have been published; but any acute abdominal crisis can probably produce a "current of injury" in the EKG.

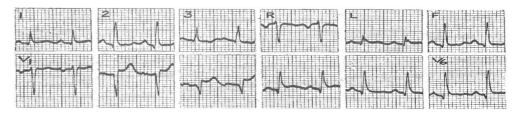

Acute hemorrhagic pancreatitis in a 61-year old gouty man with no evidence of obstructive coronary disease or myocardial infarction at autopsy three days later.

MYOCARDIAL METASTASES

When a metastatic lesion occupies the myocardium, it forms the equivalent of a "dead zone"; and is therefore not surprising that a pattern similar to that of infarction may be produced.

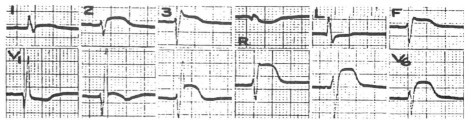

From a patient with squamous-cell carcinoma of the buccal mucosa and myocardial metastases: no infarction at autopsy.

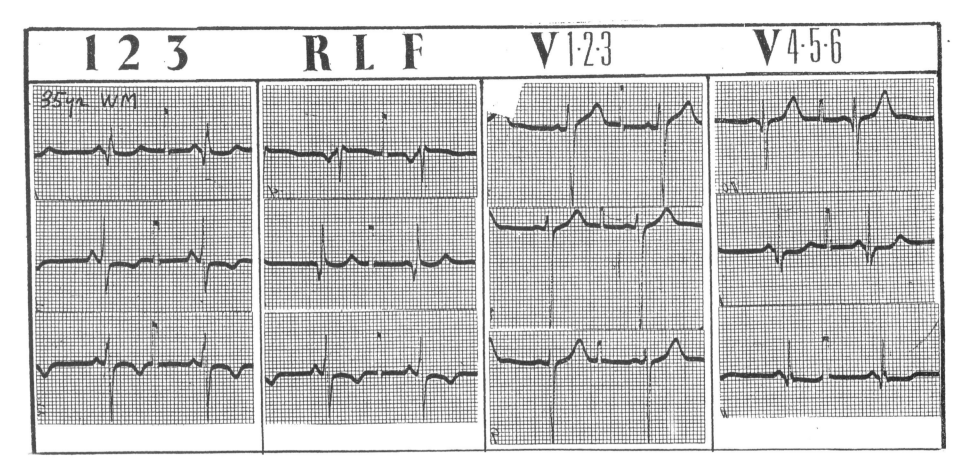

| 1 2 3 | R L F | V 1·2·3 | V 4·5·6 |

35 yr WM

This young man has "Hypertrophic Obstructive Cardiomyopathy" ("HOCOM"). When the condition was first identified, the abnormal physical findings and ventricular anatomy resulted in a label of "Idiopathic Hypertrophic Subaortic Stenosis" ("IHSS"). Understandably, the large "Q waves" in leads I, aVL, and V4-6 prompted a diagnosis of lateral wall MI. However, leads V2-3-4 are *half standardized*, indicating that there is striking QRS voltage of left ventricular hypertrophy. (Note that the S wave depth in V2 is <u>56 mm</u>!) The abnormal muscle masses of HOCOM can alter initial forces, resulting in "Q waves." The directional change in early ventricular activation may cause various patterns, mistaken as inferior, lateral, anterior, or posterior MI.

46

INFARCTION PATTERNS IN W.P.W. ACTIVATION

The presence of an accessory pathway (AP) permits abnormal activation of the ventricle. Depending on the location of the AP, initial forces may be inscribed simulating the "Q waves" of myocardial infarction. In the top tracing, the computer has missed the evident features of "preexcitation" and misinterprets the "upside down" delta waves as the Q waves due to anterior and lateral myocardial infarction. The prominent precordial R waves, due to AP activation, are mistakenly ascribed to right ventricular hypertrophy. In the bottom tracing, the early forces over the AP are misinterpreted as indicating anterior infarction. The various "patterns" seen with W.P.W. activation can mimic any of the familiar infarctions. The computer misses the majority! (Additional discussion regarding W.P.W. is presented in a separate chapter).

```
PR      137     . Sinus tachycardia, rate 72 [Remains]
QRSD    108     - Right axis deviation [Now Present]
QT      312     - RVH with ST-T abnormalities [Now Present]
QTc     424     - Old Inferior infarct [Remains]
--AXES--        - Lateral region infarct [Now Present]
P       80      - [Now Absent] Probable Posterior region wall involvement
QRS     103     - [Now Absent] Nonspecific Anterior T wave abnormalities
T       48              -ABNORMAL ECG-
```

41 YEAR OLD WOMAN
DO YOU AGREE?

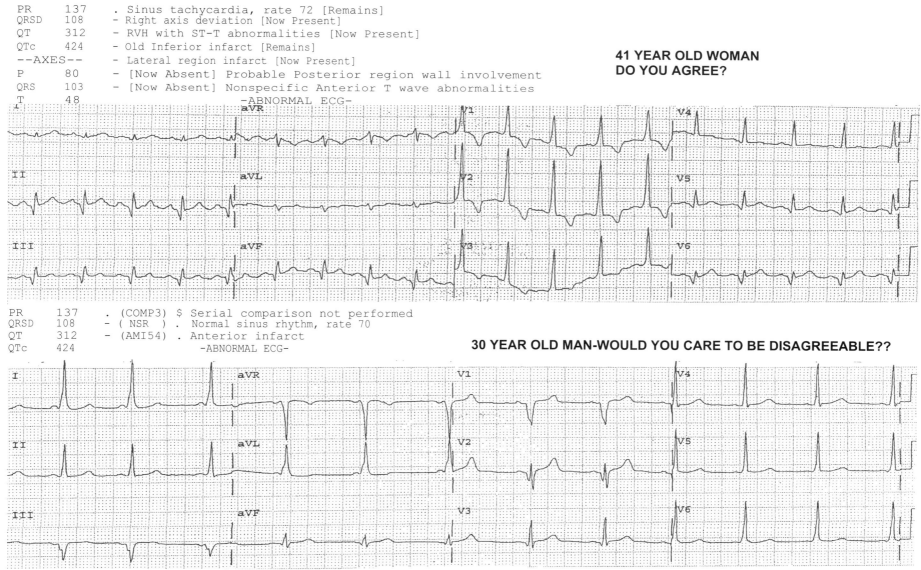

```
PR      137     . (COMP3) $ Serial comparison not performed
QRSD    108     - ( NSR  ) . Normal sinus rhythm, rate 70
QT      312     - (AMI54) . Anterior infarct
QTc     424             -ABNORMAL ECG-
```

30 YEAR OLD MAN-WOULD YOU CARE TO BE DISAGREEABLE??

60 YEAR OLD WOMAN
SEVERE COPD
ANY EVIDENCE OF MI?

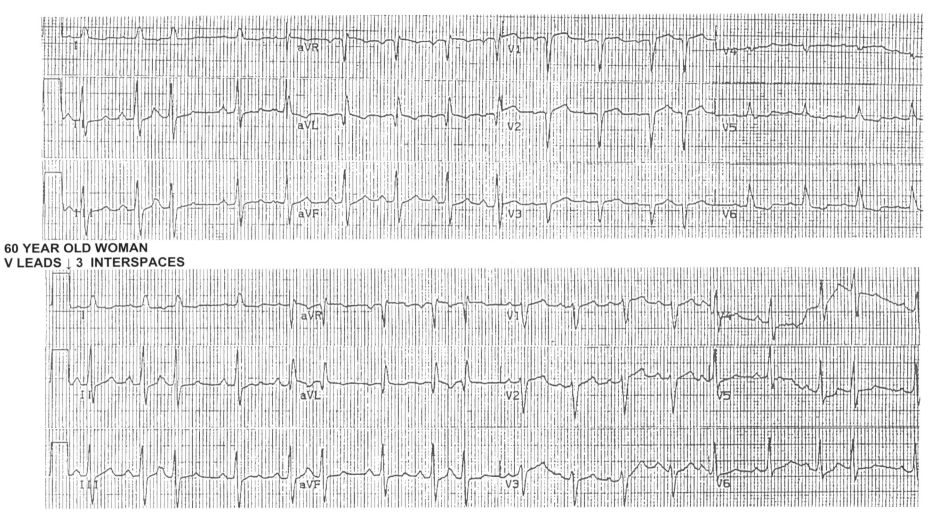

60 YEAR OLD WOMAN
V LEADS ↓ 3 INTERSPACES

Hyperinflation chronic obstructive pulmonary disease results in depression of the diaphragms, and the cardiac position becomes lower than normal. Precordial leads obtained in the standard location may be "too high," resulting in Q waves recorded in leads V1-V4, and warranting the diagnosis of anterior MI. If the chest leads are recorded in lower interspaces, a "precordial map," the initial R waves in these leads may reappear. This woman still has bad COPD but has not had an anterior infarction.

ABNORMAL VENTRICULLAR ACTIVATION
FASICULAR BLOCKS & BUNDLE BRANCH BLOCKS

The "anatomy" of electrical activation of the heart is shown in the figure.

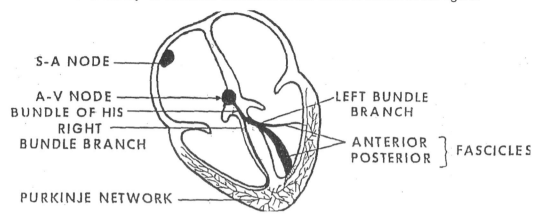

Atrial impulses start at the sinus node, cross the AV junctional bridge, traverse the common bundle of His, and enter the right and left bundle branches. The RBB continues without major branching to the apex of the right ventricle. The LBB divides into two pathways--the *left anterior (superior) fascicle* and then the *left posterior (inferior) fascicle*. Ultimately, the electrical signal reaches the Purkinje network--a myriad of rapidly conducting fibers that spreads the depolarizing impulse over the endocardium of each ventricle. The majority of the delay occurring between the inscription of the P wave and the QRS complex (PR interval) represents the time required for transmission through the AV node. It may normally require up to 200 millisec. In contrast, impulse passage from the His bundle to the myocardial cells is very rapid--normally requiring less than 55 millisec. Depolarization of the countless myocardial cells in both ventricles occurs in a flash - 80-100 millisec. is normally all that is required to complete this vital process

FASICULAR BLOCKS = "HEMIBLOCKS"

Interruption of the fascicular pathways results in changes in the normal sequence of ventricular activation. Dr. Mauricio Rosenbaum should be credited for defining the features of these conduction abnormalities. He used the term "hemiblock" - others use the term "fascicular block." Both are acceptable and will be used interchangeably; these are discussed below. The anterior fascicle runs toward the anterior papillary muscle, which is situated in the upper left region of the left ventricle (L.V.). The posterior fascicle runs toward the posterior papillary muscle in the inferior wall of the L.V. If both fascicles of the left bundle conducted with equal velocity, there would be two equal wave fronts of electrical activation. One would be oriented to the left (left anterior fascicle) and the other directed inferiorly (left posterior fascicle). The summation of these vectors is shown in the illustration, resulting in a mean QRS axis of approximately (+) 60°.

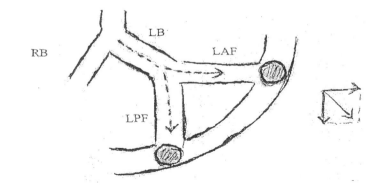

LEFT ANTERIOR FASCICULAR BLOCK--"LEFT ANTERIOR HEMIBLOCK"

When there is conduction block in the left anterior fascicle, the stimulus is directed through the remaining posterior division. The initial portion of the QRS complex becomes directed inferiorly and variably to the right. This will result in a positive deflection in leads II, III, and AVF, and a negative initial deflection in lead aVL, and commonly also in lead I. The electrical signal then travels rapidly via the Purkinje fibers in a wave front that advances leftward and superiorly as shown in figure A The summation of these multiple instantaneous vectors can be represented by single terminal vector oriented to the left and superior as depicted in figure B.

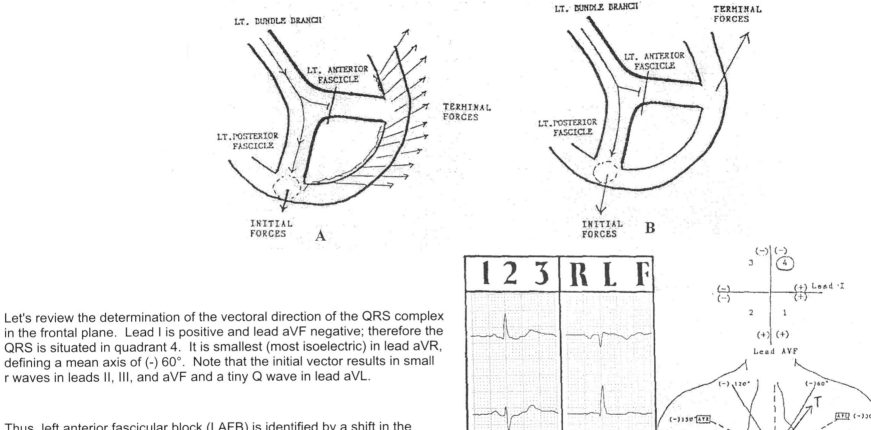

Let's review the determination of the vectoral direction of the QRS complex in the frontal plane. Lead I is positive and lead aVF negative; therefore the QRS is situated in quadrant 4. It is smallest (most isoelectric) in lead aVR, defining a mean axis of (-) 60°. Note that the initial vector results in small r waves in leads II, III, and aVF and a tiny Q wave in lead aVL.

Thus, left anterior fascicular block (LAFB) is identified by a shift in the mean QRS axis to (-) 45° or more. Note that the terminal vector, directed left and superior results in a prominent late R wave in leads aVL and especially aVR. Although there is some conduction delay with the development and LAFB, it is usually minor-0.01 or 0.02 seconds-and the total QRS duration is only slightly prolonged. The EKG to the right is a typical example of the QRS morphology of left anterior fascicular block.

71 YEAR OLD MAN – 11/11

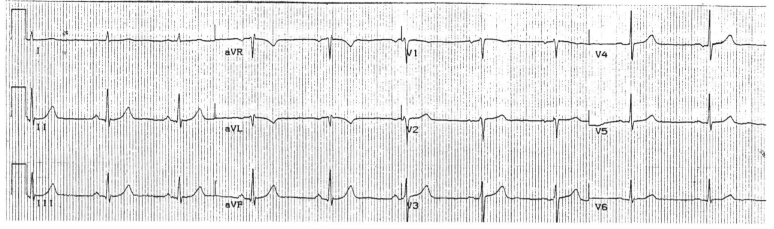

71 YEAR OLD MAN -11/14

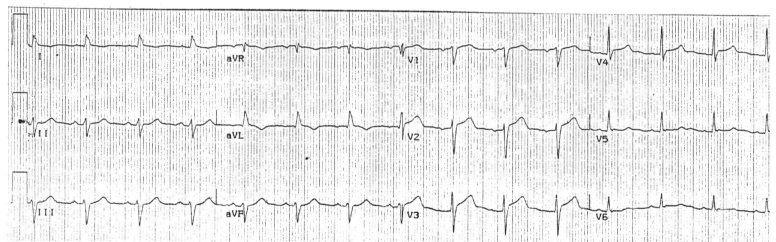

This sequence of tracings shows the transition from normal to left anterior fascicular block (LAFB). In the top tracing the frontal plane axis is in quadrant 1 (axis = approximately 75°). Three days later, the axis has shifted left and superior into quadrant 4. There is now left axis deviation of (-) 60°, which is typical of LAFB. Comparing the two tracings, note the following differences:

1. The *initial* QRS forces have become oriented inferiorly, inscribing small r waves in leads II, III, and aVF, and replacing the small q waves seen in these leads in the upper tracing. In addition, there is now a small q wave in aVL, not present in the top EKG.
2. The *late* forces are now predominantly negative in leads II, III, and aVF, resulting in the left axis deviation.
3. The QRS duration has increased slightly.
   The new ST segment elevation in V1-V4 indicates that the cause of the LAFB is an acute anterior myocardial infarction.

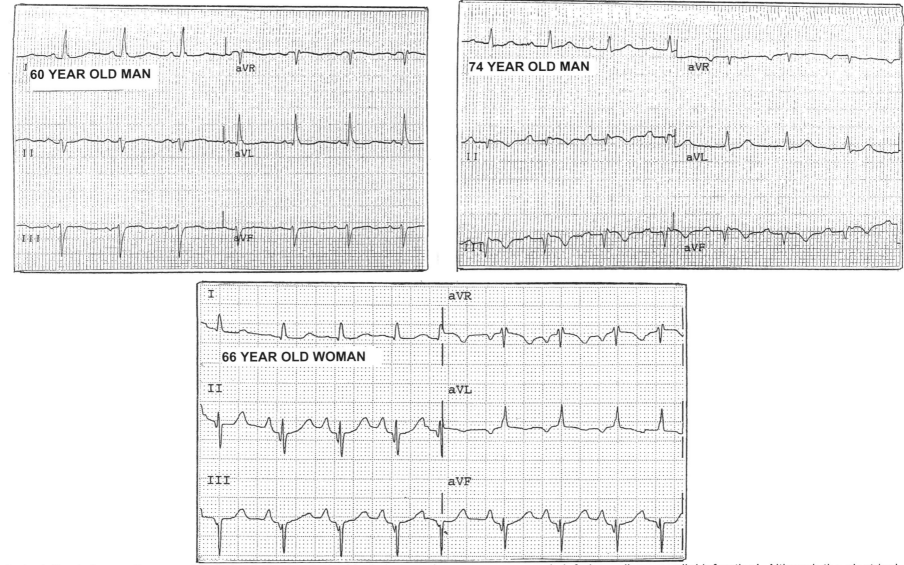

Left axis deviation is frequently caused by left anterior fascicular block, but another common cause is inferior wall myocardial infarction! Although the electrical axis may be the same, the reasons for it differ. In the 69-year-old man, LAFB results in left axis of (-) 45° because of the orientation of the <u>late</u> QRS forces. In the 74-year-old man, inferior wall infarction causes a left superior vectoral shift of (-) 45° because of the <u>initial</u> forces (Q waves). Since the two conditions alter different portions of the QRS complex, can they coexist? Note in the 66-year-old woman, with an axis of (-) 45°, that there are both the initial Q waves due to inferior M.I. and terminal S waves of LAFB.

```
PR      170    . Normal sinus rhythm, rate 90
QRSD    180    . Left axis deviation, consider LAFB
QT      344    . Early transition
QTc     421    . Nonspecific Inferior T abnormalities
--AXES--
P        45                              - ABNORMAL ECG -
QRS     -43                                                47 YEAR OLD MAN
T       -10                                                DO YOU AGREE WITH THE COMPUTER?
```

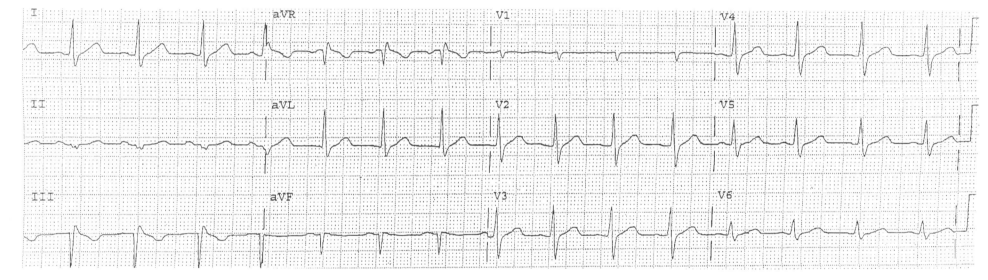

The computer has made a correct observation, but for the wrong reason! The left axis deviation results from the "Q waves" present in leads II, III, and aVF, and is due to an age undetermined inferior myocardial infarction. The "early transition" in the horizontal plane indicates an accompanying posterior infarction—often the case, and frequently ignored!

87 YEAR OLD WOMAN-4/1
YOUR OBSERVATIONS PLEASE

6/19-WHAT HAS HAPPENED TO THE INFERIOR WALL INFARCT?

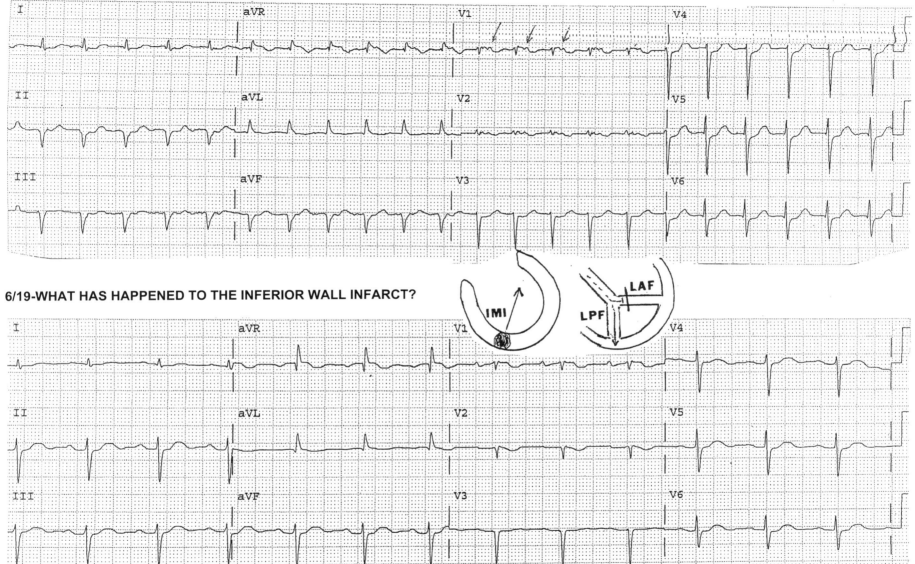

Lead V1 shows P waves that are poorly identified in other leads (arrows). They are conducted with a long PR interval. The frontal plane QRS axis is (-) 60°, with Q waves in leads II, III, and aVF, identifying an age undetermined inferior myocardial infarction. Precordial R wave progression and transition are "poor." Ten weeks later, the QRS axis remains at (-) 60°, but there are now R waves in leads II, III, and aVF. What has happened? If there is development of left anterior fascicular block, the <u>mean</u> axis is shifted to the left, but "early forces" must be conducted over the posterior fascicle, and are directed <u>inferiorly</u>. Thus, the onset of L.A.F.B. erases the Q waves of the prior inferior MI. Obviously, without serial tracings, this sequence could not be determined.

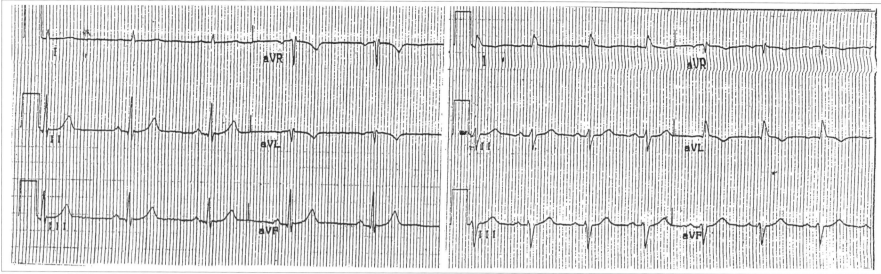

The mean QRS axis in the first tracing is normal at approximately (+) 75°. Tiny Q waves are present in leads II, III, aVF. Three days later, the mean axis has shifted to (-) 50° and II, III, and aVF now show small r waves and aVL a small Q wave. The QRS duration is obviously longer, but still normal. This is an example of the development of left axis deviation due to left anterior fascicular block.

LEFT POSTERIOR FASCICULAR BLOCK--"LEFT POSTERIOR HEMIBLOCK"

The altered sequence of depolarization due to posterior fascicular block is the opposite of LAFB. As depicted below, if the left posterior fascicle is blocked, ventricular depolarization begins in the distribution of the left anterior fascicle. Thus, initial forces are directed to the left and, variably, somewhat superiorly. This will result in an initial negative deflection (Q waves) in lead III, often in aVF, and sometimes in lead II. The electrical impulse then enters the Purkinje network and is rapidly transmitted inferiorly and to the right, the myocardial area which was deprived of its conduction limb (**A**). Terminal forces, thus, are altered to "point" to the right and inferior, resulting in S wave in lead I and aVL, and R waves in leads II, III, and aVF (**B**). The result is right axis deviation of the mean QRS vector > 90° in the frontal plane.

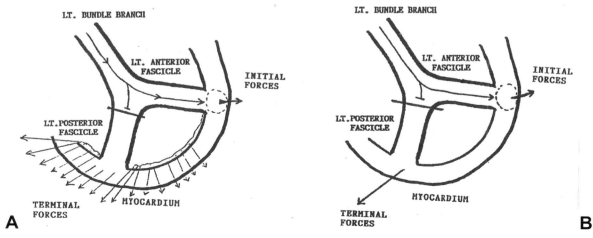

In this example of LPFB, the QRS complex is negative in lead I, positive in aVF and, thus, situated in quadrant 2. The most isoelectric lead is aVR, therefore, the mean QRS axis is (+) 120 – right axis deviation. However, Dr. Rosenbaum recognized that the most common cause of right axis is right ventricular hypertrophy, not left posterior fascicular block. Thus, for the diagnosis of LPFB there must be no evidence of RVH. One must be sure that there is no historical or physical finding, and no precordial QRS change to suggest RVH.

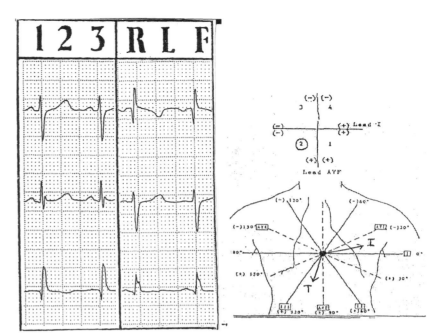

47 YEAR OLD MAN

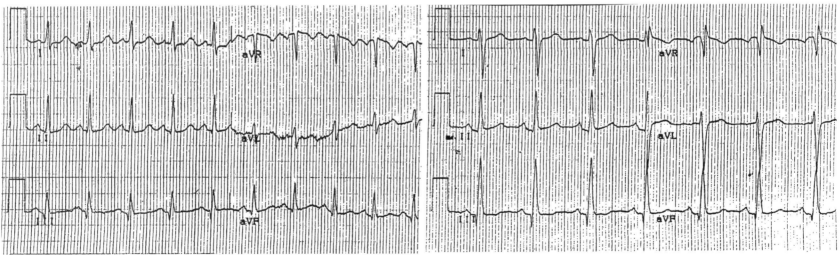

This young man was hospitalized with myocarditis. His initial EKG shows sinus tachycardia of 130/min. and a frontal plane mean QRS axis of (+) 60. Five days later, the QRS is now negative in lead I and positive in lead aVF (quadrant 2), with a mean axis of approximately (+) 120. The right axis shift cannot be due to RVH because of the short time between tracings. It must be due to left posterior fascicular block, presumably resulting from the inflammatory process. Note the increased depth of the Q waves in leads III, aVF. The significant increase in QRS voltage is due to lack of cancellation of opposing forces secondary to the conduction abnormality.

75 YEAR OLD MAN -5/29-18:46
YOUR OBSERVATIONS INCLUDE??

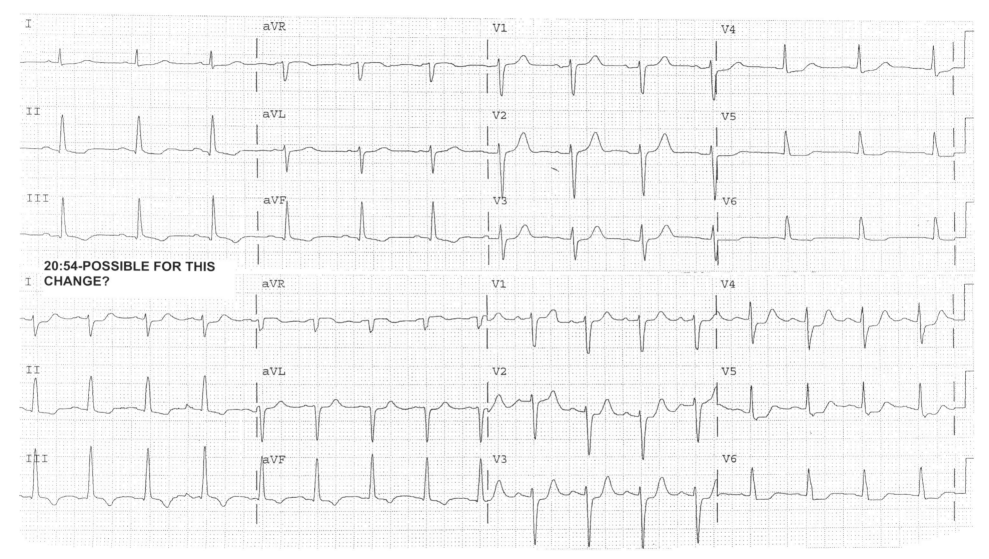

20:54-POSSIBLE FOR THIS CHANGE?

The top tracing shows a frontal plane QRS axis of 75 and nonspecific ST-T changes, likely due to ischemia. Two hours later, the axis has shifted to (+) 105° and the repolarization abnormalities are more marked. Since there is a brief time between tracings, the right axis deviation cannot be due to right ventricular hypertrophy, and must represent LPFB.

BUNDLE BRANCH BLOCKS

When one of the branches of the A-V bundle becomes blocked, the impulse travels exclusively down the other branch, first activates the ventricle on that side and then, crossing the septum, activates the ventricle on the side of the block. Thus, the ventricles are activated *consecutively* instead of simultaneously. Since the impulse has to worm its way slowly through the thickness of the septum before the second ventricle can be activated, the QRS is prolonged to 0.12 sec. or more-- an immediate alert that bundle branch block is present.

Under normal circumstances, ventricular septal activation can be simplistically depicted as occurring from left to right. In reality, it is known that there is a "right septal mass" (the cross-hatched area in the figure) and that part of septal depolarization occurs from *right to left*. The resultant opposing wave fronts result in partial cancellation of the left to right vector. Thus, the thick ventricular septum provides an initial vector that is directed left to right as well as anterior, but smaller than it would be if the right-sided contribution were not present. Subsequently, the free walls of the right and left ventricles are activated simultaneously. Since the left ventricular free wall forces are much greater than those of the thin right ventricle, the QRS complex of vector 2 is directed to the left and posterior.

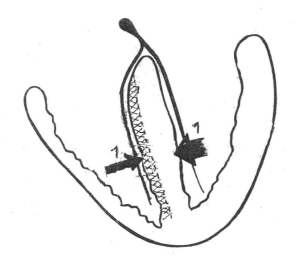 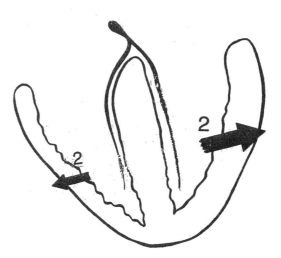

LEFT BUNDLE BRANCH BLOCK (LBBB)

If the left branch is blocked, the impulse travels down the right branch to activate the free wall of the right ventricle (RV) and the septum. Septal forces are much more powerful than the free wall forces of the minor RV; therefore right to left septal activation is dominant (**vector 1**) and writes a negative wave in V1 and a positive wave in V6. Having activated the septum, the impulse continues in the same direction (**vector 2**) to activate the free wall of the left ventricle (LV). Thus, both initial and terminal forces are traveling in the same direction, and the QRS complex tends to be monophasic, with a QS pattern in V1 and a monophasic R wave in V6. In about 30% of LBBB's an initial r wave is inscribed in V1 and this suggests that in these cases activation begins in the free wall of the RV slightly sooner than in the septum. In general, the QRS's in lead 1, aVL, and V6 have similar shapes. Since LBBB alters the depolarization forces--initial, middle, and terminal--usually little else can be interpreted. Repolarization events will be abnormal with sagging ST segments and inverted T waves in leads with (+) QRS complexes. Thus, the vector of the ST-T is +/- 180° from the QRS vector.

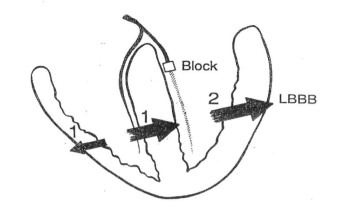

The 2 powerful forces in left bundle-branch block (LBBB) are the septal (**1**) and the LV free-wall (**2**) forces, both of which are traveling in the same direction, from right to left; hence the complexes of LBBB tend to be monophasic.

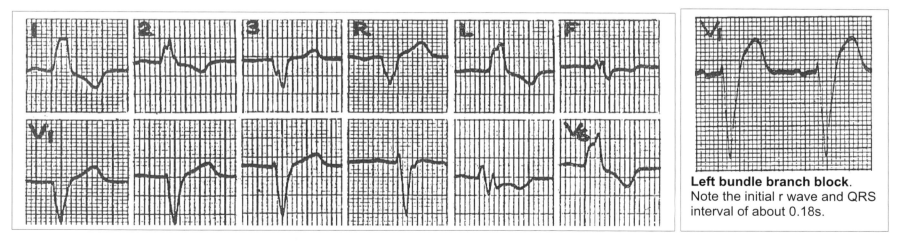

Left bundle branch block. Note the initial r wave and QRS interval of about 0.18s.

Left bundle branch block. Not the wide QRS interval (0.15), tendency to monophasic complexes, prolonged ventricular activation time, QRS complex in V1, axis of about 0°, and similarity of the QRS in leads I, aVF, and V6.

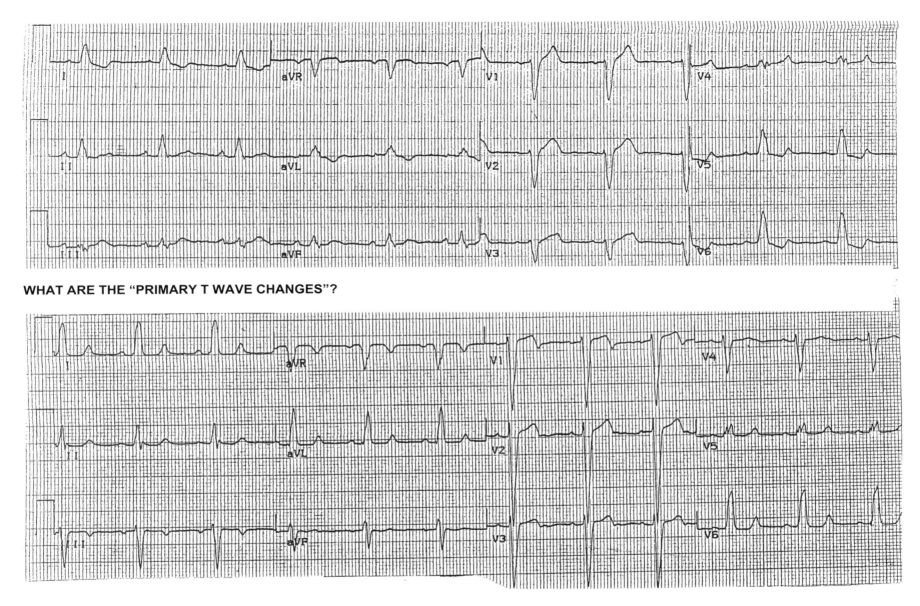

WHAT ARE THE "PRIMARY T WAVE CHANGES"?

Comparing repolarization abnormalities in two patients with LBBB. The top tracing shows ST-T changes with a vectoral direction <u>opposite</u> that of the QRS. This is appropriate "secondary" repolarization. In the bottom EKG, the QRS has a similar morphology, but in contrast to the top tracing, repolarization has the <u>same</u> general direction. The T waves are (attractively) upright in most leads-an example of a <u>primary</u> T wave abnormality which has negated the repolarization expected with LBBB. The significance of this requires clinical correlation, but can indicate ongoing myocardial ischemia.

57 YEAR OLD MAN
DO YOU AGREE WITH THE REVIEWER?

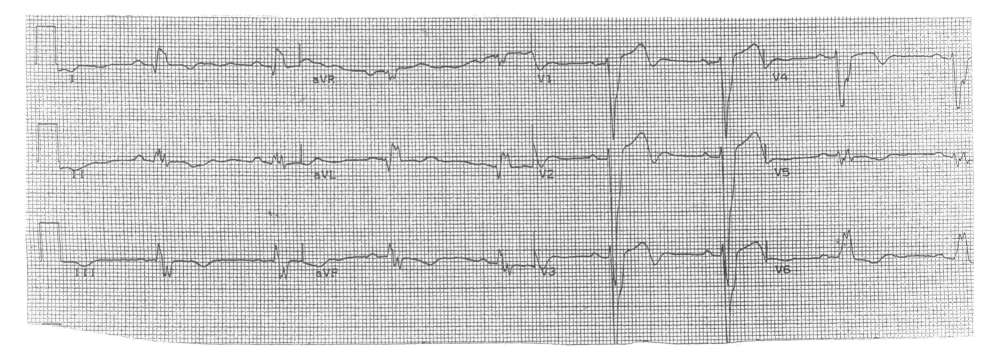

It is acknowledged that the depolarization abnormality of left bundle branch alters the entire QRS complex. A frequent question posed is, can one interpret myocardial infarction from the QRS changes when LBBB is present? A validated and logical criterion is sometimes present. Recall: in normal activation, the ventricular septum is depolarized predominately from left to right and can cause small q waves in leads I, aVL, and V 5-6. These have been termed "septal Q waves." In uncomplicated LBBB, since the septal activation is from *right to left*, these cannot be present. As in this example, if the EKG shows LBBB with initial q waves in leads I, aVL, and/or V 5-6, there is excellent correlation with this pattern and <u>extensive</u> anteroseptal MI. This abnormality indicates the presence, but not the timing, of the infarction.

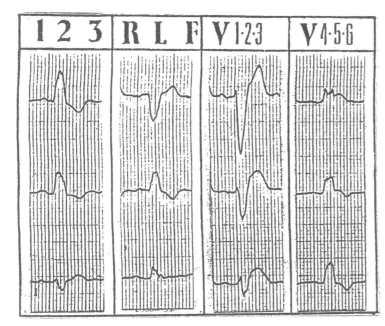

EKG Dx of M.I. with L.B.B.B.

IS THERE ST SEGMENT ELEVATION => 1mm IN ANY
LEAD THAT IS *CONCORDANT* WITH THE QRS COMPLEX?

IS THERE ST SEGMENT DEPRESSION IN LEAD V1 or V2 or V3?

IS THERE ST SEGMENT ELEVATION => 5mm THAT IS
  DISCORDANT WITH THE QRS COMPLEX?

Sgarbossa et. al.   N. Eng. J. Med. 334: 481, 1996

As previously mentioned, the depolarization abnormality of LBBB results in significant, but expected, repolarization abnormality. The diagnosis of acute MI in the presence of LBBB can be provided by the "GUSTO criteria." (reference cited above). They reflect *inappropriate* repolarization indicating the presence of an "injury current." In the upper left example, note the ST segment elevation in leads V4-5, concordant with the QRS complexes. In the upper right tracing, the ST segment is depressed in V1-2-3, leads in which the QRS is negative and the ST segment should be elevated. The lower right example shows exaggerated ST segment elevation in leads V1-3 > 5 mm, as well as concordant ST elevation in lead V4. Any of these patterns is consistent with acute MI.

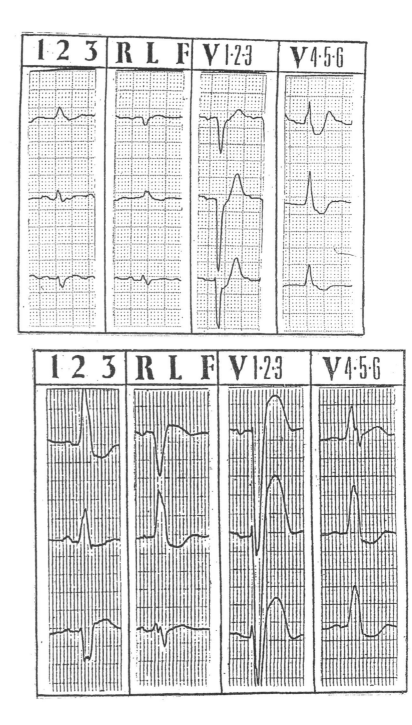

PR   187   +   Normal sinus rhythm, rate 71 [Remains]
QRSD   128   +   Left bundle branch block [Remains]
QT   392   .   No previous tracing
QTc   426
--AXES--
P   54   - ABNORMAL ECG -

69 YEAR OLD MAN-2/7
A TYPICAL EXAMPLE OF ____ ?

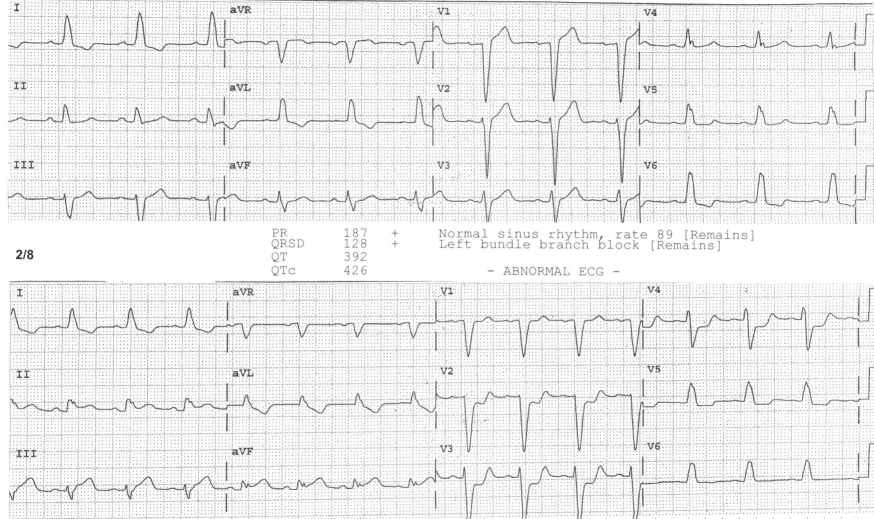

2/8

PR   187   +   Normal sinus rhythm, rate 89 [Remains]
QRSD   128   +   Left bundle branch block [Remains]
QT   392
QTc   426   - ABNORMAL ECG -

The interpretation of the top tracing is correct, but the next day it is sorely lacking. Note the concordant ST segment elevation in leads II and aVF, and the ST segment depression in the precordial leads--"GUSTO criteria"--indicating an acute inferoposterior M.I. in the presence of left bundle branch block.

```
PR     195   .  No further analysis attempted for this ECG - not enough leads could be measured
QRSD   161   -  [Now Absent] Atrial fibrillation with V. response of 99
QT     342   -  [Now Absent] Left bundle branch block
QTc    454

--AXES--                                    - DEFECTIVE ECG -
P      74
QRS    71                                                        RIGHT CHEST LEADS
T      268      80 YEAR OLD WOMAN -6/30
```

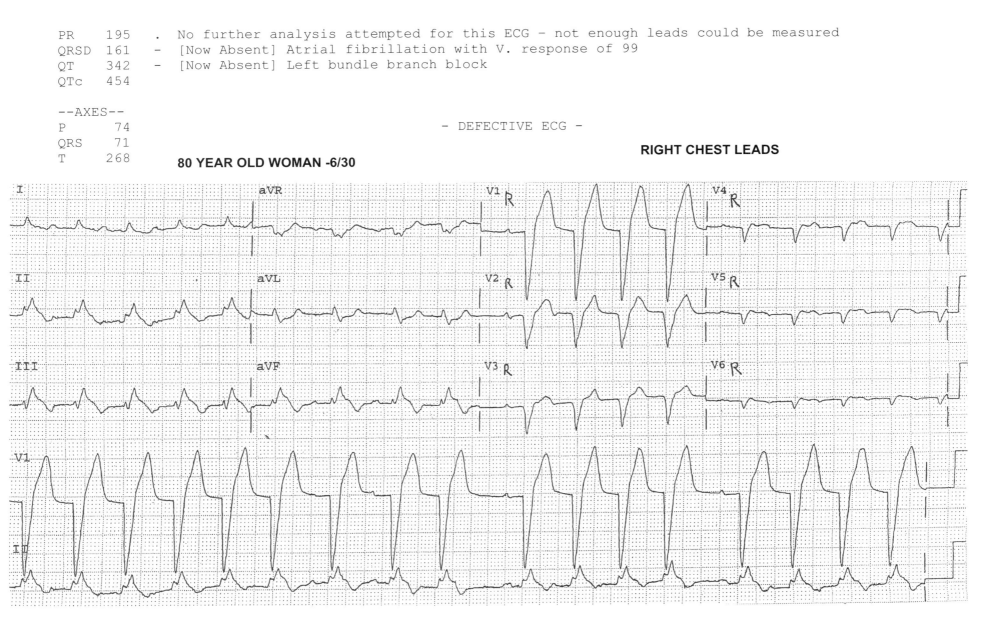

The computer decided not to work today! Although the P waves are few and far between, there must be a sinus mechanism but the P-P cycle is unclear. The pauses indicate second-degree AV block; the shortening R-R intervals between pauses supports Wenckebach A-V block. The QRS morphology indicates LBBB and the concordant ST elevation in leads II, III, and aVF is consistent with acute inferior MI. ST segment elevation in the right chest leads (V4R, V5R and V6R) provides evidence that the infarction also involves the right ventricle.

PR   208   +   Bigeminy pattern. Mean ventricular rate = 58 [Now Present]
QRSD 102   -   Left atrial enlargement [Remains]
QT   430   -   Left ventricular hypertrophy [Remains]
QTc   422   -   Poor R-wave progression, possibly due to LVH [Remains]
                                         - ABNORMAL ECG -

59 YEAR OLD MAN
-**"A FUNNY KIND OF BIGEMINI"??**

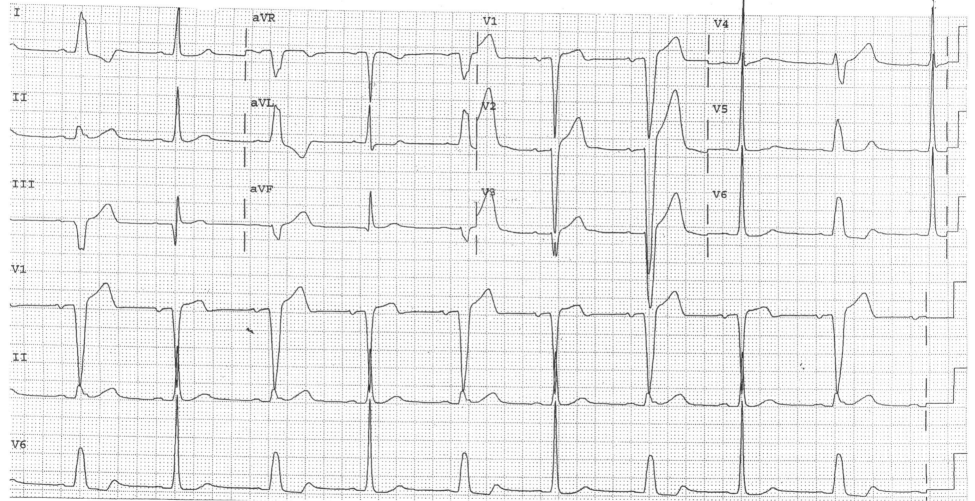

"Gemini" means twin and obviously, "bigemini" means two twins. In this instance, one QRS twin shows complete LBBB morphology and the other incomplete. Perhaps the variable conduction is due to minor changes in cardiac rate? Another possible explanation is that, since the impulse blocks in the left bundle branch, it is not depolarized. This results in increased time available for repolarization of the LBBB, allowing the abnormal left bundle branch to become available to transmit the next atrial stimulus?

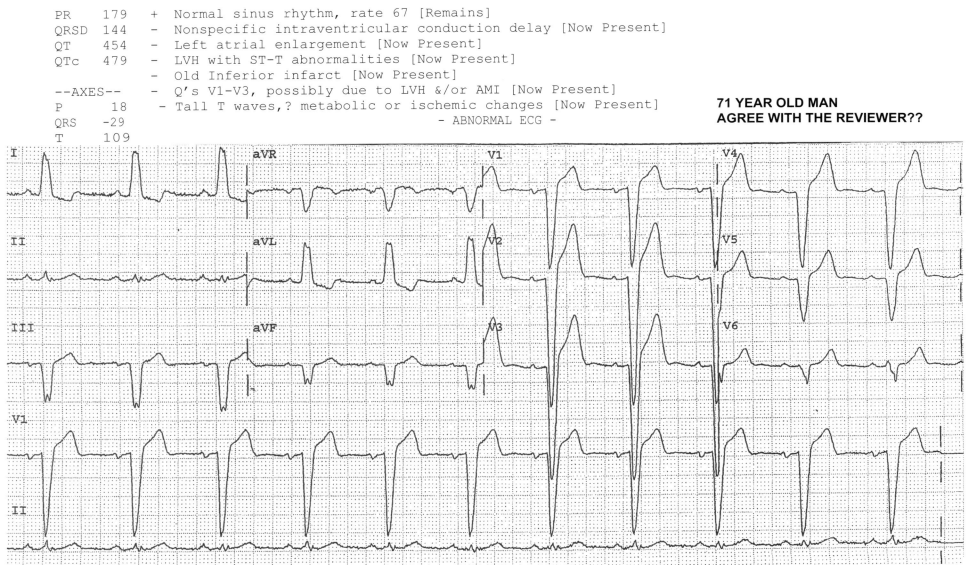

```
PR    179   +  Normal sinus rhythm, rate 67 [Remains]
QRSD  144   -  Nonspecific intraventricular conduction delay [Now Present]
QT    454   -  Left atrial enlargement [Now Present]
QTc   479   -  LVH with ST-T abnormalities [Now Present]
            -  Old Inferior infarct [Now Present]
--AXES--    -  Q's V1-V3, possibly due to LVH &/or AMI [Now Present]
P      18    - Tall T waves,? metabolic or ischemic changes [Now Present]
QRS   -29                              - ABNORMAL ECG -
T     109
```

71 YEAR OLD MAN
AGREE WITH THE REVIEWER??

Let's accept the rhythm diagnosis and evidence of left atrial enlargement, and erase everything else! Once the interpretation is complete LBBB, the majority of other diagnoses are either impossible or poorly validated. LBBB may be associated with a frontal plane axis that is normal or with left axis deviation. The <u>significance</u> of LAD complicating LBBB is more evident than its <u>cause</u>. When LAD is present, the LBBB is associated with a higher incidence of myocardial dysfunction, more advanced disease of the conducting system, and an earlier mortality than is LBBB with a normal axis. Infrequently, LBBB may be associated with right axis deviation. The combination of LBBB with right axis suggests a congestive cardiomyopathy.

RIGHT BUNDLE BRANCH BLOCK (RBBB)

If the right branch is blocked, the impulse spreads down the left branch and activates the septum, as it does normally, from the left (vector 1). Thus, the initial part of the QRS complex in right bundle branch block (RBBB) is usually unchanged compared with the normal complex. This initial septal activation produces the usual r in V1 and q in V6. As has been discussed, in the *normal* heart, with both branches functioning, soon after the forces enter the left side of the septum, right-sided forces also enter the septum and counteract the left to right forces. This leaves the free wall forces of the LV unopposed so that they inscribe a deep S wave in V1. Not so in RBBB: if the right branch is blocked, counteracting forces cannot enter the septum from the right side, and therefore the left to right septal forces are available to oppose the LV free wall forces (vector 2) and the S wave in V1 shrinks. After both the septum and the free wall of the LV have been activated, there remains only the RV to be depolarized. The flimsy RV, which contributes virtually nothing to the normal EKG, now comes into its own (vector 3). Since it is unopposed, it writes a large terminal deflection--an R' in lead V1 and a broad shallow s wave in V6. The morphology in V1 may vary depending on the *early portion* of the QRS complex. Some examples are shown below and others will be seen later.

Emphasis: The delayed activation of the RV in RBBB provides an abnormal late vector which is "added on" to the preceding QRS complex. Thus, in order to *meaningfully* determine the frontal plane QRS axis, the delayed RV forces must be discounted. This may be termed the "pre-blocked axis," and the calculation of it becomes mandatory if one is to understand the combination of RBBB and fascicular blocks.

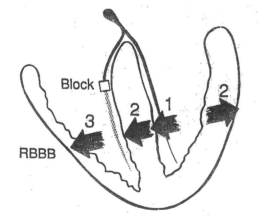

The main forces in RBBB are (**1**) early, normal septal forces, (**2**) LV free-wall forces, to a large extent counteracted by the continuing trans-septal forces, and the (**3**) delayed, unopposed RV free-wall forces. With the two changes in direction, first to the right, then to the left, and then to the right again, there is a tendency to write triphasic complexes.

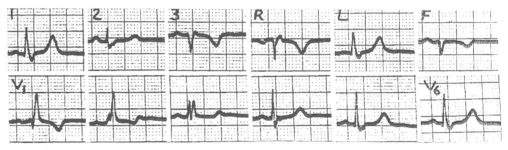

Right bundle branch block. Note the wide, QRS interval (0.12 sec.), tendency to triphasic complexes with rSR' pattern in V1, and similarity of the QRS in leads I, aVL, and V6.

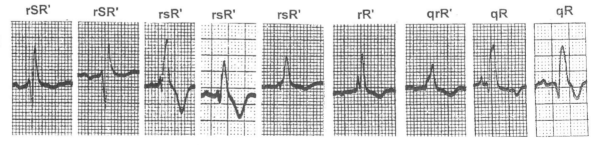

| rSR' | rSR' | rsR' | rsR' | rsR' | rR' | qrR' | qR | qR |

Various patterns of right bundle branch block in V1

Critical Rate. The cardiac rate may be an important determinant of intra-ventricular conduction. Just as in A-V block, an increase in rate with consequent shortening of the cycle often reveals evidence of block, so increase in the sinus rate may result in the stimulus sampling the refractory period of a bundle branch and cause block. The role of rate is so important--and so often overlooked--that it is well to stress an admonition: *Never evaluate the significance of any sort of block without taking rate into consideration.*

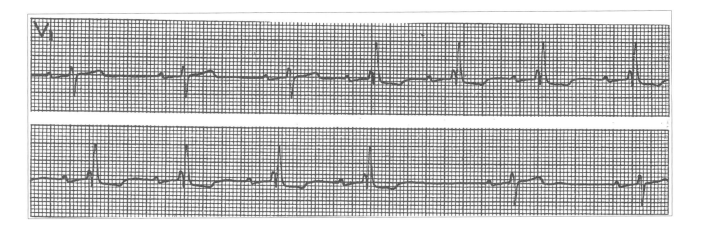

Rate-dependent right bundle branch block (RBBB). As the cycle shortens in the top strip, RBBB develops; when the cycle lengthens toward the end of the bottom, normal conduction resumes.

Emphasis: RBBB provides a <u>late</u> contribution to the QRS and does not alter the <u>early</u> forces. Thus, abnormalities of the initial vector remain valid (e.g.--the "Q waves" of myocardial infarction). Ectopic beats arising in the left ventricle can have a morphology similar to RBBB, but usually the initial forces are different.
Contrast typical RBBB with LV ectopy in the figure.

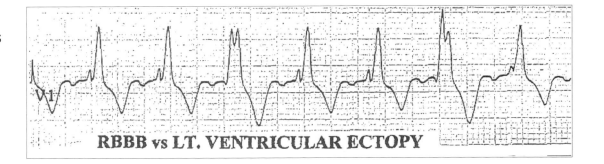

RBBB vs LT. VENTRICULAR ECTOPY

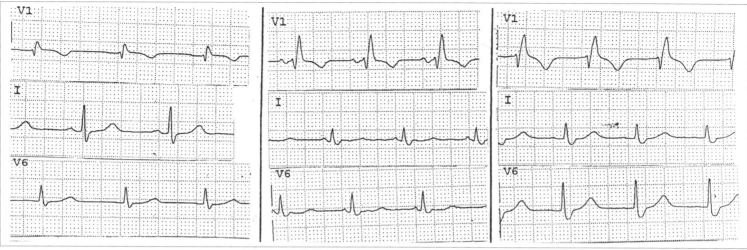

Contrasting "degrees" of RBBB in three subjects. Note the increasing duration of the R' in V1 and terminal s waves in leads I and V6.

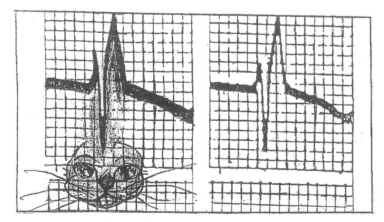

Years ago, an alert CCU nurse provided the observation that there was similarity of RBBB morphology and "rabbit ears." This analogy quickly spread across the country and is in common usage today. In typical RBBB, the "left ear" does not approach the height of the "right ear."

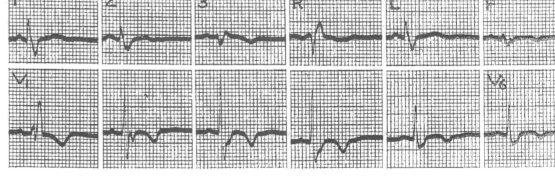

Right bundle-branch block. Note the primary T wave changes: in aVF and V2-V6 the T wave is pointing in the same direction as the latter half of the QRS complex.

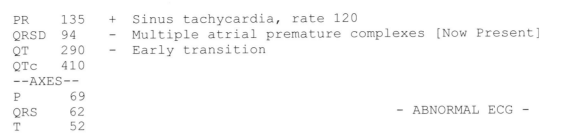

```
PR     135   +  Sinus tachycardia, rate 120
QRSD    94   -  Multiple atrial premature complexes [Now Present]
QT     290   -  Early transition
QTc    410
--AXES--
P       69
QRS     62                              - ABNORMAL ECG -
T       52
```

78 YEAR OLD WOMAN
HOW MANY OBSERVATIONS??

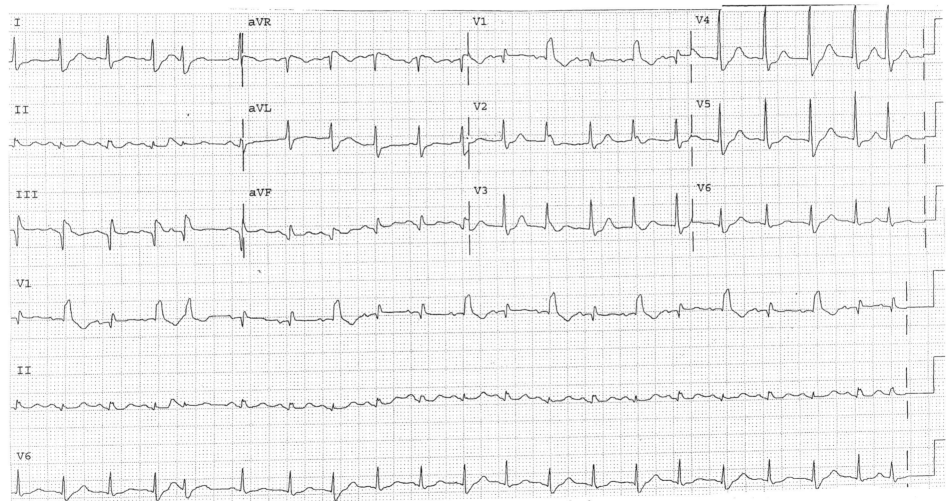

The computer interpretation is correct--but sorely incomplete! All the atrial stimuli--sinus and APCs--are conducted with variable right bundle branch block some with incomplete RBBB, many with complete RBBB. The observation of "early transition" ignores the Q waves in leads II, III, and aVF. The combination of the frontal plane Q waves and the prominent initial R waves in V2 and V3 indicates an inferior-posterior MI of indeterminate age.

```
PR     209    + Sinus tachycardia, rate 65
QRSD   138    -   Multiple atrial premature complexes [Now Present]
              - Consider RVH with ST-T abnormalities
QT     395    - Nonspecific intraventricular conduction delay
QTc    411
--AXES--
P       64
QRS     66                          - ABNORMAL ECG -
T
```

70 YEAR OLD WOMAN
DO YOU AGREE WITH COMPUTER?

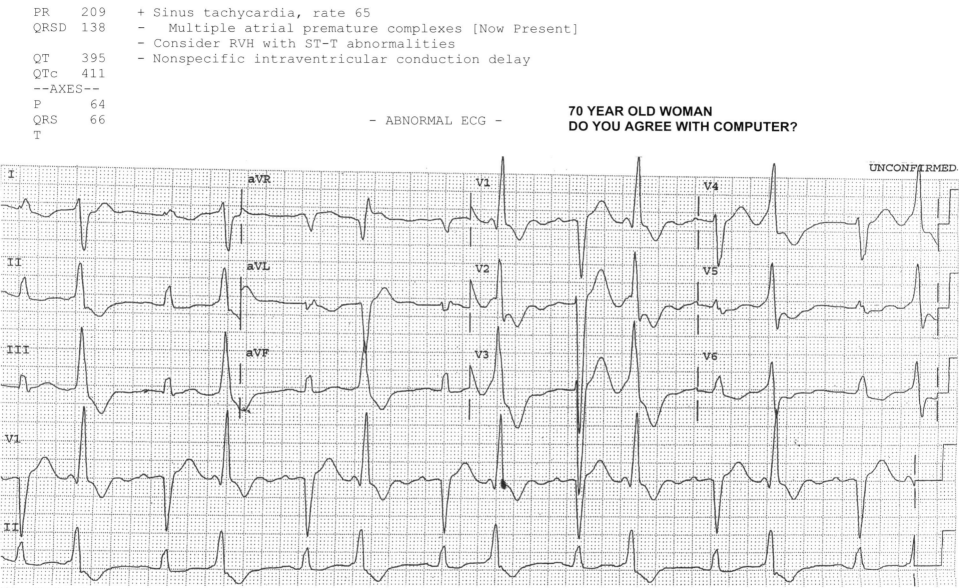

We will all make errors of omission and commission, but the computer commits both with this tracing. The sinus impulses are conducted with <u>LBBB</u> and are wedded to bigeminal <u>VPCs</u>. The morphology of these simulates "RBBB" with right axis deviation, and prompts the computer to "consider RVH."

BIFASCICULAR BLOCKS

Our trifascicular conducting circuit consists of the right bundle branch and the two fascicles of the left bundle branch. Obviously, "bifascicular block" is a loss of two of the three fascicles--a frequent EKG abnormality. The most common is a combination of RBBB and left <u>anterior</u> fascicular block; less frequent is RBBB and left <u>posterior</u> fascicular block. A number of examples of both varieties will be presented.

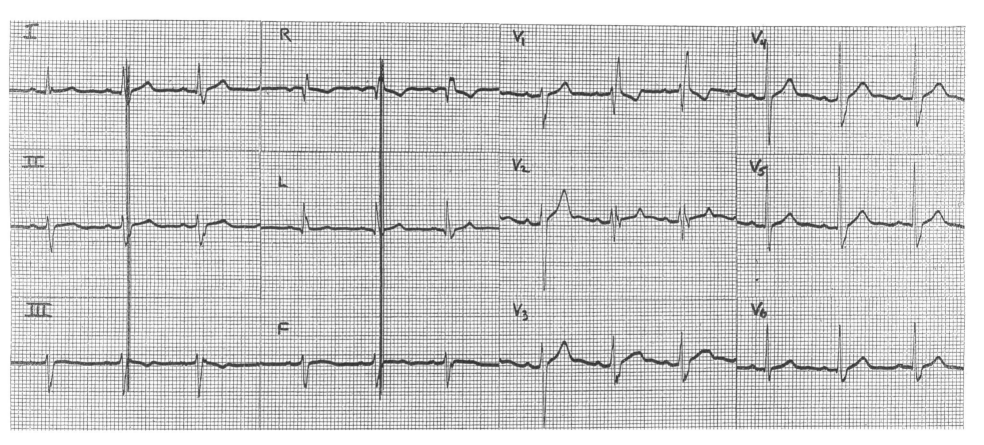

This is an informative example of an intraventricular conduction abnormality in a 20-year-old man. The <u>first</u> QRS complex in each lead set is narrow and has a frontal plane axis of (-) 60°--representing left axis deviation secondary to left anterior fascicular block. The second and third complexes show LAFB + RBBB. In the middle QRS in the frontal leads, the delayed RBBB contribution is inked-out to emphasize that the *initial* QRS forces of LAFB are unchanged. Although this is true in both planes, note the change in the middle portion of the QRS in leads V2-3. The explanation for this was provided earlier in the Chapter (p. 58).

```
PR     206    + Normal sinus rhythm, rate 82
QRSD   147    - Bifascicular block: RBBB & LPFB
QT     392    - Left atrial enlargement
QTc    458    - Borderline ST elevation, inferior leads
--AXES--
P       20
QRS    209                        - ABNORMAL ECG -     77 YEAR OLD WOMAN
T        8                                             DO YOU AGREE WITH COMPUTER?
```

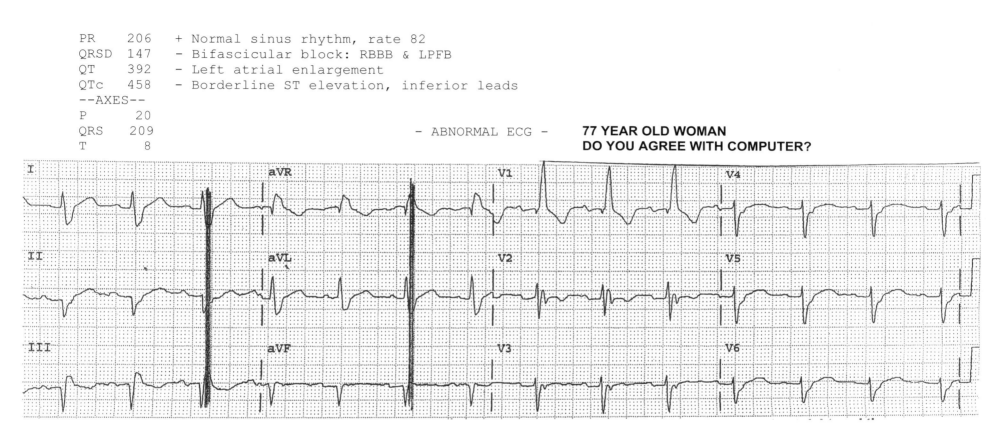

A serious computer error. There is right bundle branch block, but the pre-blocked axis is <u>left</u> at (-) 60° and not right, and thus, not LPFB. The left axis deviation is due to an age undetermined <u>inferior MI</u> which is ignored by the computer.

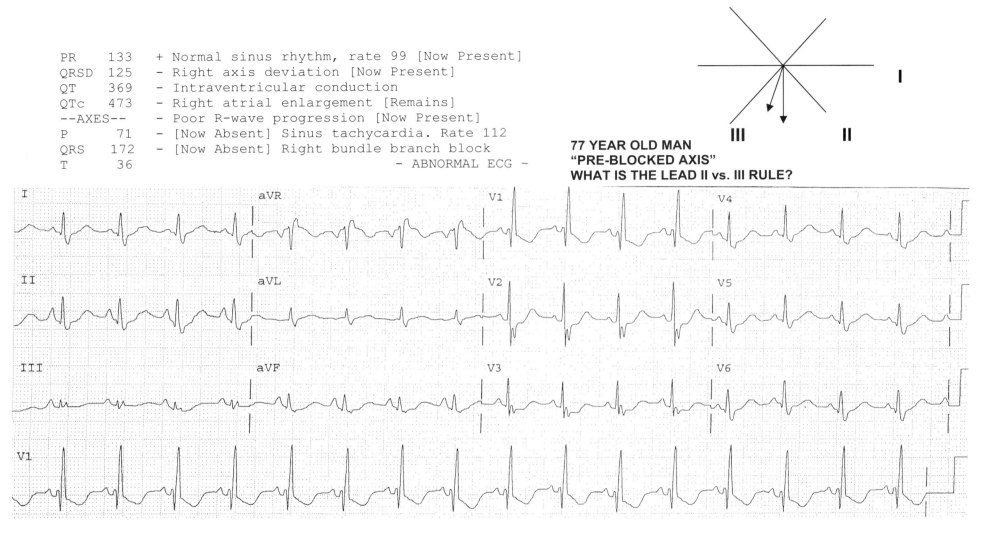

```
PR      133     + Normal sinus rhythm, rate 99 [Now Present]
QRSD    125     - Right axis deviation [Now Present]
QT      369     - Intraventricular conduction
QTc     473     - Right atrial enlargement [Remains]
--AXES--        - Poor R-wave progression [Now Present]
P        71     - [Now Absent] Sinus tachycardia. Rate 112
QRS     172     - [Now Absent] Right bundle branch block
T        36                              - ABNORMAL ECG -
```

77 YEAR OLD MAN
"PRE-BLOCKED AXIS"
WHAT IS THE LEAD II vs. III RULE?

The wide QRS complex and rsR' pattern in V1 identify RBBB. The "pre-blocked axis" is (+) 30°--not right axis deviation as indicated by the computer. Right atrial abnormality and increased QT duration are additional observations. An easy rule to confirm (or deny) right axis is shown in the diagram. This is the "lead III versus lead II rule." If the mean QRS axis is 90°, the amplitude of the R wave in leads II and III will be identical; if it exceeds 90°, the R wave in lead III will always be larger than in lead II; if it is not, the axis is *less* than 90° and, therefore, <u>not right axis deviation</u>!

74

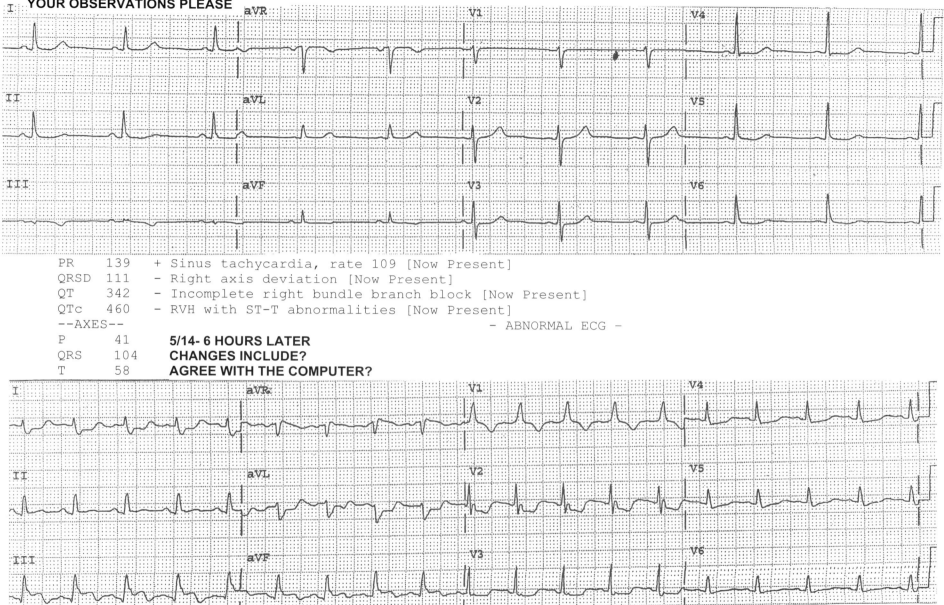

60 YEAR OLD WOMAN -5-14-07:29
YOUR OBSERVATIONS PLEASE

PR	139	+ Sinus tachycardia, rate 109 [Now Present]
QRSD	111	- Right axis deviation [Now Present]
QT	342	- Incomplete right bundle branch block [Now Present]
QTc	460	- RVH with ST-T abnormalities [Now Present]

--AXES--   - ABNORMAL ECG -

P	41	**5/14- 6 HOURS LATER**
QRS	104	**CHANGES INCLUDE?**
T	58	**AGREE WITH THE COMPUTER?**

The top tracing shows a QRS axis of (+) 30° and "nonspecific" ST segment sagging, but is unimpressive. The marked changes in the bottom EKG include complete RBBB and a pre-blocked axis of (+) 105°. The right axis shift is due to left posterior fascicular block, due to acute inferior-posterior myocardial infarction. The computer has combined the prominent R waves in lead V1 and the right axis deviation and concluded "right ventricular hypertrophy," an unlikely possibility in six hours!

```
PR      155    + Tachycardia of undetermined origin, rate 105
QRSD    162    - Right axis deviation
QT      346    - Right bundle branch block
QTc     457    - Consider left atrial enlargement
--AXES--       - Anterior infarct, age indeterminate                - ABNORMAL ECG -
P       IND
QRS     116
T        37
```

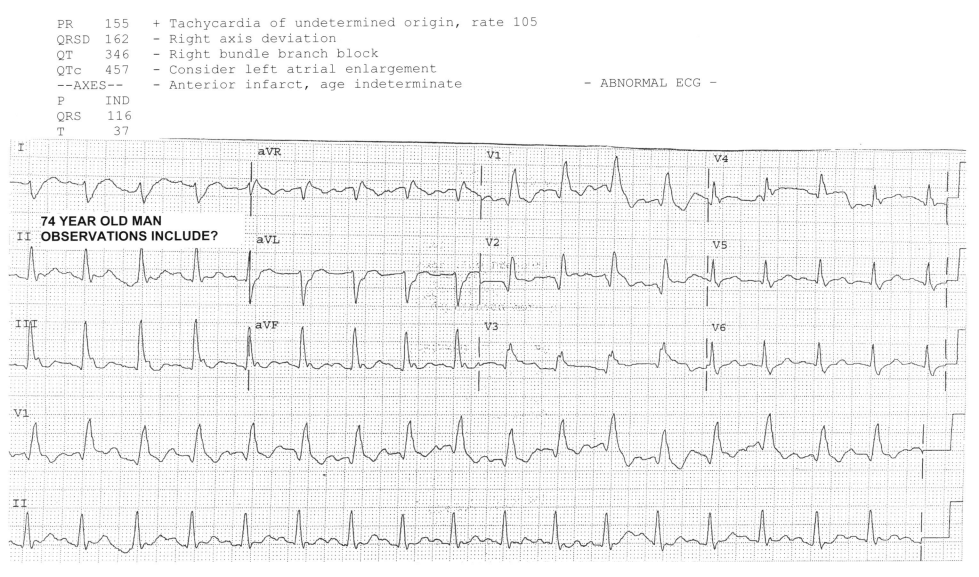

**74 YEAR OLD MAN
OBSERVATIONS INCLUDE?**

Let's make some corrections to the computer interpretation. Sinus tachycardia at 105/min. is present. The right bundle branch block is accompanied by right axis deviation of the "preblocked forces" due to the left posterior fascicular block (bifascicular block). The anterior MI is identified, but the ST segment elevation in leads V1-V4 indicates it is an acute process and is not "age undetermined." The conduction abnormality, in the presence of acute anterior MI, is ominous, warning of possible complete AV block (which occurred shortly thereafter).

```
PR     167    + Normal sinus rhythm, rate 63 [Remains]
QRSD   161    - Right axis deviation [Remains]
QT     458    - Right bundle branch block [Remains]
QTc    469    - Left atrial enlargement [Remains]
--AXES--      - Nonspecific Lateral region T wave abnormalities [Now Present]
P       50    - Cannot exclude ischemia
QRS    133    - [Now Absent] Nonspecific Lateral region T wave abnormalities
T      -36                    - ABNORMAL ECG -
```

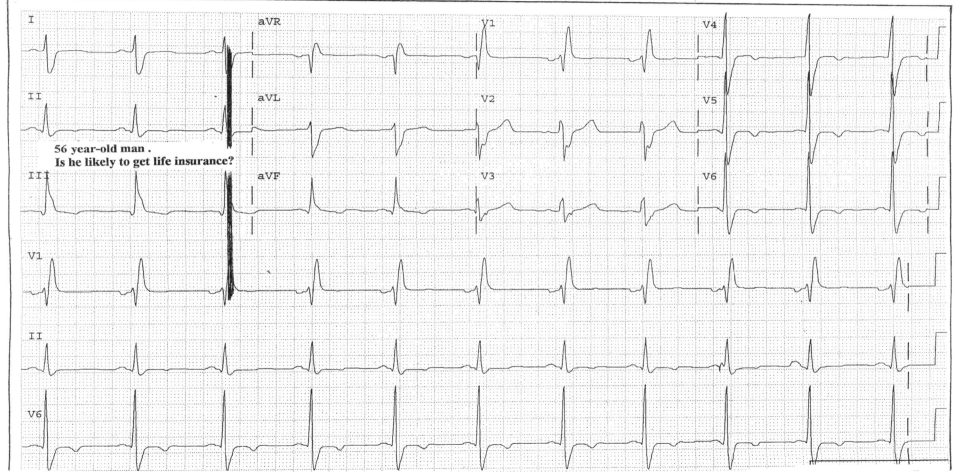

The interpretation is correct--as far as it goes. The frontal plane pre-blocked axis is (+) 100° and it <u>must</u> be due to left posterior fascicular block. Why? Since RBBB adds a *late* component to the QRS duration, the right ventricle cannot be contributing to the *early* (pre-blocked) forces and, thus, RVH cannot be the cause of the right axis deviation and it must be due to LPFB. Bifascicular block accompanied by left atrial enlargement and ST-T abnormality would likely make this man ineligible for life insurance.

79 YEAR OLD MAN -12/12
"I KEEP PASSING OUT-WHY"?

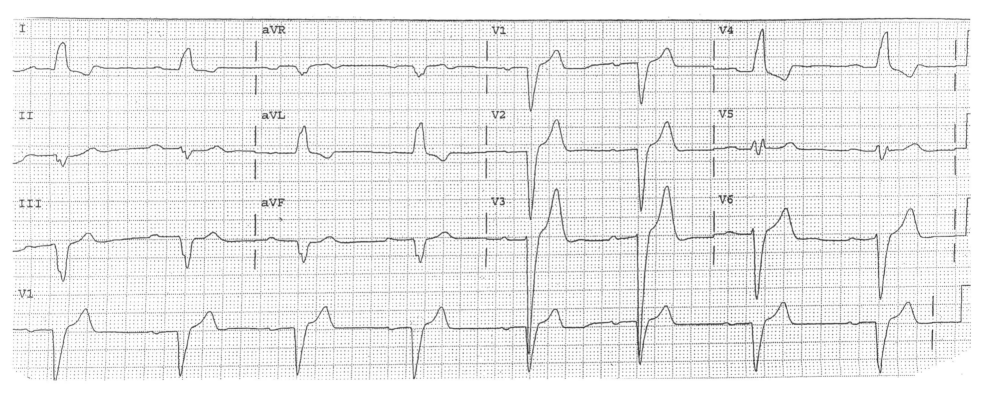

Let's agree with the computer, with concerns about the validity of the last diagnosis in the presence of left bundle branch block. Can you anticipate the next EKG and the reason for his "passing out"?

```
PR     179   - Sinus bradycardia, rate 47
QRSD   165   - Right axis deviation
QT     607   - Right bundle branch block
QTc    537   - Left atrial enlargement
--AXES--
P       73
QRS    125
T      -15                        - ABNORMAL ECG -
```

79 YEAR OLD MAN -12/12
DOES THIS PROVIDE AN EXPLANATION?

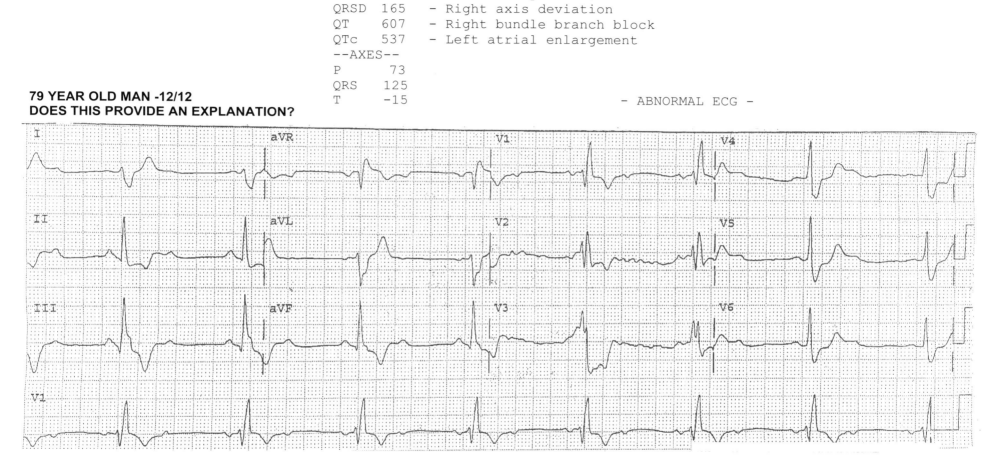

Later in the same day, the sinus rate has increased to 94/min. and there is 2:1 A-V block. In addition there is now <u>RBBB</u> with right axis deviation due to left posterior fascicular block. Obviously this man has serious infranodal conduction system disease and will need an electronic pacemaker. If you anticipated these changes -congratulations.

ABNORMALITIES OF THE CARDIAC CHAMBERS

Atrial Abnormalities

Since the sinus node P wave arises in the roof of the right atrium, the signal must cross to the left atrium. It does so over a specialized conducting path-- Bachman's bundle--requiring a transit time of only 40 msec. If one could record the P waves within the atria (**A**), they would be recorded with an initial right and, 40 msec. later, a left atrial P wave. However, on the body surface (**B**), in the electrocardiographic frontal plane, the normal P wave has a rounded summit, with an amplitude < 2.5 mm and a duration <100 msec. If there is an increase in the right atrial portion (**C**), the P wave increases in height and becomes pointed. Left atrial abnormality results in a broader P wave (**D**), often with a notch between components. When both are abnormal (**E**), the morphology includes an initial sharp and subsequent broad configuration. In the frontal plane, both right and left atrial components have the same general vectoral direction. However, in the horizontal plane, the initial right atrial P wave is directed anteriorly, and is recorded <u>positive</u> in lead V1, while the left atrial event is oriented left and posterior and is recorded as <u>negative</u> in lead V1 (**F**). If the right atrial component is increased (**G**), the initial (+) part of the P wave in V1 is increased, exceeding 1 mm. When the left atrial P wave is increased, the terminal trough of the P wave (**H**) exceeds 1 mm deep and 1 mm wide. (The "P terminal force").

Terminology varies regarding abnormal P waves but since they need not indicate chamber *hypertrophy* or *enlargement*, we will use the less specific term "*atrial abnormality.*"

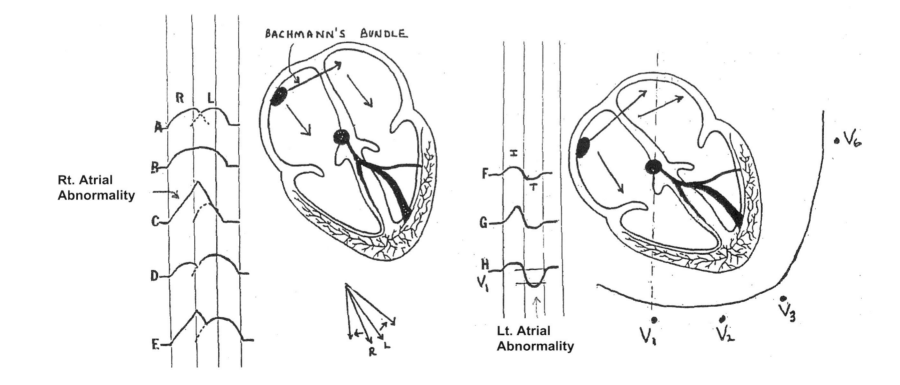

65 YEAR OLD WOMAN
WHAT IS "P-MITRALE"?

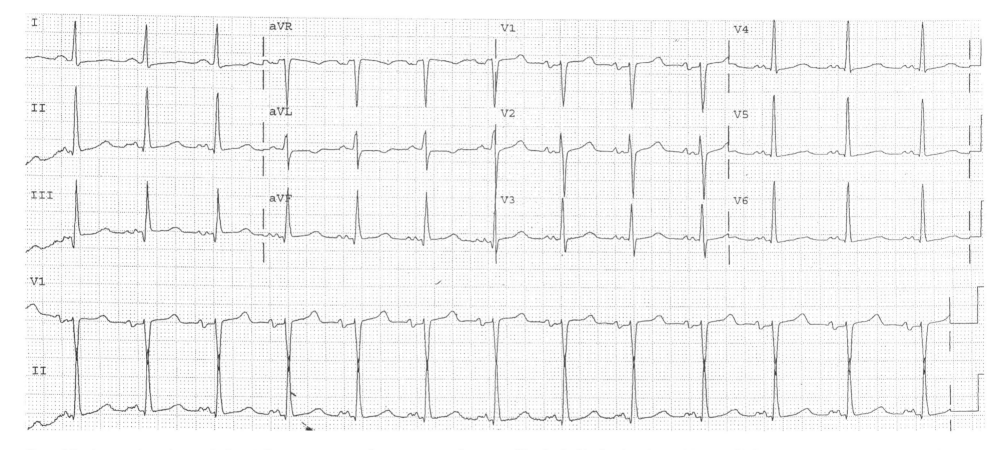

One of the terms when rheumatic heart disease was prevalent, was prevalent, was "P mitrale," indicating that evidence of left atrial abnormality was most often due to mitral valve disease. Obviously, there are other causes, but the P wave morphology remains characteristic. Note the notched P wave in lead II and most of the precordial leads, and the "P terminal force" in V1. Unfortunately, no clinical information is available regarding this woman.

LEFT VENTRICULAR HYPERTROPHY

Despite decades of study, the EKG criteria for the diagnosis of LVH remain elusive. Many have been recommended, but although the specificity is excellent, the sensitivity is poor. We will select only the best-known and often cited criteria. From the outset, it is evident that the most important diagnostic feature is <u>excess QRS voltage</u>.

Since the original leads were limited to the bipolar limb leads I, II, and III, the first criterion was based on these leads. Gubner and Ungerleiter indicated that if the <u>R wave in lead I plus the S wave in lead III</u> equaled or exceeded <u>25 mm</u>, LVH was present.

The unipolar leads aVR, aVL, and aVF arrived years later. Lead aVL was selected as the lead in which amplitude should be considered. The criteria recommended varied, ranging from 7mm to 13mm. Let's compromise with an <u>aVL amplitude of 11 mm or more</u> required to diagnose LVH.

When the precordial leads arrived on the scene, additional criteria appeared. Sokolow and Lyons recommended the addition of the <u>S wave in lead V1 plus the R wave in V5 or V6</u>. If the combination equaled <u>35 mm</u>, and the patient was older than 45 years, LVH voltage was present.

Romhilt and Estes provided a composite of elements that might provide accuracy in the diagnosis of LVH. In addition to QRS voltage, they added repolarization changes, electrical axis, delayed QRS activation, and presence of left atrial abnormality and assigned a point score.

1. R or S in the limb leads	20mm or more	
S in V1-V2-or V3	25mm or more	→ 3 points
R in V4-V5-or V6	25mm or more	
2. Any ST shift (without digitalis)	3 points	With a maximum of 13 points, 5 indicates LVH
3. Lt. axis of (-) 15° or more	2 points	and 4 points probable LVH
4. QRS interval of 0.09 sec. or more	1 point	
5. Ventricular activation time in V5-V6 of 0.04 sec.	1 point	
6. Lt. atrial abnormality		
(P-terminal force in V1 more than 0.04 sec.)	3 points	

Later, a criterion was recommended combining both frontal and horizontal plane elements-the <u>Cornell voltage</u>. This adds the <u>R wave in aVL and the S wave in V3</u>. If the combination is <u>28 mm or greater in men, or 20 mm in women</u>, LVH voltage is present. The presence of left atrial abnormality is additional evidence, as it is in all other criteria.

LVH with Repolarization Abnormalities

Change in repolarization is often present with excessive depolarization voltage. In leads V5 + V6, with tall R waves, the ST segments become depressed with an upward convexity and the final downward curve blends into an inverted T wave. In leads were the QRS is predominantly negative, as in V1, the ST segment is reciprocally elevated with an upward concavity. The term "strain" has been applied to these changes and is a useful, if non-committal term. The exact mechanism that produces this pattern is not completely settled, but there are several factors believed to contribute to it. It is known to be related to the duration with which LVH is present, and correlates well with increasing left ventricular mass as determined by echocardiography. Myocardial ischemia and slowing of intraventricular conduction are probably additional factors.

Since echocardiography came on the scene and provided a safe, noninvasive, and accurate method of assessing chamber size without having to wait for autopsy correlation, investigators have flocked to better the EKG criteria for the diagnosis of LVH. Abundant as are the criteria now available to choose from, it is disappointing that, despite the ingenuity and variety of the offerings, improvements are minor.

Just as one size of shoe will not fit all, one criterion for LVH may be present while another doesn't apply. In the examples of LVH to follow, select the diagnostic criteria which "fit best."

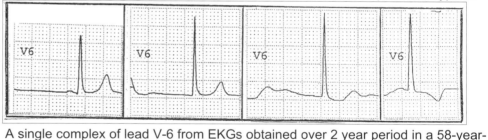

Left ventricular hypertrophy. Note the huge amplitude of the QRS in V5 and V6, with high voltage in all chest leads. The axis is + 40°, and the ST-T pattern is typical.

A single complex of lead V-6 from EKGs obtained over 2 year period in a 58-year-old man, with poorly controlled hypertension. The QRS amplitude increases, the T-wave voltage decreases, the ST segments becomes sagging and, ultimately, typical "LVH with strain" appears.

Some observations and reservations

1. With the current mode of recording multiple leads, an initial approach should be to glance at the precordial leads. If the QRS complexes are so large that they overlap, LVH is almost certainly present. (An exception is children and young adults)

2. Importantly, the frontal plane criteria do not consider variations in the QRS axis. For example, if the axis is (+) 60°, the QRS would be isoelectric in lead aVL and it would be a poor lead to select for amplitude measurement. Also, since the technician's placement of precordial leads often lacks precision, it seems unwarranted to insist on particular lead combination (e.g. S in V1 + R in V 5-6). A reasonable compromise is to combine the *deepest S wave and the tallest R wave*. If the sum is 35 mm or more, and the patient is over the age of 45, LVH voltage is present. If a patient is 35 years or less, a sum of 45 mm can be allowed.

3. It seems reasonable that, because of the anatomical location of the left ventricle, LVH should cause left axis deviation in the frontal plane. Although this has been accepted for years, the reality is that the majority of EKGs with evident LVH voltage have a <u>normal axis</u>. When left axis accompanies LVH, it is usually because left anterior fascicular block is present.

4. Another sobering fact is that, although the interpreter is provided the patient's age and gender, usually little other information is available. It is obvious that body build and presence or absence of "surface insulators" (air or fat) are considerations that can change transmitted voltage.

52 YEAR OLD MAN
YOUR OBSERVATIONS INCLUDE?

R1 + S3 = 25 mm or more
aVL = 11 mm or more
SV1 + R V5 or V6 = 35 mm or more

R or S limb leads = 20 mm or more
R or S chest leads = 25 mm or more
R aVL + S V3 = 28-men 20-women

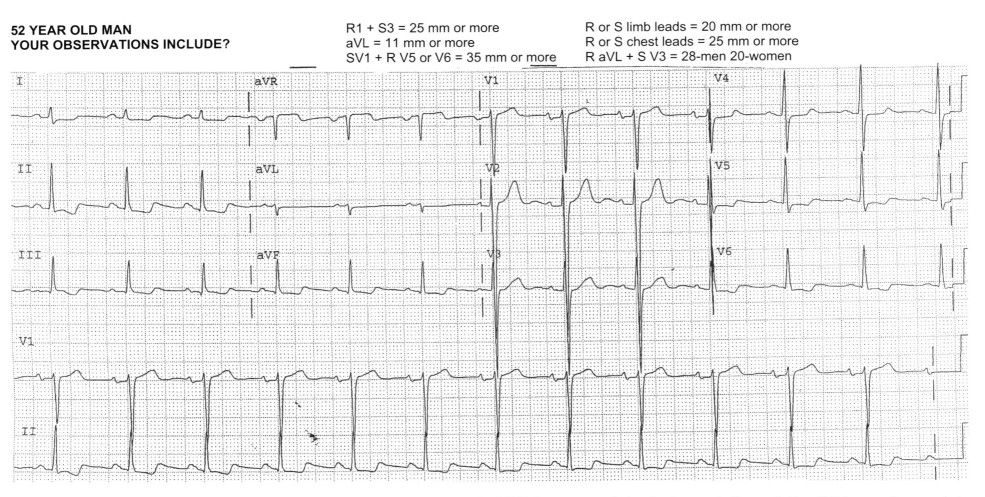

The axis is (+) 70°. QRS voltage in the frontal plane leads is normal, although the ST-T changes are obviously abnormal. Precordial lead V2 has an S wave of at least 30 mm. The P wave duration and morphology in lead II is consistent with left atrial abnormality. Let's diagnose LVH with repolarization abnormality.

84

24 YEAR OLD MAN
WOULD YOU DIAGNOSE L.V.H.?

R1 + S3 = 25 mm or more
aVL = 11 mm or more
SV1 + R V5 or V6 = 35 mm or more

R or S limb leads = 20 mm or more
R or S chest leads = 25 mm or more
R aVL + S V3 = 28-men or 20-women

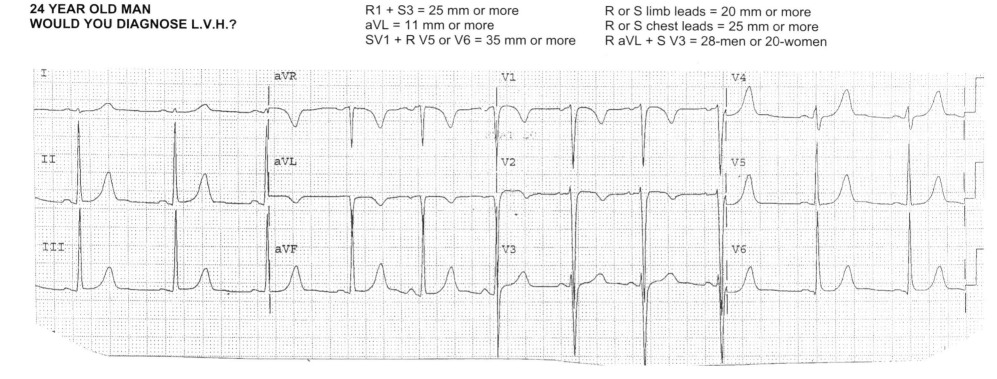

Young and healthy men often have QRS voltage that exceeds the usual criteria and is often marked. Since the diagnosis of LVH can jeopardize insurability, it should not be rendered too quickly. However, it is important that clinical information be considered. This man had a significantly obstructive bicuspid aortic valve. The QRS amplitude is >20 mm in the limb leads and the sum of the "deepest S and tallest R wave" in the precordial leads is > 50 mm. A diagnosis of LVH voltage is warranted.

66 YEAR OLD WOMAN
ANY EVIDENCE OF L.V.H.?

R1 + S3 = 25 mm or more
aVL = 11 mm or more
SV1 + R V5 or V6 = 35 mm or more

R or S limb leads = 20 mm or more
R or S chest leads = 25 mm or more
R aVL + S V3 = 28-men or 20-women

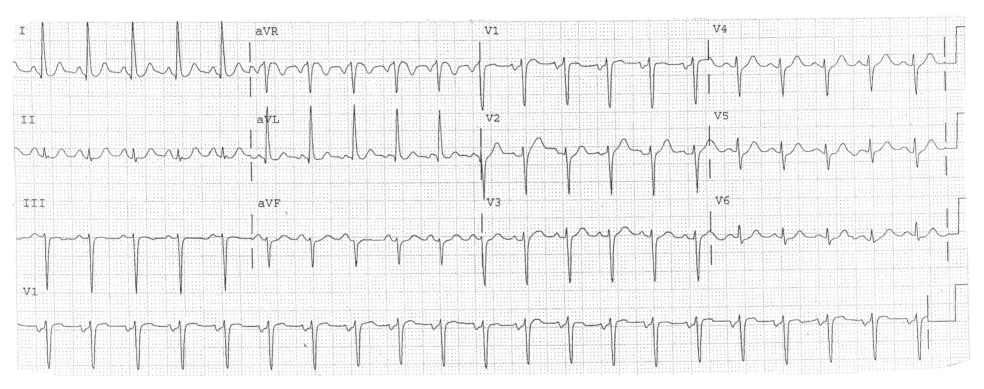

In this woman, the voltage of LVH is better defined in the frontal then in the horizontal plane. The left atrial abnormality provide supporting evidence.

45 YEAR OLD MAN
HOW MANY L.V.H. "POINTS"?

R1 + S3 = 25 mm or more
aVL = 11 mm or more
SV1 + R V5 or V6 = 35 mm or more

R or S limb leads = 20 mm or more
R or S chest leads = 25 mm or more
R aVL + S V3 = 28-men or 20-women

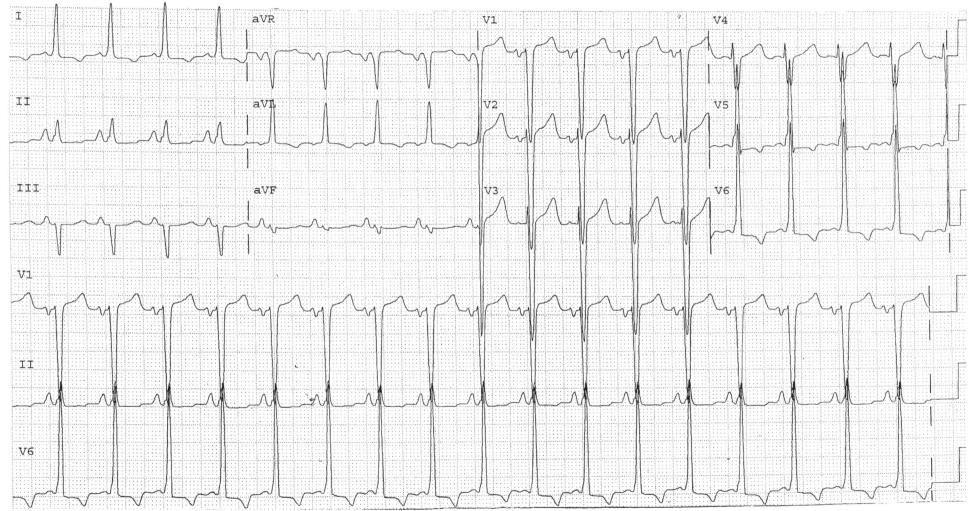

As left ventricular hypertrophy progresses, the thickened LV wall requires additional time to complete depolarization. A helpful and simple measurement is "ventricular activation time" (VAT). This is the time from the beginning of the R wave to its summit. If this is 40 msec. or more, the diagnosis of LVH receives major support. In this man, there are QRS voltage criteria, ST-T changes, and left atrial abnormality (biatrial enlargement) accompanying the VAT.

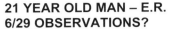

21 YEAR OLD MAN – E.R.
6/29 OBSERVATIONS?

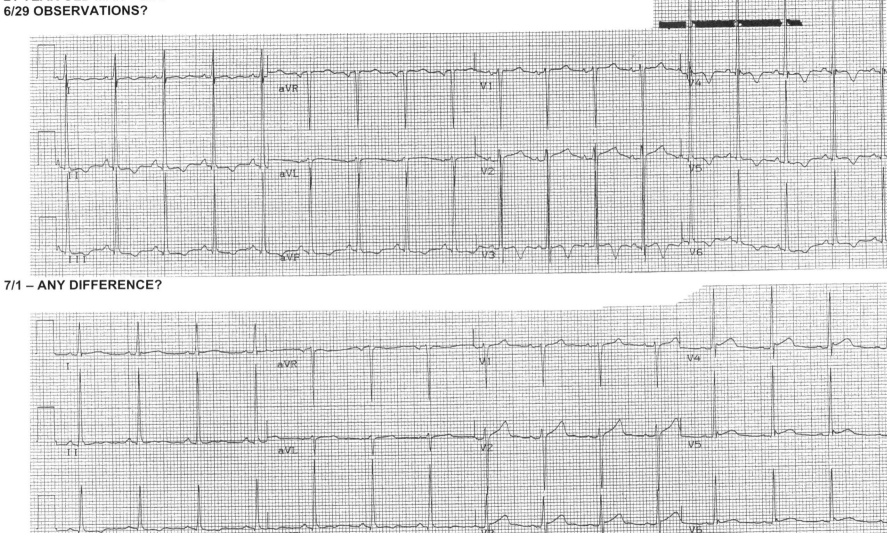

7/1 – ANY DIFFERENCE?

An interesting sequence of tracings with an unexpected change. The top tracing was obtained in this young man, intoxicated with "crack cocaine." He was seriously hypertensive, and his EKG showed striking evidence of LVH with strain pattern. Two days later his blood pressure normalized and the QRS voltage has regressed and the ST-T abnormalities have disappeared. This EKG would not be sufficient to diagnose LVH at age 21 years. How could this occur? There is evidence that if the left ventricular "*transmyocardial wall tension*" is increased; the depolarization voltage generated is significantly increased. This is probably the explanation of the decrease in QRS voltage frequently seen in patients responsive to treatment of hypertension and for the alleged "regression of LVH."

```
PR     183    + Normal sinus rhythm, rate 64 [Remains]
QRSD    87    - Vertical axis, unusual for age [Now Present]
QT     468    - Probable LVH with ST-T abnormalities [Now Present]
QTc    483    - Poor R-wave progression, possibly due to LVH [Now Present]
--AXES--      - Probable Inferior injury [Now Present]
P       73    - [Now Absent] Nonspecific Lateral region T abnormalities
QRS     84
T       87              - ABNORMAL ECG -
```

80 YEAR OLD WOMAN
CHANGES FOR THE COMPUTER?

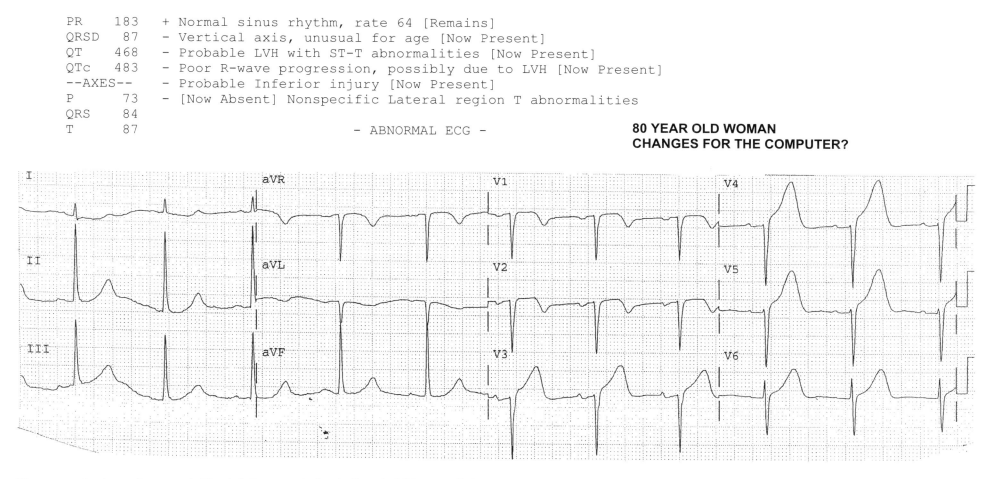

The computer is partly correct. The tall R waves in leads II and aVF are sufficient to diagnose left ventricular hypertrophy, and the computer acknowledges this. A frequent problem in patients with LVH results from the hypertrophied left ventricular *free wall*. Its electrical forces cause a posterior-lateral direction of the precordial QRS complexes, resulting in "poor R wave progression." This raises concern for a possible anterior myocardial infarction and requires clinical correlation. The concern is certainly justified in this woman. The ST segment elevation across the precordial leads and the absent R waves in V1-V4 indicate an <u>acute</u> anteroseptal MI, not recognized by the computer. The motion artifact in the first complex in lead III is misinterpreted as "inferior injury."

```
PR      226  + Sinus rhythm, rate 66 [Remains]
QRSD     94  - First degree AV block [Remains]
QT      415  - Left atrial enlargement [Remains]
QTc     435  - Left ventricular hypertrophy [Now Present]
--AXES--     - [Now Absent] QT interval long for rate
P        29  - [Now Absent] Anterolateral region ST-T abnormalities
QRS      52
T        62                    - ABNORMAL ECG -
```

**77 YEAR OLD WOMAN
IS THE HEART ALLOWED TO MAKE A U TURN?**

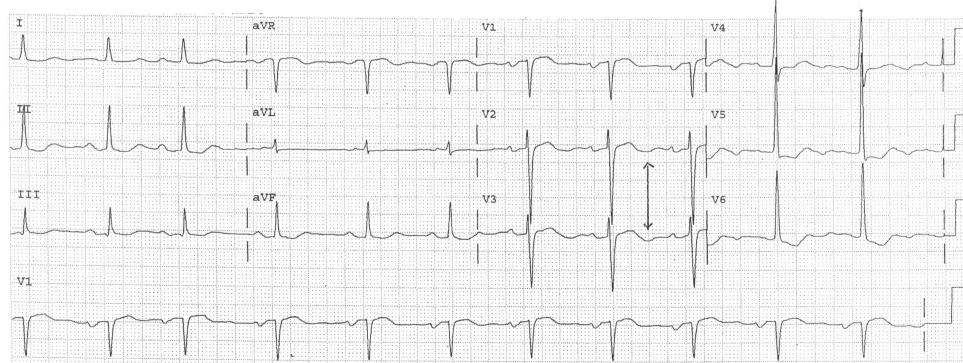

The rhythm is sinus with a prolonged PR interval and evident left atrial abnormality. Although the frontal plane QRS amplitude is normal, the precordial leads show clear-cut LVH voltage, with repolarization abnormality. A particularly concerning thing is the additional repolarization event- the negative U waves, well seen in leads V2 - V3 (arrows). There presence often indicates ongoing myocardial ischemia, but could represent hypokalemia.

RIGHT VENTRICULAR HYPERTROPHY

In infancy, childhood, and for variable periods of young adult life, the right ventricle is the electrically dominant chamber. In the older adult, the right ventricle recedes and the left ventricle assumes command, and will be the dominant "driving force" for the rest of one's life. This helps to understand why it may be difficult for the adult to overcome the LV and demonstrate right ventricular hypertrophy. Nonetheless, there are validated criteria for the diagnosis of RVH, but they are insensitive and other abnormalities share some of the features.

The anatomical location of the right ventricle dictates the best criteria for the diagnosis of RVH.
1. Right axis deviation in the frontal plane (in the adult (+) 90° or more).
2. Excess anterior force in the horizontal plane
   (R to S ratio in V1 greater > 1 or R in V1 = 7 mm or more).
3. Too little posterior force in lateral chest leads (R to S ratio in V5 or V6 < 1).

RVH is commonly accompanied by right atrial abnormality, and by repolarization abnormality ("strain"). In the example below, there is right axis deviation of + 120°, right atrial abnormality, tall R waves in V1, and deep S waves in V6. This unfortunate man had progressing pulmonary fibrosis, with resulting pulmonary hypertension and right ventricular hypertrophy.

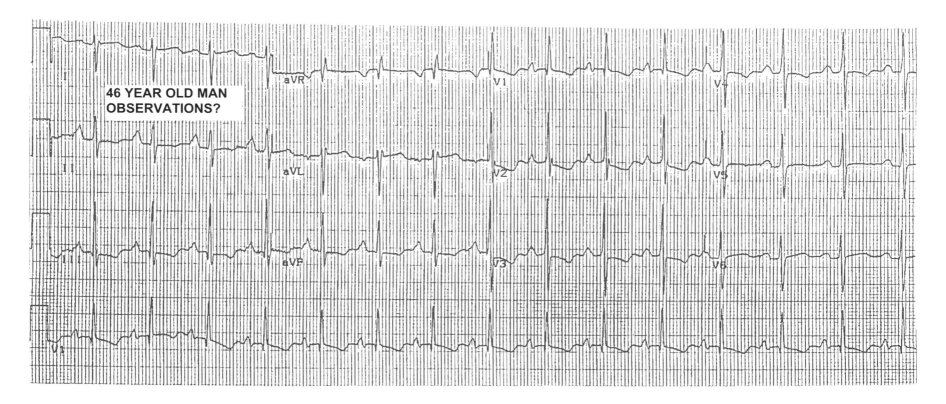

46 YEAR OLD MAN OBSERVATIONS?

```
PR                 + Check patient history - mismatch with previous race
QRSD     94        - Atrial fibrillation with rapid ventricular response of 139 [Now Present]
QT       285       - Right axis deviation [Now Present]
QTc      433       - Probable RVH with ST-T abnormalities [Now Present]
--AXES--           - Probable Anteroseptal region MI, age
P                  - [Now Absent] Anterolateral region ST-T abnormalities
QRS      112
T        -54                    - ABNORMAL ECG -
```

30 YEAR OLD WOMAN-PROBABLE Dx

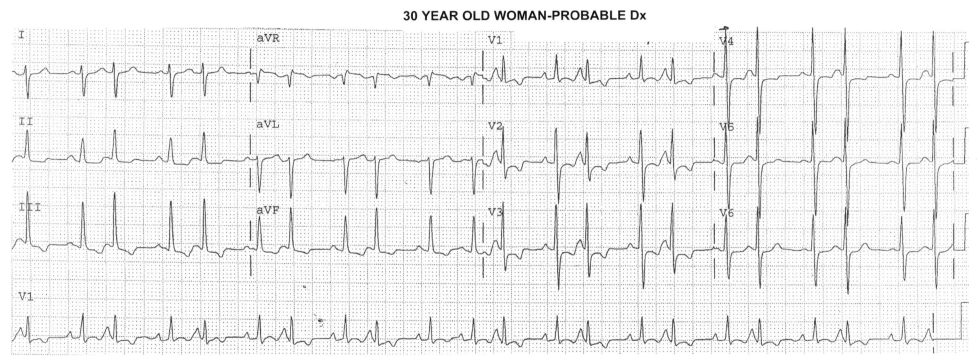

The rhythm is predominantly atrial bigemini, which the computer has misinterpreted as atrial fibrillation. There is right axis deviation in the frontal plane of (+) 110°, with an R/S ratio in V1 >1 and an R/S ratio in V5 <1. P waves are consistent with right atrial abnormality. The combination indicates excess RV forces and the ST-T changes in V1-V4 permit a diagnosis of right ventricular hypertrophy with "strain." There is no basis for the computer call of "anteroseptal MI." This unfortunate young woman had primary pulmonary hypertension and did not survive the year.

49 YEAR OLD WOMAN
OBSERVATIONS?? – CLUE:
WKS/MONTH X MONTHS/YR X 10 =?

WHO IS JOE IN THE DICKENS' STORY??

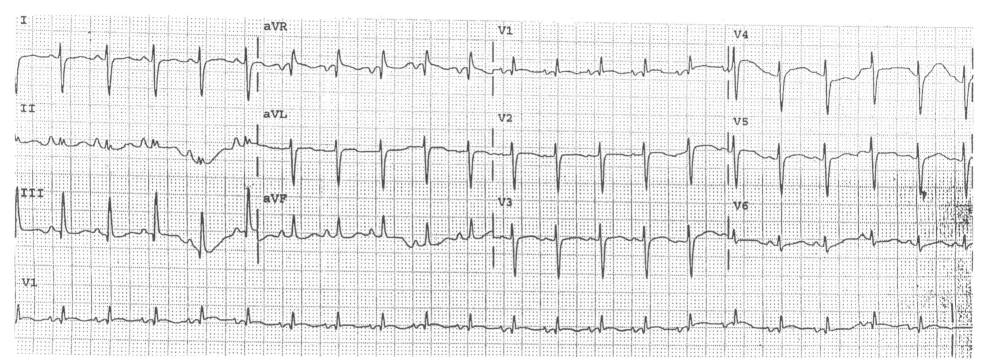

If you powered up your pocket calculator, you would quickly determine that 4 X 12 X 10 = 480. This is the patient's weight and makes it evident that she is a candidate for the "obesity-hypoventilation syndrome." The right axis deviation, right atrial enlargement, and the precordial pattern combine to indicate that the tracing represents right ventricular hypertrophy and that she has significant pulmonary hypertension. This is an example of the "Pickwickian Syndrome." The eponym arises from the Charles Dickens' book "The Pickwick Papers." Joe was the character in the story that Dickens provided a picturesque description of "*Joe, the wonderously fat boy.*" He was a delivery boy who would fall asleep while standing at a customer's door.

```
PR      249  + Sinus rhythm, rate 87 [Remains]
QRSD    101  - First degree AV block [Remains]
QT      363  - Right axis deviation [Remains]
QTc     437  - Consider right atrial enlargement [Now Present]
--AXES--     - Probable RVH with ST-T abnormalities [Now Present]
P        74  - Consider left atrial enlargement [Remains]
QRS     106
T       -44                          - ABNORMAL ECG -
```

87 YEAR OLD MAN
DO YOU AGREE WITH COMPUTER?

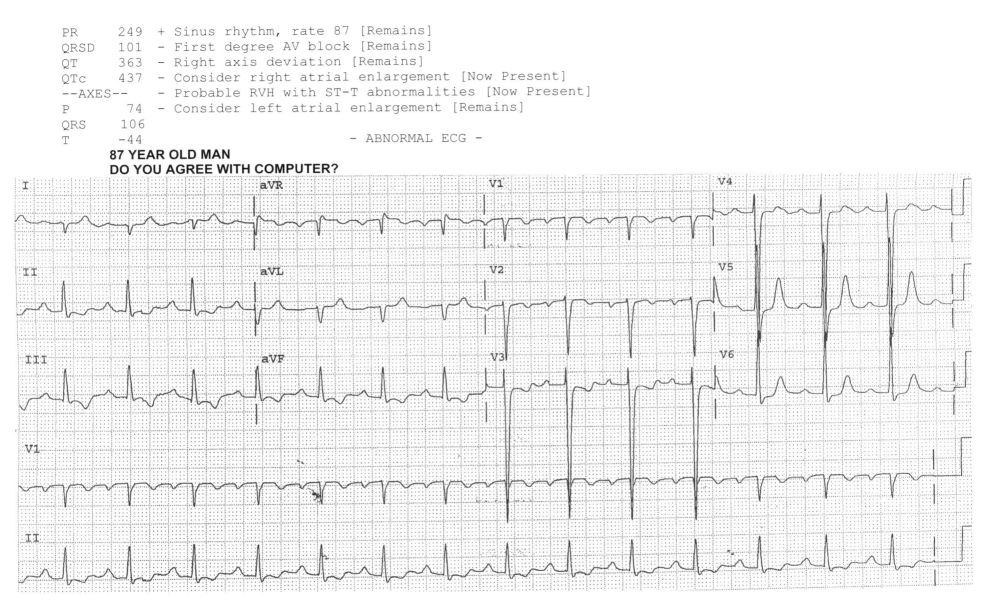

Of the six computer diagnoses, five are correct. Pretty good batting average--but the diagnosis of RVH is a strikeout! There is biatrial abnormality and a prolonged PR interval. Note the broad Q waves in leads I and aVL indicating that *lateral wall myocardial infarction* is the cause of the right axis deviation. The computer has used the right axis as the basis for the interpretation of "RVH." The precordial leads deny this and, instead, indicate left ventricular hypertrophy is present.

```
PR      192  + Normal sinus rhythm, rate 94 [Remains]
QRSD     90  - Right axis deviation [Remains]
QT      365  - Right atrial enlargement [Remains]
QTc     456  - Consider left atrial enlargement [Now Present]
--AXES--
P        72
QRS     113
T       -34                        - ABNORMAL ECG -
```

61 YEAR OLD MAN
YOU SUSPECT WHAT PROBLEM??

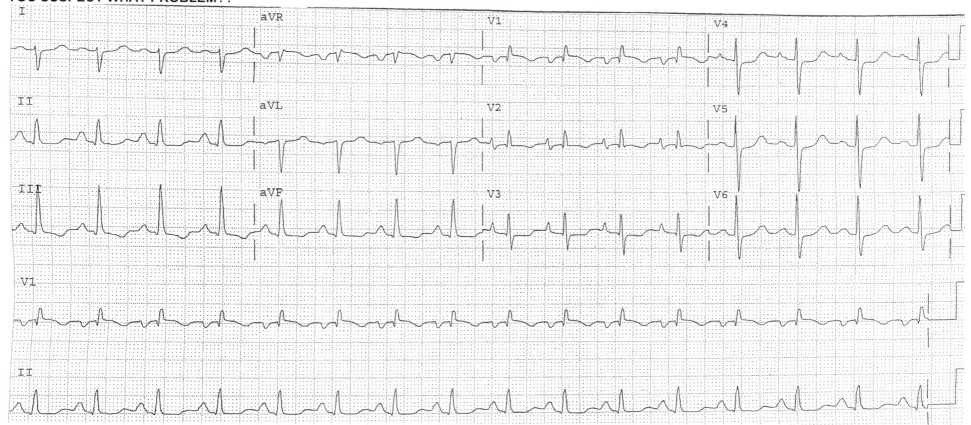

The computer interpretation is correct, but is lacking a conclusion. The right axis deviation and the prominent terminal R wave in V1 are secondary to right ventricular hypertrophy. The small Q waves in V1-2-3 may represent an anterior M.I., but can be seen with marked RV hypertrophy. Right atrial enlargement typically accompanies RVH, but the evident left atrial enlargement should not. This is the important clue to the patient's problem--which is <u>mitral stenosis</u> with "backup" pulmonary hypertension.

33 YEAR OLD MAN
5'2" – Eyes of blue – 300#

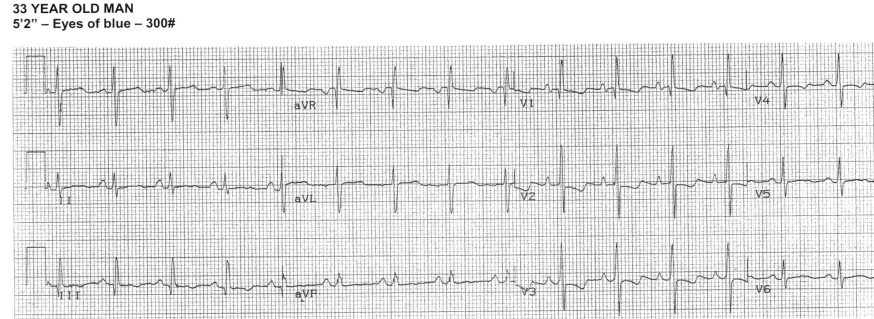

This young man has a combination of problems: obesity-hypoventilation syndrome; recurrent pneumonia; and repetitive pulmonary emboli. The result is serious pulmonary hypertension resulting in a classical example of RVH. The EKG shows right atrial abnormality and right axis deviation of (+) 120°. The tall R wave in lead V1 is not due to delayed RV activation (RBBB), but is caused by "too much" anterior right ventricle. The repolarization abnormality seen in V1-V4 reflects right ventricular "strain" and the initial q wave in V1 suggest that RV pressure is near or at systemic levels.

```
PR      145   + Sinus tachycardia, rate 120
QRSD     90
QT      295
QTc     417
--AXES--
P        82
QRS      25
T        30                        - OTHERWISE NORMAL ECG -
```

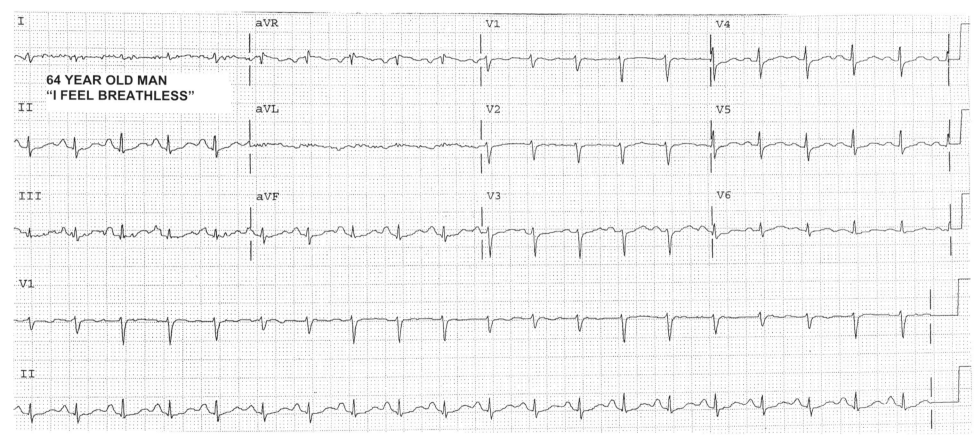

64 YEAR OLD MAN
"I FEEL BREATHLESS"

When does RVH not look like RVH? In patients with advanced COPD, the heart follows the low-lying diaphragm and becomes "vertical." The frontal plane QRS axis assumes this direction and is isoelectric in lead I. The lack of precordial QRS transition and the low QRS voltage reflect both the lower cardiac position and the insulation effect of the hyperinflated lungs. The undulating pattern in the V1 rhythm strip ("dyspnea pattern") and the right atrial prominence are additional features.

```
PR      167    + Sinus tachycardia, rate 109
QRSD     97    - Superior axis
QT      326    - Right ventricular hypertrophy
QTc     439    - Nonspecific Lateral region ST depression
--AXES--
P        82
QRS     268
T        14          - ABNORMAL ECG -    77 YEAR OLD MAN
                                         DO YOU AGREE WITH THE REVIEWER?
```

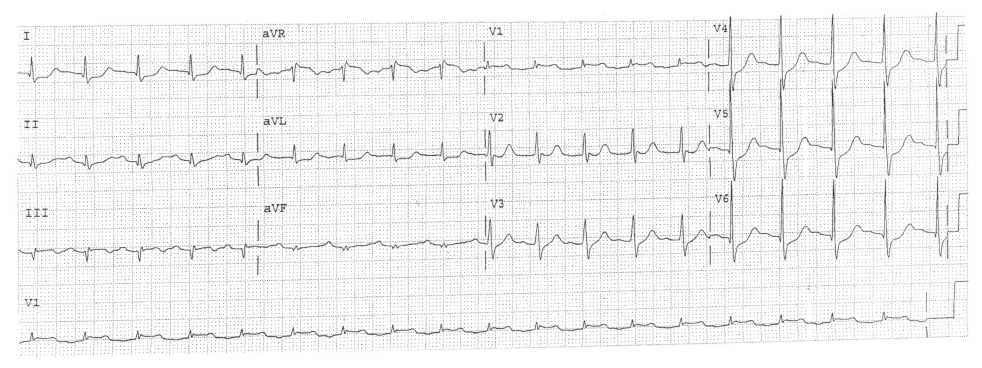

Although the computer has noted RVH, there is, in fact, no evidence of that. There is no right axis deviation and the r' in V1 and the terminal S waves in leads I and V6 indicate *incomplete* RBBB. The QRS voltage is smallest in lead aVF and, therefore, the frontal plane axis is 0°. Q waves in limb leads, and V5-6, indicate an age- undetermined inferolateral MI, and the early transition and broad R waves in V1-V3 implicate an accompanying posterior infarction. ST segment elevation in aVR should raise the concern of a <u>left main</u> coronary artery lesion.

76 YEAR OLD WOMAN
IS THERE EVIDENCE OF R.V.H.?

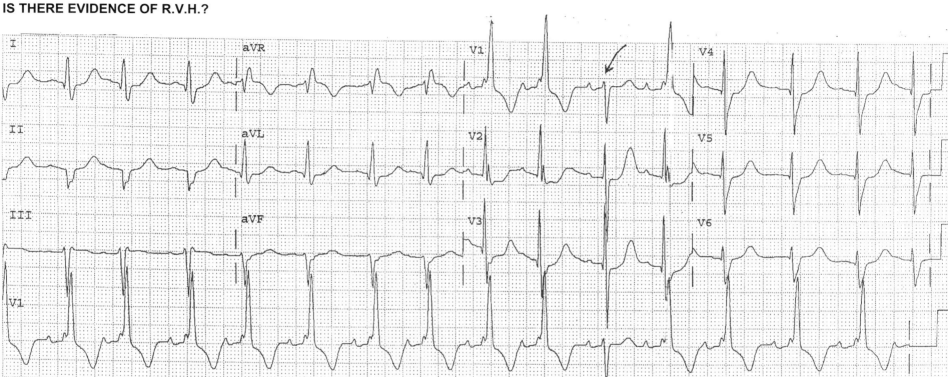

Sinus impulses are conducted with right bundle branch block and left axis deviation of the preblocked forces, due to left anterior fascicular block. It has been suggested that, in the presence of RBBB, if the R' in V1 is 15 mm or more, a diagnosis of RVH is warranted. This is an interesting example that provides doubt for this criterion. Note that, for a single complex (arrow), normal ventricular activation is present, with nothing to suggest RVH. The Q waves in V2-V6 are concerning for an anterolateral infarction of unknown age.

82 YEAR OLD MAN-7/31-23:24
YOUR OBSERVATIONS INCLUDE??

PR	192	+ Normal sinus rhythm, rate 76 [Remains]
QRSD	98	- Consider left atrial enlargement [Now Present]
QT	380	- Inferolateral region ST-T abnormalities
QTc	427	- Borderline intraventricular conduction delay
--AXES--		- Nonspecific anterolateral region ST-T abnormalities
P	43	
QRS	79	
T	-25	- ABNORMAL ECG -

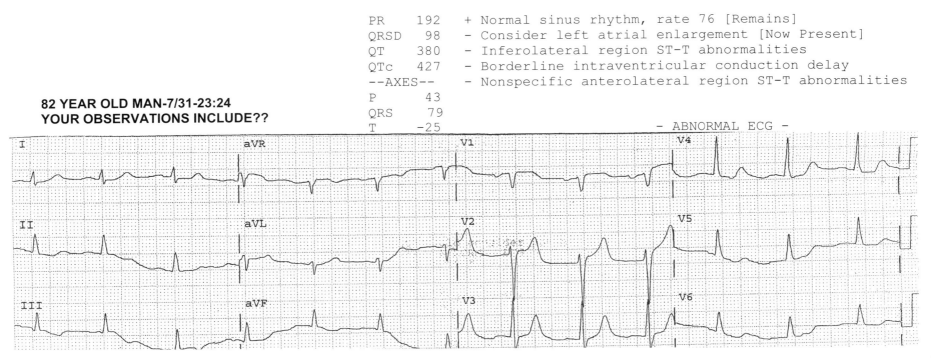

Interpretation of the upper tracing is correct, but the computer analysis of the lower EKG--obtained *four minutes later*--is bizarre! The wide QRS complexes show typical RBBB with a "preblocked axis" of (+) 110°. The right axis deviation cannot be due to RVH developing in four minutes and must be secondary to *left posterior fascicular block*. The subtle ST segment elevation in leads V1-V3 is concerning for an acute anterior MI as cause for the conduction abnormality.

- Normal sinus rhythm, rate 77 [Remains]
- Nonspecific intraventricular conduction delay [Remains]
- Right ventricular hypertrophy [Now Present]
- [Now Absent] Nonspecific Anterolateral region ST-T abnormalities

7/31-23:28

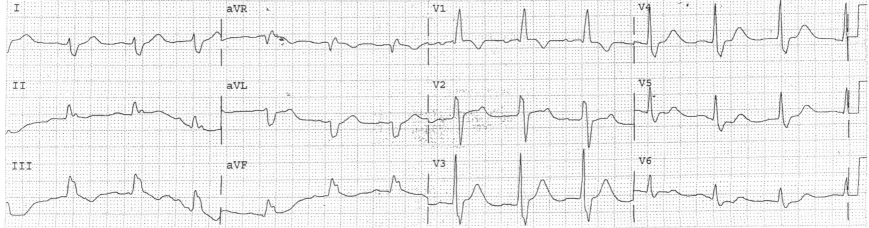

BIVENTRICULAR HYPERTROPHY

48 YEAR OLD WOMAN

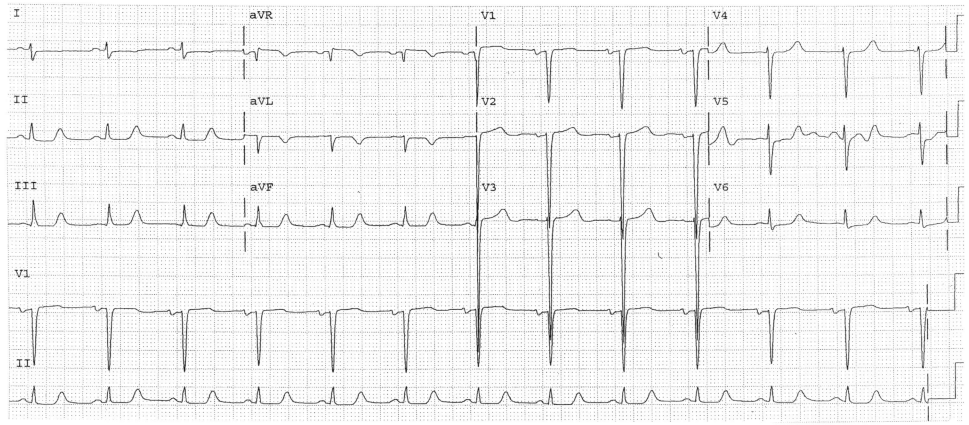

The precordial leads show LVH voltage, associated with a P wave in lead V1 consistent with left atrial abnormality. The peculiar thing about this EKG is that the frontal plane axis is (+) 100°. This is an example of <u>biventricular hypertrophy</u>. The criteria are: evidence of LVH voltage in the horizontal plane leads, with *right axis deviation* in the frontal leads. This woman has advanced rheumatic heart disease with aortic and mitral valve lesions.

When the QRS duration is normal, the most common cause of right axis deviation and early precordial QRS transition is a right ventricular hypertrophy. The tables below identify other causes that are encountered, and examples of some are presented in the following pages.

CAUSES OF RT. AXIS DEVIATION	CAUSES OF EARLY TRANSITION
Normal in youth	Normal in youth
Right ventricular hypertrophy	Left ventricular hypertrophy
Lateral myocardial infarction	Posterior myocardial infarction
Lt. posterior fascicular block	Accessory Pathway (W.P.W.)
Pulmonary embolism	Technician error
Accessory pathway (W.P.W.)	
Technician error	

65 YEAR OLD WOMAN 3/1
OBSERVATIONS? AXIS?   A

3/1-AXIS SHIFT REPRESENTS?   B

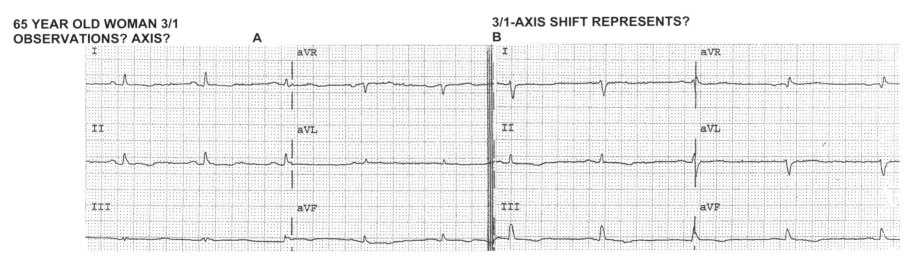

Right axis deviation, thought due to left posterior fascicular block, requires assurance that the cause is not due to right ventricular hypertrophy, since it is the most common cause of this abnormal QRS direction. Clinical correlation, if available, helps solve the problem. Lacking this, serial tracings may allow judgment. The first set of limb leads (**A**) in this woman shows a QRS axis of (+) 45°. The axis in a tracing *later in the same day* (**B**) has shifted to (+) 120°. Obviously, the change in axis in this short time cannot be due to RVH, and a diagnosis of LPFB is warranted.

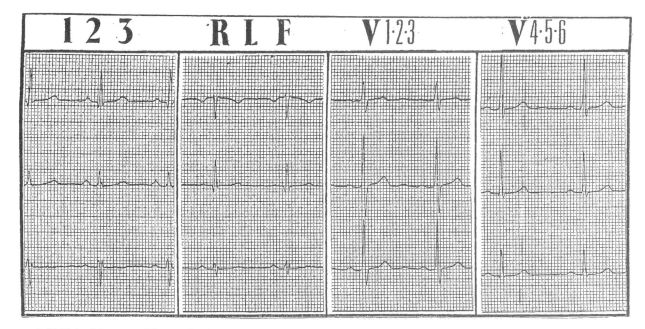

1 2 3	R L F	V 1·2·3	V 4·5·6

"Oh, to be young again!" This 18-year-old man had a tracing as part of a research project. His prominent R wave in lead V1 and early transition reflect the residual right ventricle present from childhood and is normal at his age.

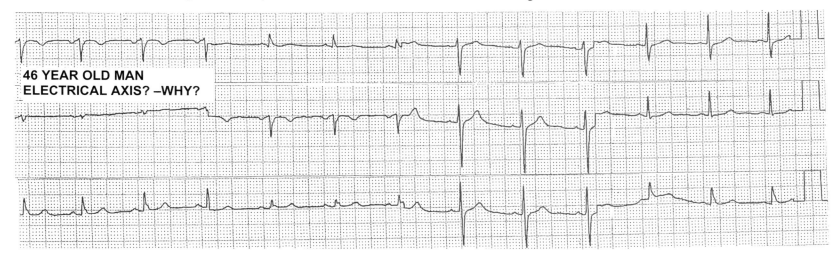

**46 YEAR OLD MAN
ELECTRICAL AXIS? –WHY?**

A frequent technician error is to interchange the right and left arm electrode. This reverses the polarity of lead I, resulting in a spurious right axis deviation. The "tip-off," at a glance, is that the P wave is negative in lead I.

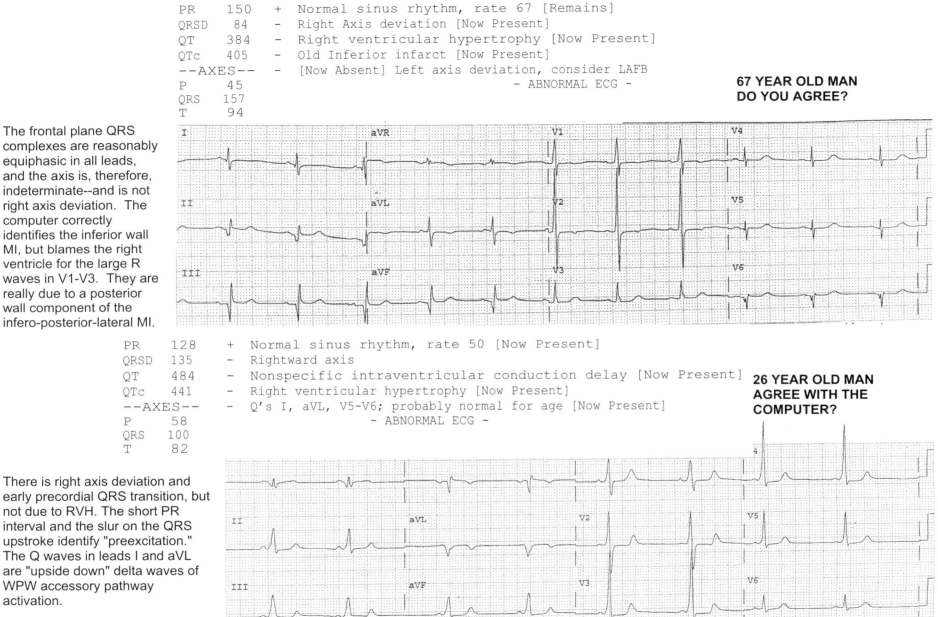

```
PR      150    +  Normal sinus rhythm, rate 67 [Remains]
QRSD     84    -  Right Axis deviation [Now Present]
QT      384    -  Right ventricular hypertrophy [Now Present]
QTc     405    -  Old Inferior infarct [Now Present]
--AXES--       -  [Now Absent] Left axis deviation, consider LAFB
P        45                          - ABNORMAL ECG -
QRS     157
T        94
```

**67 YEAR OLD MAN
DO YOU AGREE?**

The frontal plane QRS complexes are reasonably equiphasic in all leads, and the axis is, therefore, indeterminate--and is not right axis deviation. The computer correctly identifies the inferior wall MI, but blames the right ventricle for the large R waves in V1-V3. They are really due to a posterior wall component of the infero-posterior-lateral MI.

```
PR      128    +  Normal sinus rhythm, rate 50 [Now Present]
QRSD    135    -  Rightward axis
QT      484    -  Nonspecific intraventricular conduction delay [Now Present]
QTc     441    -  Right ventricular hypertrophy [Now Present]
--AXES--       -  Q's I, aVL, V5-V6; probably normal for age [Now Present]
P        58                          - ABNORMAL ECG -
QRS     100
T        82
```

**26 YEAR OLD MAN
AGREE WITH THE
COMPUTER?**

There is right axis deviation and early precordial QRS transition, but not due to RVH. The short PR interval and the slur on the QRS upstroke identify "preexcitation." The Q waves in leads I and aVL are "upside down" delta waves of WPW accessory pathway activation.

104

```
PR    128    +  Normal sinus rhythm, rate 97 Normal
QRSD  91     -  Consider right ventricular hypertrophy [Now Present]
QT    315    -  Borderline low voltage in frontal leads [Remains]
QTc   400    -  [Now Absent] QT interval long for rate
--AXES--     -  [Now Absent] Nonspecific Anterior T wave abnormalities
P     60              - ABNORMAL ECG -
QRS   38
T     52
```

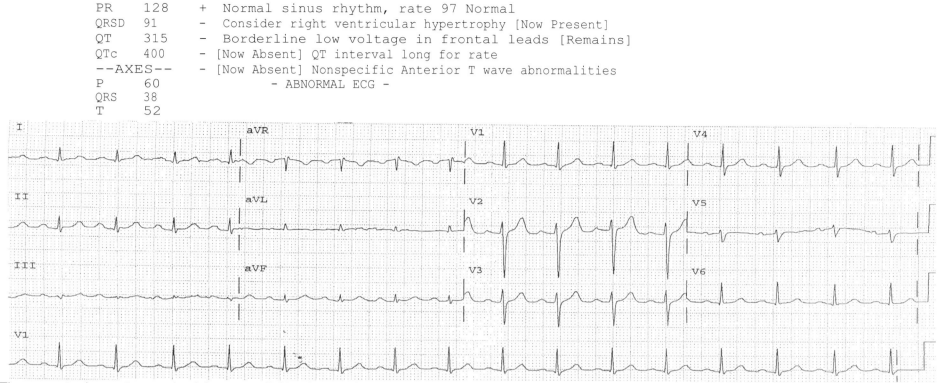

The computer has not recognized the precordial lead error of the "treacherous technician." Look carefully: lead V5 is really V1, V3 is V2, V2 is V3, V4 is correct, V1 is V5, and V6 is correct...With this rearrangement, the precordial leads are normal and there is no evidence of RVH.

The early transition accompanies decisive Q waves in leads I, aVL, V5-6, and is the pattern of a posterolateral MI.
The ST segment changes are concerning for an acute process.

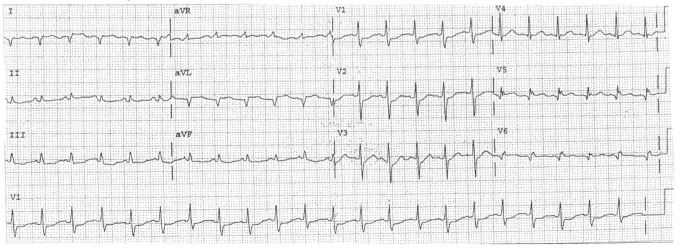

LOW QRS VOLTAGE

At the opposite extreme of excessive left ventricular voltage are tracings showing low voltage QRS complexes. The criteria include: frontal plane total QRS amplitude of 5 mm or less, and precordial lead showing voltage of 10 mm or less.
Causes include:

1. Decrease in the left ventricle "generator strength" (e.g. myocardium replaced by non-electrical tissue, such as amyloid deposition, cardiac tumor, or most frequently, scar tissue due to multiple infarctions).
2. An increase in "insulators" on the surface or surrounding the heart (e.g. excess fat, or air, and fluid accumulation in the pleural or pericardial space).
3. A combination of causes (e.g. hypothyroidism resulting in decrease in myocardial electrical generation, often associated with pericardial effusion).

Examples of the common causes follow.

67 YEAR OLD WOMAN

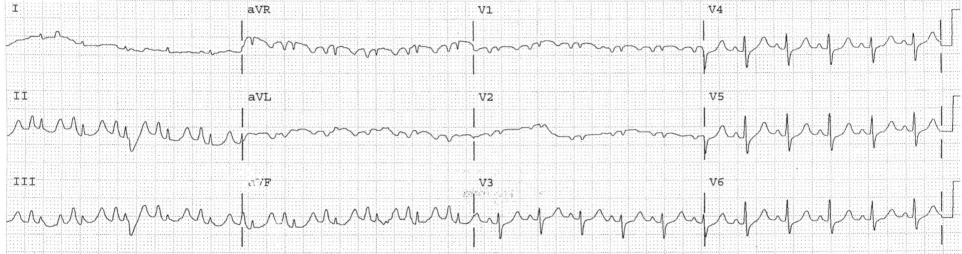

Perhaps the commonest cause of low QRS voltage is chronic obstructive pulmonary disease. The QRS axis of (+) 90°, the gigantic P waves in the frontal plane, and the lack of precordial QRS transition are characteristic features identifying this cause.

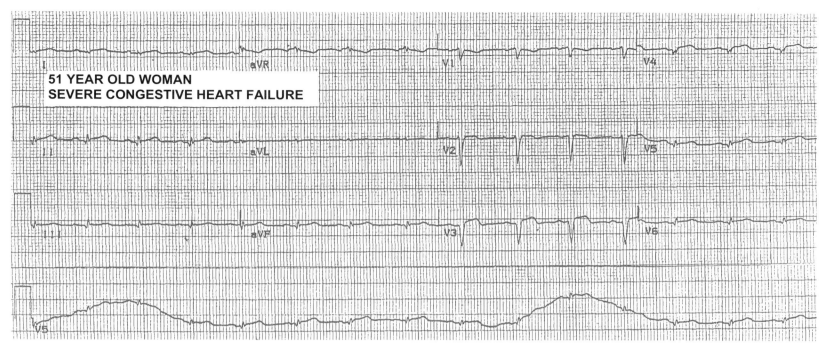

**51 YEAR OLD WOMAN
SEVERE CONGESTIVE HEART FAILURE**

A sad case! This woman has sustained in inferior and extensive anteroseptal-lateral infarction, and is now left with little functioning myocardium. The low QRS voltage is due to a loss of much of her "electrical generator." A gold star will be awarded if you noticed that the rhythm strip of lead V5 has two large baseline artifacts. These reflect the fact that she is being breathed by a respirator set at 12 breaths /minute.

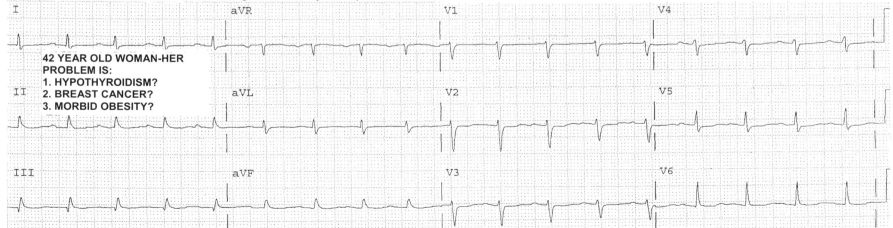

**42 YEAR OLD WOMAN-HER
PROBLEM IS:
1. HYPOTHYROIDISM?
2. BREAST CANCER?
3. MORBID OBESITY?**

The rhythm is sinus at 115/minute. The axis is (+) 60° and there are diffuse repolarization changes. The low-voltage QRS complexes might be due to any of the 3 choices. Right axis deviation would be expected if #3 was the cause, so let's eliminate that choice. Hypothyroidism usually results in sinus bradycardia, and this patient's heart rate would be against that diagnosis. The correct answer is #2. This unfortunate woman has a breast malignancy with pericardial metastases and a pericardial effusion with tamponade. 1000 ml of fluid was removed by a pericardiocentesis with return of normal QRS voltage.

107

- BRADYCARDIA OF UNDETERMINED ORIGIN, RATE 43
- FIRST DEGREE AV BLOCK
- LOW VOLTAGE THROUGHOUT
- NONSPECIFIC ANTEROLATERAL REGION T ABNORMALITIES – ABNORMAL ECG-

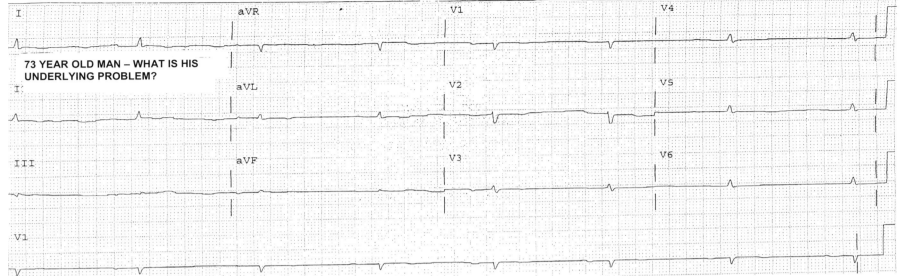

73 YEAR OLD MAN – WHAT IS HIS UNDERLYING PROBLEM?

The computer interpretation is correct, but does not suggest a possible cause for the marked low QRS voltage. This tracing is characteristic of "hypothyroid heart disease." Clues include the low voltage, not only of the QRS, but of the T waves and the P waves, and the presence of marked bradycardia. The diagnosis is important because, unlike many other causes of low-voltage, these abnormalities will regress with treatment of the underlying condition.

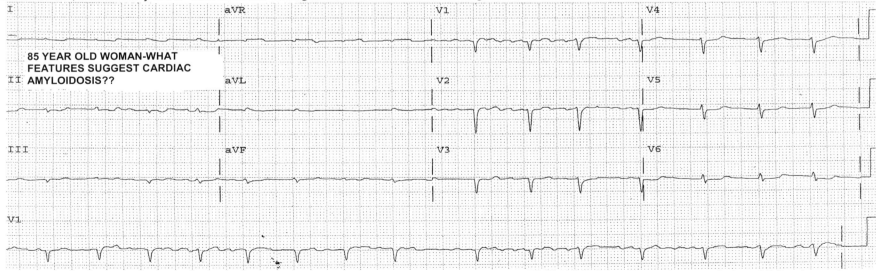

85 YEAR OLD WOMAN-WHAT FEATURES SUGGEST CARDIAC AMYLOIDOSIS??

Amyloid deposition in the myocardium usually occurs in the elderly, with involvement of both ventricles and atria. There is not only low QRS voltage, but commonly, atrial fibrillation. Since amyloid is not electrically active, deposits may lead to a "dead zone" effect, and simulate myocardial infarction. Such is the case in this woman.

108

SUPRAVENTRICULAR ORIGIN OF WIDE QRS BEATS

An impulse arising in the atria may activate the ventricles in an abnormal matter with a "wide QRS" complex resulting. This is a common and important arrhythmic phenomenon. Possible causes for this include:

A. *Fixed* intraventricular conduction disturbances-such as would be seen with established right or left bundle branch block.

B. *Intermittent* intraventricular conduction disturbances. Two varieties are encountered:

    1. "Functional" - due to aberrant ventricular conduction.

    2. "Nonfunctional" - occurring when bundle branch block develops as the atrial rate increases to a "critical rate." An example will be shown below. Rate-related bundle branch block should only be considered when "new" BBB is encountered. The rate related nature is usually due to tachycardia, and less often occurs with decrease in rate.

C. Alternate A-V pathways-the "preexcitation syndrome" -Wolff-Parkinson-White pattern. An example will be shown.

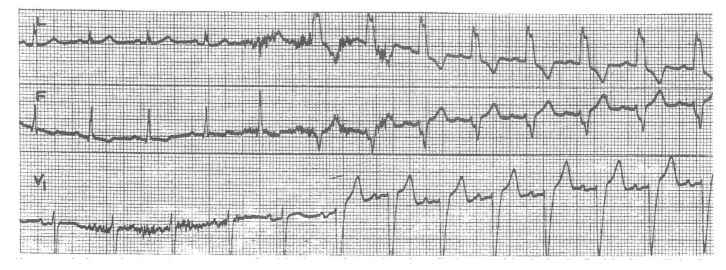

Illustrated above is the phenomenon of *critical rate-dependent bundle branch block*. And a "critical rate," the inability of the left bundle branch to conduct the impulse becomes evident. Note the onset of complete LBBB as the sinus rate increases from 90-95/min. to 100/min. Whenever sinus tachycardia was present, the abnormal conduction appeared.

When an accessory pathway is present, the atrial stimulus has an option. It may conduct over the normal A-V bridge or use the accessory pathway (AP) for ventricular activation (or conduct over both, with a ventricular fusion complex resulting). In the example shown, the first two P waves are conducted normally, and the third uses the AP. The shorter PR segment and "slur" in the initial part of the QRS complex ("delta wave") identifies typical "W.P.W" activation. More on this subject will be presented in a later chapter.

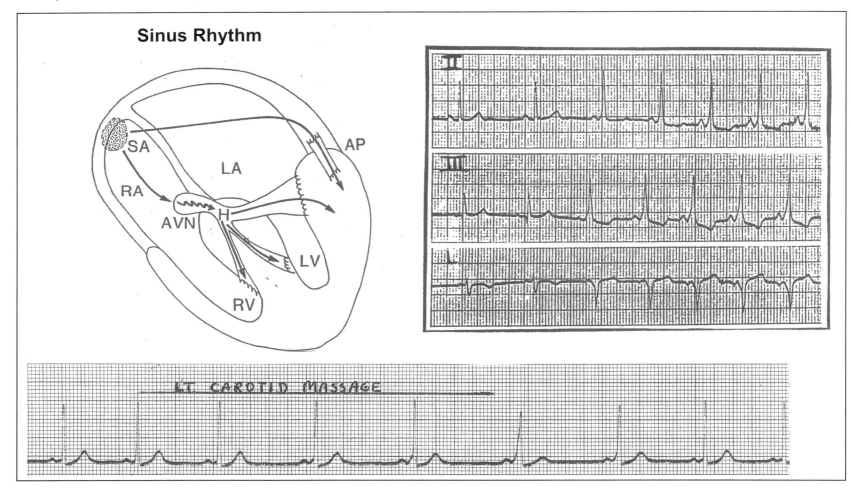

This 35-year-old man carried a diagnosis of "intermittent bundle branch block." The slight delay in the QRS upstroke raised the possibility of "preexcitation." To clarify the issue, a vagatonic maneuver (carotid sinus massage) was done during EKG recording. Note the evident decrease in the PR segment and increase in the delta wave (and QRS duration) proving the presence of an accessory pathway. The maneuver has decreased AV nodal transmission, and forced the atrial stimulus to use the accessory pathway, proving that he has *intermittent WPW* complexes and not bundle branch block. Administration of adenosine, which produces transient A-V block, may also be utilized to unmask conduction over an accessory pathway.

110

"FUNCTIONAL" CAUSES

A premature impulse arising in the atria or A-V junction may attempt transmission to the ventricles while a portion of the intraventricular conducting network is completely or partially refractory. Thus, the impulse may be conducted either not at all or in an abnormal matter. This concept is illustrated below.

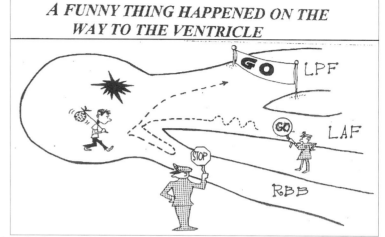

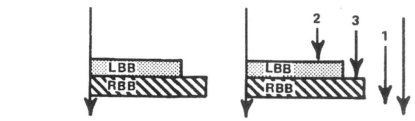

Ventricular depolarization is indicated by the vertical arrows and the refractory period (recovery time) of the intraventricular pathways—left and right bundle branches—are depicted as horizontal bars. The numbered arrows represent atrial stimuli which are premature in the previously established cycle. Stimulus #1, although premature, would find both bundle branches "recovered" and would be normally conducted. (Terminology: atrial premature beat, normally conducted). Stimulus #2 is so premature that neither bundle branch has repolarized and it would not be conducted to the ventricles. (Terminology: atrial premature beat, nonconducted). As depicted in the figure, in the normal individual, the RBB has a somewhat longer refractory period than the LBB. Stimulus #3 is critically timed to find the left bundle branch responsive but the right branch still refractory. It succeeds in its conduction into the ventricle via the LBB and is propagated as though there were right bundle branch block. (Terminology: atrial premature beat, aberrantly conducted with right bundle branch block).

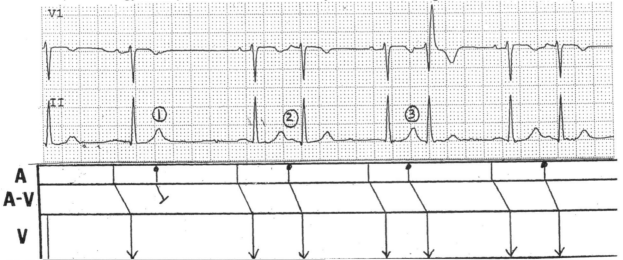

An example of this concept. Multiple premature atrial stimuli are present with only slight variation in their timing. APC #1 is hiding in the T-wave and is early enough that it is not conducted. APC #2 arrives slightly later and is normally conducted. APC #3 is critically timed to find the left bundle recovered but the right bundle still refractory, and it is conducted with RBBB aberration.

111

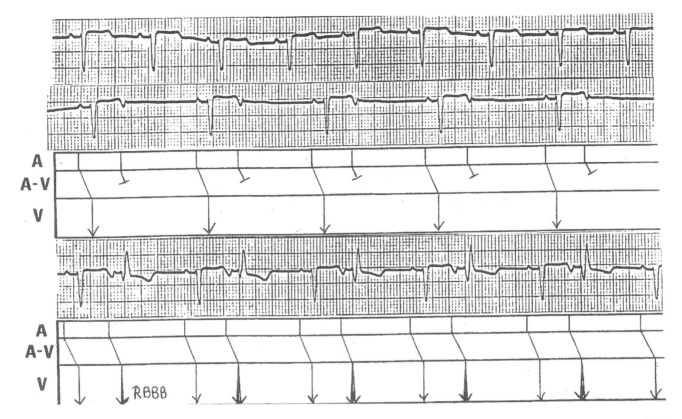

The strips are from a monitor chest lead and are not continuous. The top recording shows sinus rhythm at a rate of 72/min. It is useful because it demonstrates the underlying sinus cycle and the morphology of the ST-T waves. In the middle strip, it is obvious that there are P waves partially concealed in the T wave. They are sufficiently premature that they cannot be conducted. Although ineffective for ventricular activation, the ectopic P wave discharges the sinus node, forcing it to "reset," with a resulting pause. Premature P waves follow each sinus node discharge, occurring in a *bigeminal rhythm*. The result is to slow the *effective* rate to 45/min. A fancy--but accurate--designation of this strip would be "sinus rhythm with non-conducted atrial bigemini."

APCs are a common "cause of a pause." The diagnosis in the bottom strip should be fairly evident. The bigeminal APCs succeed in AV conduction, but find the RBB refractory and are aberrantly conducted, with RBBB morphology. A four word description of this strip would be "aberrantly conducted atrial bigemini."

This variety of aberrant ventricular conduction, typical RBBB, is the most common encountered. Although the P wave responsible for the aberrantly conducted complex may be obvious, it frequently attempts to "hide" in the T wave of the preceding beat, and may not be apparent. Often, there may be only a subtle distortion of the previous T wave to reveal its presence. Nonetheless, before deciding that a premature "wide QRS beat" is a VPC, and particularly if it shows typical RBBB morphology, the preceding T wave should be carefully examined, in multiple, in multiple leads, for a tell-tale P wave that may be the culprit.

112

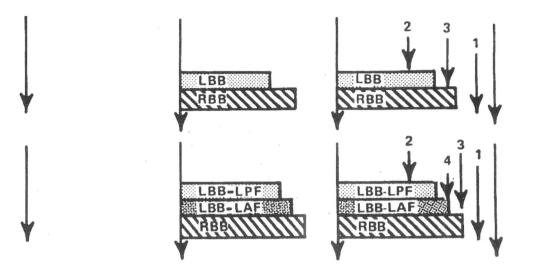

You have seen the upper portion of this diagram. In the lower part, the left bundle branch is displayed to show the differing refractory periods of its divisions-the left anterior fascicle (LAF) and the left posterior fascicle (LPF). "Recovery time" of the LAF is usually somewhat longer than that of the LPF. In this illustration, premature stimuli #1, #2, and #3, as previously discussed, would result in normal conduction, non-conduction, or aberrant conduction. The only additional element is premature stimulus #4. Note that its timing finds the LPF responsive, while the LAF and RBB remained refractory. The stimulus would, thus, be conducted via the left posterior fascicle and be distributed as though there were *left anterior fascicular block and right bundle branch block*. A combination of LAFB and RBBB is frequently seen as a pattern of ventricular aberration. An example of this is shown.

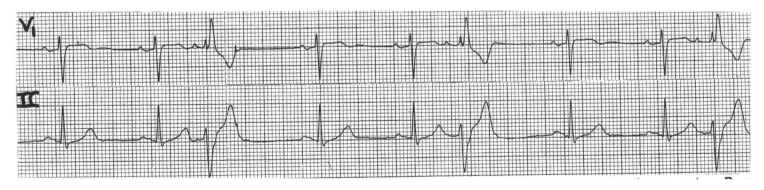

Simultaneous segments of the leads V1 and II are shown. Note the merit of having both leads, since the premature P wave is obvious in lead V1, but not evident in lead II. Lead V1 shows rSR' morphology characteristic of complete RBBB. Lead II shows a deep S wave consistent with LAFB. Thus the diagnosis is: multiple atrial premature complexes which are aberrantly conducted with LAFB and RBBB.

113

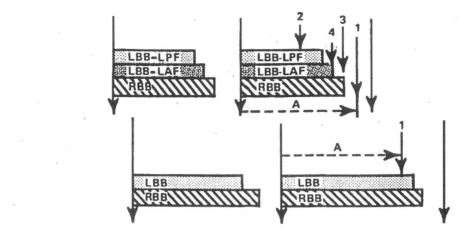

We have discussed the upper part of this illustration. The additional concept is diagrammed in the lower part and indicates the effect of a change in heart rate ("cycle length") on the recovery periods. In general, when the cycle length is prolonged so is the refractory period. In the EKG, the recovery time is indicated by QT interval and it is contingent on the heart rate, shortening as the rate speeds and lengthening as the rate slows. In the bottom part of the figure above, the vertical arrows, representing ventricular depolarization, are further separated to depict slowing of the heart rate. As a result, the recovery time is prolonged. Note in the top strip that stimulus #1 (separated by the preceding depolarization by interval A) is *normally* conducted. As the rate slows and the recovery time prolongs, a premature stimulus with the same timing (interval A) finds neither the LBB nor the RBB "recovered" and thus is *non-conducted*.

The concept that the changing cycle lengths determine the recovery period of conduction pathways was described many years ago by Dr. (Ph.D.) Richard Ashman who was Professor of Physiology at Louisiana State University Medical School. The term "Ashman phenomenon" is a valid and useful eponym to apply to this effect. In his writings, Dr. Ashman emphasized the frequent occurrence of this phenomenon in patients with atrial fibrillation. It should be obvious why the markedly variable cycles occurring in this arrhythmia could lead to aberrant conduction. Since there are no discrete atrial stimuli in atrial fibrillation, it is essential to be alert to this possibility; otherwise every "wide-QRS complex" may be mistaken for a VPC!

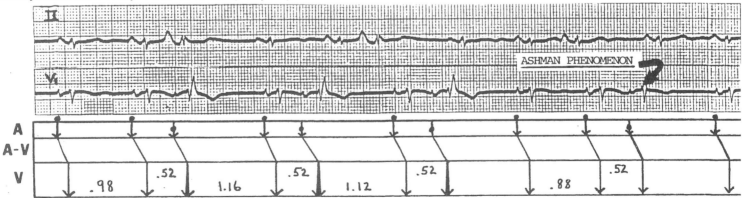

Note the numerous premature P waves--better seen in the lead II strip that in the V1 lead. These identically timed atrial premature complexes (APCs) have the same separation of the resulting ventricular depolarization and the preceding QRS (0.52 sec.) and are three times aberrantly conducted. Note the typical RBBB morphology in lead V1. Why is the fourth APC conducted normally? Observe that the cycles preceding the first three APCs are relatively long (0.98 sec., 1.16 sec., and 1.12 sec.) whereas the cycle preceding the fourth APC is significantly shorter (0.88 sec.). The shortened cycle length results in a decrease in the refractory period of the conduction pathways, permitting the last APC to be normally conducted, while the previous ones were aberrantly conducted.

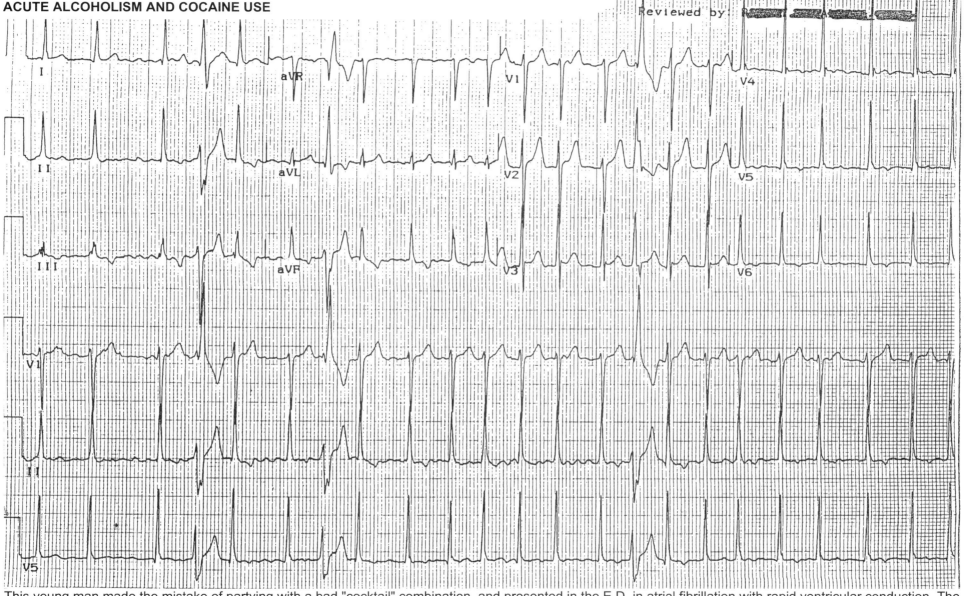

Reviewed by:

This young man made the mistake of partying with a bad "cocktail" combination, and presented in the E.D. in atrial fibrillation with rapid ventricular conduction. The three abnormal complexes represent "Ashman beats." Dr. Ashman emphasized that if the R-R cycle prolongs, the refractory period of the conducting pathway is lengthened. Because of the preceding longer R-R interval, three of the atrial fib. stimuli find that the right bundle branch and left anterior fascicle have not recovered, and the impulses are aberrantly conducted with RBBB and LAFB.

```
PR                + Atrial fib. w/rapid ventr. Response, rate=166
QRSD    83        - Paired ventricular premature complexes
QT      234       - Diffuse ST-T abnormalities
QTc     389       - Possible ischemia

--AXES--
P       69                              - ABNORMAL ECG -
QRS     46
T       258
```

83 YEAR OLD WOMAN
CARE TO CORRECT THE COMPUTER?

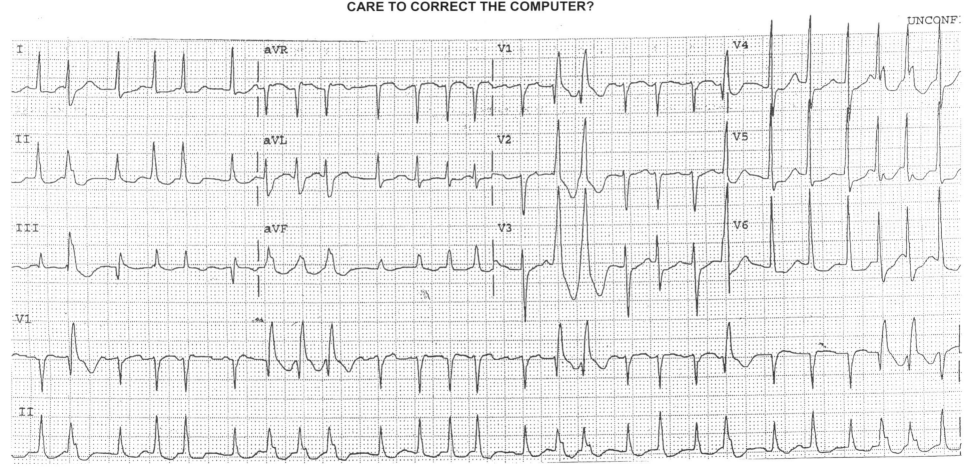

An important computer error. The rhythm is atrial fibrillation with a rapid ventricular response--but the wide-QRS complexes are not VPC's. Instead, many of the atrial stimuli are aberrantly conducted with typical RBBB configuration. The aim should be better rate control, and it would be unwise to direct therapy to suppress the *alleged* ventricular ectopy.

116

67 YEAR OLD WOMAN
CAUSE OF THE PAUSES?
CAUSE OF THE F.L.B.?

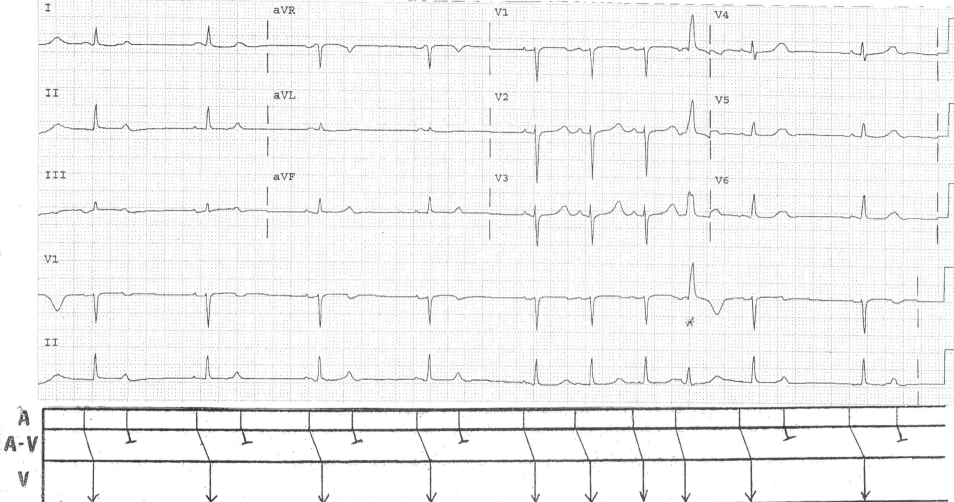

If you compare the character of the majority of the "T waves" with that at the arrow, you will conclude that there are hidden P waves. Most of the non-conducted P waves result in pauses; one is aberrantly conducted with right bundle branch block morphology (*); and several are normally conducted.

70 YEAR OLD MAN
"PALPITATIONS"

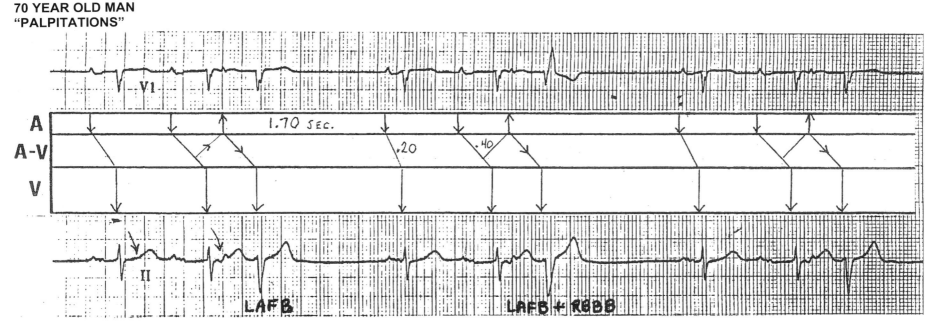

Suggestion: Begin by looking at the strip of lead II and note the difference in the ST segments of the first two beats (arrows). Clearly there is an APC present and its morphology indicates that it is a retrograde conducted impulse. The ladder diagram now becomes a little more palatable. There is a sinus pacemaker at 75/min. conducted with prolonging PR intervals. At a critical PR interval, the penetrating impulse is able to turn-tail and return to the atria. It then echoes and returns to the ventricle. Its prematurity results in aberrantly conducted complexes-LAFB or LAFB + RBBB.

A-V DISSOCATION

Atrial ventricular dissociation (A-V dissociation) represents the circumstances in which the atrial are activated by one pacemaker and the ventricles by another-- the two pacemakers competing for control of ventricular activation. It is evident that, in the resulting duel, the one with the fastest rate will dominate the overall rhythm. Lack of normal ventricular activation is *not* due to AV *block* because, although disturbed A-V conduction commonly coexists, in A-V dissociation there must always be the <u>potential</u> for conduction between the atria and ventricles. Several points deserved emphasis: A-V dissociation can occur in a normal person and its presence need not imply heart disease. A-V dissociation is never a "*primary*" rhythm disturbance. It is always due to "something." A-V dissociation is frequently due to drugs and it should be an alert to drug toxicity. A-V dissociation and A-V block are not synonymous terms or concepts! The competition of pacemakers for atrial and ventricular activation can be due to an entirely different mechanism with different treatment implications.

I. A-V DISSOCIATION DUE TO DEFAULT

This concept is shown in the ladder diagram below. Depicted is a decrease in sinus rate from 75/min. (P-P interval = 0.80 sec.) to a rate of 54/min. (P-P interval = 1.10 seconds). At a critical degree of sinus slowing, a rescue mechanism takes over. An auxiliary pacemaker in A-V junction, with an inherent rate of 57/min. (1.05 seconds) "escapes" and activates the ventricles. The appearance of this junctional focus is said to be due to the "default" of the sinus node and is the *result of sinus bradycardia*. The onset of dissociation can be identified by noting the PR interval. When the PR shortens (arrow) compared to its previous interval, dissociation has developed. Notice that the slower sinus node discharge will occur later and later in the wake of the junctional focus and may reach a point that the junctional tissues are responsive, and be conducted, resulting in a "capture beat."

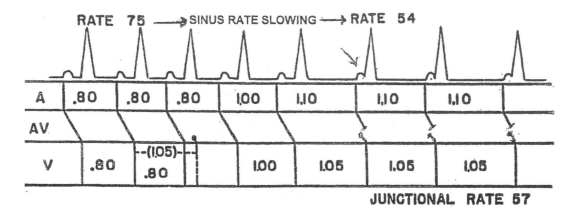

Important Concepts
1. A-V dissociation by "default" of the sinus node can be seen in normal people.
2. The escape focus may be located in the A-v junction or, less commonly, in the ventricle. Thus, the QRS complex may be normal or wide.

119

II. A-V DISSOCIATION DUE TO USURPATION

Although there may be adequate function and appropriate rate of the sinus node discharge, if there is an increase in the firing rate of an ectopic pacemaker, the "lower" site of impulse formation may assume dominance and activate the ventricles, leaving the sinus node responsible for atrial excitation. The ectopic pacemaker represents an *accelerated* focus and is usually located in the AV junction, but can arise in the ventricle. A diagrammatic example is presented below.

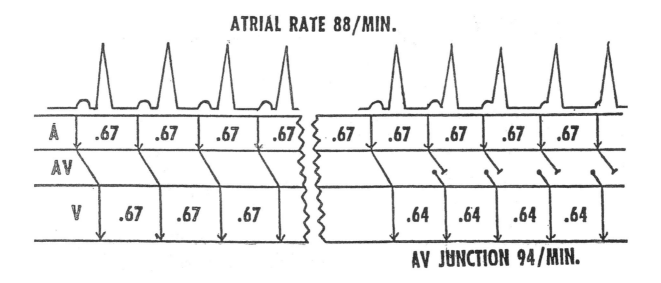

The ladder diagram depicts an initial sinus rate of 88/min. (P-P cycle = 0.67 sec.). In the second portion of the illustration, and despite the continuing sinus rate of 88/min., there is the appearance of an enhanced A-V junctional focus at a rate of 94/min. (R-R interval = 0.64 sec.). Because of its faster rate, the accelerated focus will take command of ventricular excitation and providing the stimulus is not conducted retrograde to the atrium, A-V dissociation will occur. Note that the slower sinus rate causes the P waves to appear at later intervals after the depolarization due to the A-V junctional discharge. They may reach a point where they find the junctional pathway responsive and succeed in anterograde conduction to "capture" the ventricles, proving that the A-V bridge is intact.

The appearance of accelerated A-V junctional or ventricular foci may be due to "ischemia," excess sympathetic activity, or to drug effect (particularly digitalis excess). Although there is no absolute limit to the allowable rate of the normal A-V junctional pacemaker, a limit of 60 impulses/min. would seem reasonable. Rates above this level can be considered increased automaticity of an auxiliary focus, representing an effort by a lower impulse site to "usurp" pacemaker function. This is in sharp contrast to the appearance of such foci at slower rates (such as 40-50/min.) functioning as "escape" pacemakers.

The tracing below is an example of AV dissociation due to a usurping junctional pacemaker.

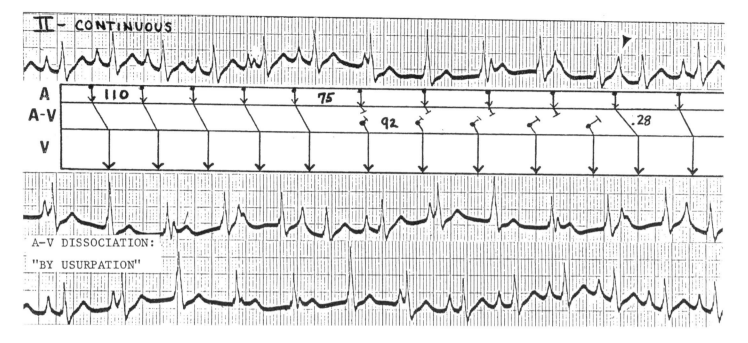

There is a variability in the sinus rate, and whenever it slows to the critical degree, an "enhanced" pacemaker at a rate of 92/min. appears in the A-V junction and activates the ventricles. The slower sinus P waves gradually march through the QRS complex, and when they reach an appropriate time in the refractory period of the preceding beat, the sinus impulse (arrow) is conducted (with a somewhat longer P-R interval of 0.28 sec.). The successful penetration of the sinus impulse momentarily extinguishes the forming impulse in the A-V junction and allows the sinus pacemaker to temporarily regain control of ventricular activation. Subsequent sinus slowing, however, permits the junctional focus to reappear with the P waves "leapfrogging" the QRS and T until the A-V junction is responsive, permitting another "capture beat." This phenomenon is repetitively seen in the second and third strips. Notice the interesting coincidental effect of the P waves merging with the QRS complexes--adding to their height or somewhat changing their morphology.

In this patient, the accelerated junctional focus was due to digitalis intoxication, and the correct interpretation was obviously important. When the drug was stopped, sinus activity continued and the enhanced junctional pacemaker disappeared.

III. A-V DISSOCIATION DUE TO A-V BLOCK

Separate pacemaker for atria and ventricles may occur because of an *abnormality in junctional transmission--*<u>A-V dissociation "due to AV block.</u>" Such a circumstance is always seen during <u>complete</u> heart block, because, in order for life to continue, a stimulus must be available for ventricular activation. If none of the atrial impulses can succeed in activating the ventricles (complete heart block), there is <u>always</u> dissociation of atrial and ventricular events. If <u>incomplete</u> AV block is present, the total number of impulses capable of crossing the A-V bridge may be less than that of an auxiliary pacemaker, resulting in the latter site activating the ventricles.

A-V dissociation due to incomplete A-V block is illustrated in the ladder diagram below.

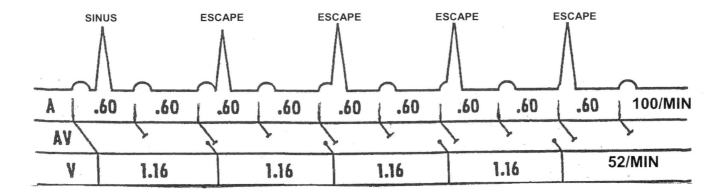

The circumstance depicted is depression of A-V conduction, such that only alternate atrial impulses can be transmitted (2:1 A-V block). Thus, despite the presence of numerous P waves at a rate of 100/min. (P- P interval = 0.60 sec.), the effective ventricular rate is a function of the number of conductible impulses-- 50/min. In this setting, an auxiliary pacemaker somewhere in the AV junction may surface to provide ventricular activation. In the ladder diagram provided, an A-V junctional focus at a rate of 52/minute assumes command, appearing as an "escape" pacemaker, when an inadequate number of stimuli cross the A-V bridge. It is evident that the rate of the auxiliary pacemaker as well as the conductible rate of the atrial stimuli are additive factors in determining whether AV dissociation will occur.

122

Try your hand at ladder diagram analysis of the tracing below--but be careful (clue-beware of hidden P waves).

Which of the following statements are correct?

1. There is a sinus discharge rate of approximately 70/min. with frequent atrial and ventricular complexes.
2. There is a stable atrial tachycardia of approximately 130/minute with variable second-degree A-V block.
3. AV block promotes the appearance of a subsidiary pacemaker which emerges with a discharge rate of 68/min. This is thus, AV dissociation due to AV block.
4. The changed QRS morphology, due to the discharge of the ectopic pacemaker, indicates that it arises below the level of the bundle of His and is, therefore ventricular in origin.
5. The competition of penetrating atrial impulse and ventricular ectopic focus results in fusion beats.

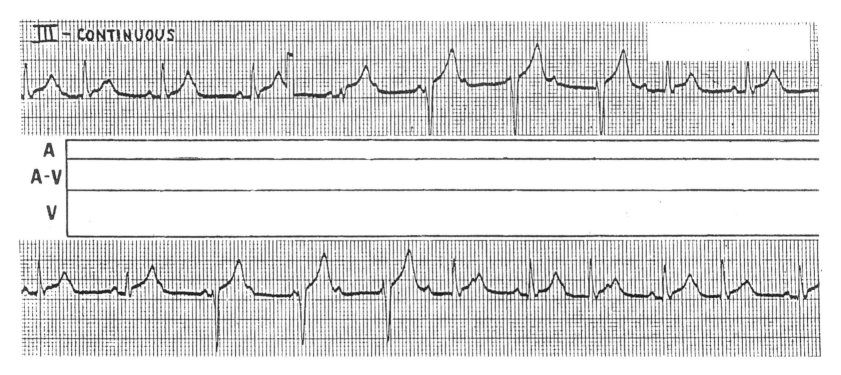

The artistic "official solution" to this interesting and rather difficult tracing is shown below.

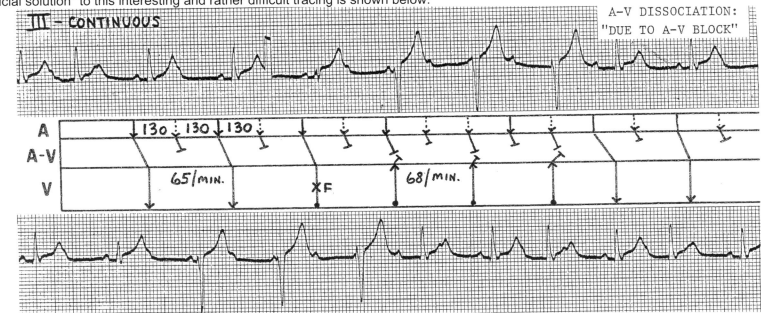

Although P waves are evident, it takes more than a casual glance to determine that the true atrial rate is 130/min, and that, initially, the atrial stimuli are conducted 2:1 to the ventricle. Thus, the effective rate is 65/min. Lurking in the ventricle is an ectopic pacemaker with a firing rate of 68/min. A little reflection should make it obvious who will win this duel! The ventricular focus assumes command with a fusion complex (F), indicating the participation of both atrial and ventricular impulses in cardiac excitation. The ventricular focus remains in charge for the next three beats, then the dissociated P wave finds a critical time in the refractory period established by the ventricular focus, and "captures" the ventricle. This phenomenon is repeated in the bottom strip. Of interest, it ends with an interlude of 3:2 Wenckebach A-V block.

There are several abnormalities and considerations to emphasize in this EKG:
1. It is evident that *some degree of AV block* must be present or all of the atrial stimuli would be conducted.
2. The rate of the ventricular focus--68/minute--is certainly abnormal and it must be an accelerated discharge site.
3. The fusion complex proves that the ectopic pacemaker is arising in the ventricle.
   Thus, AV block sets the stage where an accelerated ventricular focus can surface to cause A-V dissociation.

If you completed your ladder diagram, it should be evident in all but the first are correct.

Thus, causes of A-V dissociation include:

1. "Default" of the atrial focus (usually the sinus node).
2. "Usurpation" by an accelerated pacemaker.
3. "A-V block."
4. Combinations of the above. A common combination is "some degree" of A-V block which results in a decrease in the conductible atrial impulses, allowing an appropriate or accelerated pacing site to assume command.

Numerous examples will be presented.

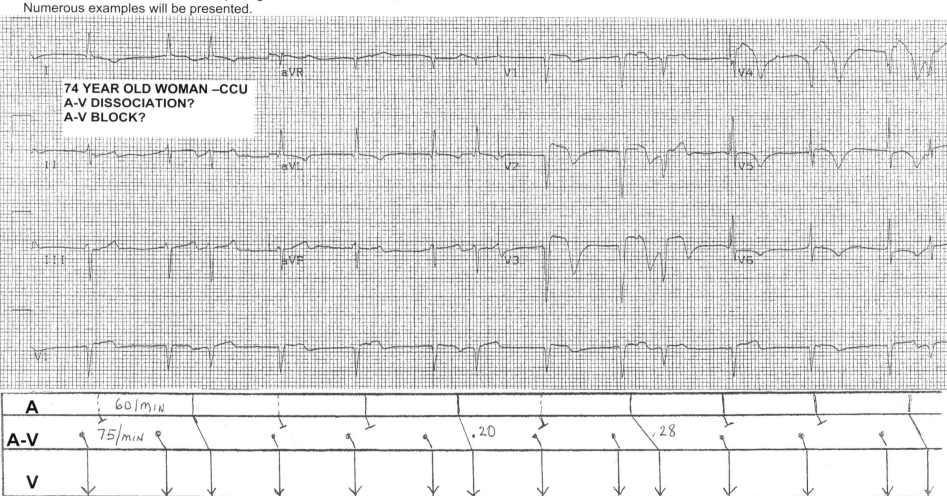

74 YEAR OLD WOMAN –CCU
A-V DISSOCIATION?
A-V BLOCK?

It is evident that this arrhythmia is occurring in the setting of an acute anteroseptal M.I. There is an atrial pacemaker at 60/min, competing with, and dissociated from, an accelerated junctional focus firing at 75/min (A-V dissociation by "usurpation"). The occurrence of the P waves, beyond the absolute refractory period following the junctional discharge, permits passage of the atrial impulses, capture-beats resulting. The timing of the successful P wave determines its PR interval, i.e. the earlier the arrival of the P wave in the relative refractory period, the longer will be the PR interval, and vice versa.

125

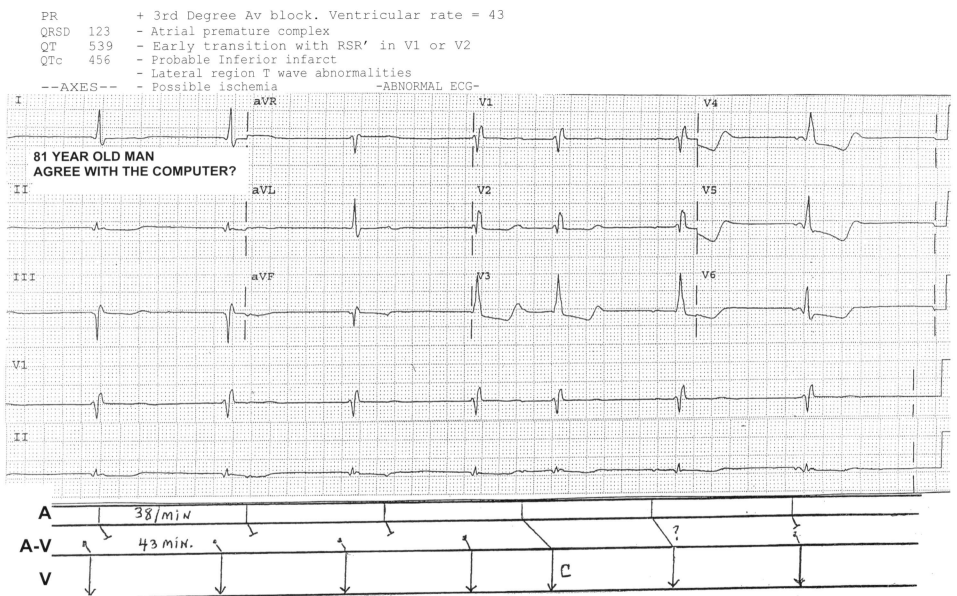

```
PR          + 3rd Degree Av block. Ventricular rate = 43
QRSD   123  - Atrial premature complex
QT     539  - Early transition with RSR' in V1 or V2
QTc    456  - Probable Inferior infarct
            - Lateral region T wave abnormalities
--AXES--    - Possible ischemia           -ABNORMAL ECG-
```

81 YEAR OLD MAN
AGREE WITH THE COMPUTER?

A   38/min

A-V   43 min.

V

The computer is partly correct--but provided an incorrect rhythm judgment! The atrial rate is slow, but regular at 38/min., and is competing with a slightly faster junctional focus at 43/min. A-V dissociation develops due to the default of the atrial site. The trailing P waves gradually progress beyond the refractory period of the junctional discharge, and one crosses the A-V bridge to "capture" (**C**) ventricular activation. Perhaps the next P wave is also conducted? The "capture beat" is easily identified because it underlines shortens the R-R cycle previously established. It is important because it demands an intact A-V bridge, and denies *complete* AV block. The incorrect diagnosis of third-degree AV block carries an evident treatment implication--an electronic pacemaker. In this man, bradycardia was due to excessive beta blocker therapy and disappeared on its withdrawal.

126

74 YEAR OLD MAN

AV DISSOCIATION
LOW VOLTAGE QRS
ST & T WAVE ABNORMALITIES, CONSIDER ANTERIOR ISCHEMIA
ABNORMAL ECG

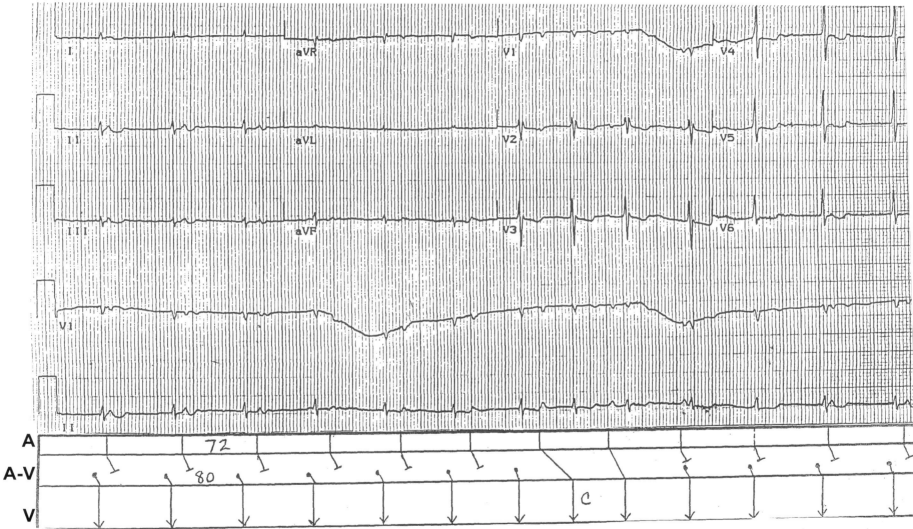

The computer diagnosis is correct, but incomplete. A junctional pacemaker at a rate of 80/min. coexists with a sinus pacemaker at 72/min. The rate disparity allows the junction to remain in command--AV dissociation "by usurpation." The independent P wave marches through the refractory period of the junctional discharge, until a capture beat (C) occurs with a long PR interval. The next sinus P wave is conducted with a normal PR interval and then the junctional focus resumes command. When the right timing exists, the atrial signal can be conducted with <u>no A-V delay</u>. The problem obviously is due to the enhanced junctional focus.

127

**37 YEAR OLD MAN
DRUG OVERDOSE**

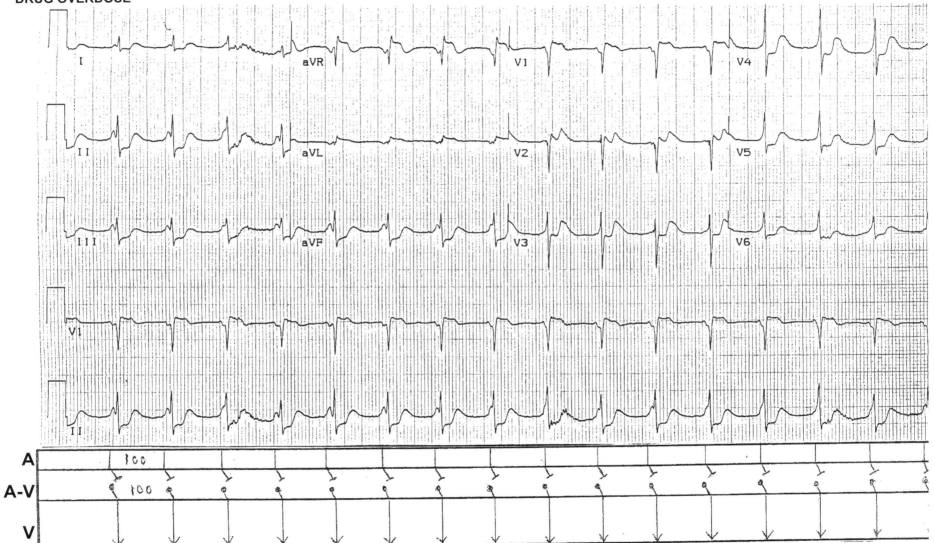

A sad story. Over the course of several days, this young man repetitively smoked "crack" cocaine. The resulting "high" prevented sleep, so he attempted to "come down" by taking a large dose of morphine. He quickly slipped into the arms of Morpheus, and it wasn't until he stopped breathing that his friend became concerned and called EMS. He was intubated in the field but was "brain-dead" on arrival at the hospital. The ladder-diagram depicts his rhythm disturbance. An accelerated junctional focus is competing with sinus rhythm. The rates of the two are virtually identical, and the rhythm represents so-called isochronic A-V dissociation. The accelerated junctional discharge was probably due to the sympathomimetic effect of cocaine.

64 YEAR OLD WOMAN
AV DISSOCIAITON? BOTH? AV BLOCK?

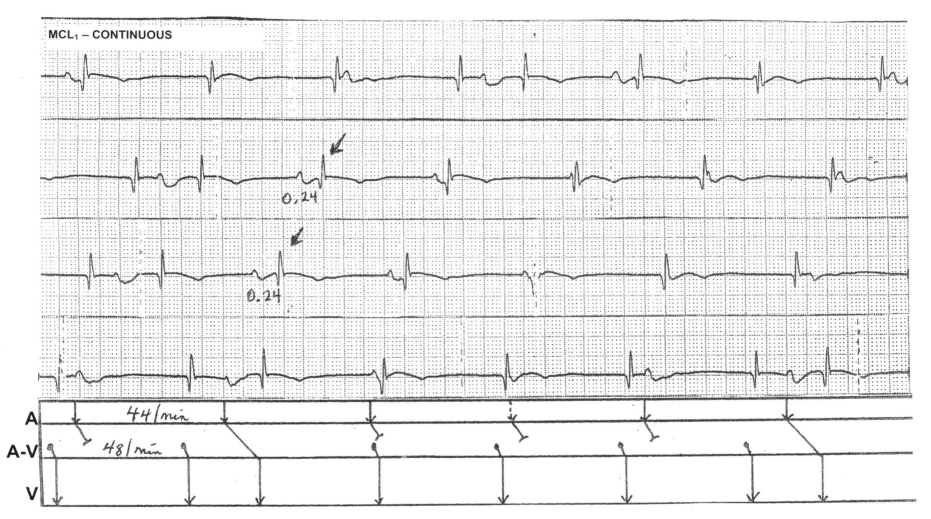

MCL$_1$ – CONTINUOUS

0.24

0.24

A   44/min

A-V   48/min

V

The most obvious thing about this tracing is the bradycardia! The sinus pacemaker is lazily firing at 40/min, permitting a junctional focus at 48/min to take command. The result is A-V dissociation due to the "default" of the sinus node. When the timing is right, the dissociated atrial impulse is able to cross the A-V bridge and "capture" the ventricle. The arrow on the tracing indicate a sinus-conducted impulse which is well-beyond the refractory wake of the previous capture beat (**C**). The PR interval of 0.24 sec indicates that there is a "little" A-V nodal suppression accompanying the A-V dissociation. Clearly the major problem is the marked sinus bradycardia and not A-V transmission. Drugs that suppress the sinus node must be considered.

```
PR    207   +  3rd degree Av block with junctional escape rhythm
QRSD   69   -  Low voltage throughout [Now Present]
QT    405   -  ST elevation, inferior leads
QTc   424   -  [Now Absent] Atrial premature complex
            -  [Now Absent] Nonspecific Inferior T wave abnormalities
--AXES--                                           - ABNORMAL ECG -
```

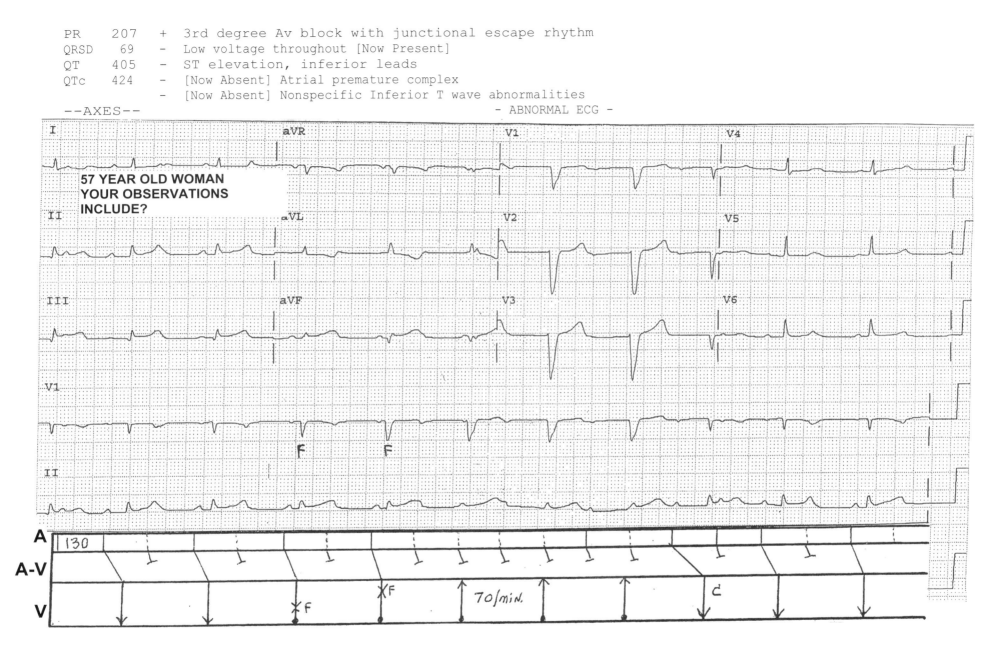

**57 YEAR OLD WOMAN
YOUR OBSERVATIONS
INCLUDE?**

The interpretation is seriously mistaken. The atrial rate is 130/min., transmitted with a 2:1 ratio. The *conductible* rate, therefore, is 65/minute. An auxiliary pacing site in the ventricle has a rate of 70/min. and since it is faster than the conductible rate, it assumes command. Two fusion complexes (**F**) prove the ventricular origin of the competing beats. When the dissociated P wave finds the A-V bridge responsive, a capture beat (**C**) occurs and the atrial stimuli take charge. This example of AV dissociation is due to both the AV block and a usurping ventricular focus, and occurred during an acute inferior wall infarction.

130

```
PR      152    + Check patient history - inconsistent with previous age of 28 years
QRSD     80    - Sinus tachycardia, rate 106 [Now Present] Normal P axis
QT      314    - Diffuse ST-T abnormalities, [Now Present] ST-T negative
QTc     390    - Supraventricular tachycardia
               - [Now Absent] Incomplete right bundle branch block
--AXES--       - [Now Absent]   Left atrial enlargement
P        69                                                          - ABNORMAL ECG -
QRS       8
T       -22
```

27 YEAR OLD MAN - INFECTIVE ENDOCARDITIS
HIS CURRENT PROBLEM IS??

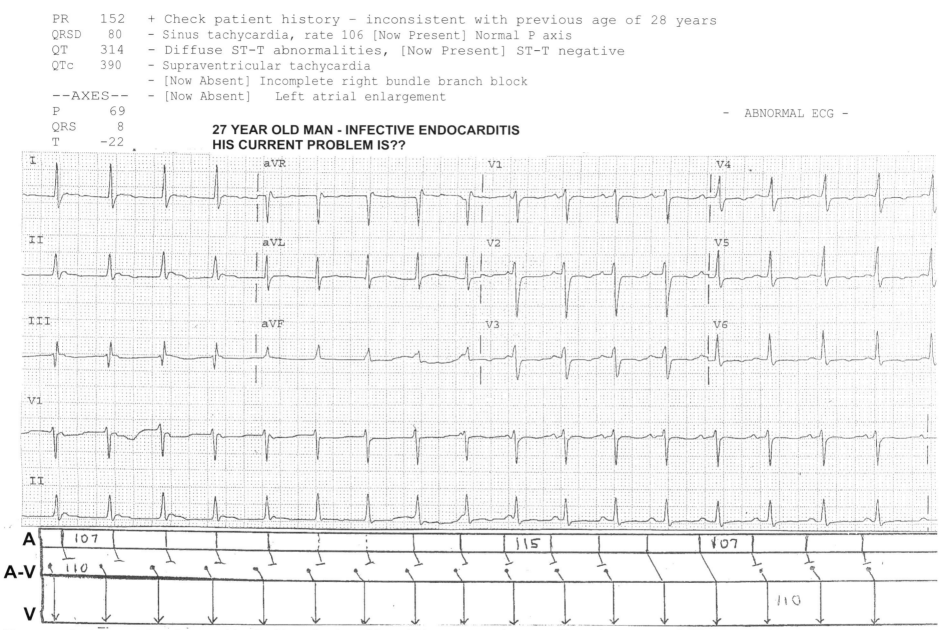

The computer interpretation does not identify this patient's problem. This young man's severe illness has prompted diffuse repolarization abnormality, sinus tachycardia, and an abnormally accelerated junctional focus. The ladder diagram presents the interplay of the two pacemakers. Obviously, in this competition, the focus with the faster rate will dominate. For the most part, the junction is in command and the P waves lag behind (*A-V dissociation due to "usurpation"*). However, note that when the sinus rate reaches 115/min., it temporarily is in charge. As its rate slows, the junction once again takes over.

131

```
PR     137   + Sinus bradycardia, rate 34 [Now Present]
QRSD   142   - Multiple atrial premature complexes [Now Present]
QT     493   - Right axis deviation [Now Present]
QTc    371   - Right bundle branch block [Now Present]
             - Consider right atrial enlargement [Now Present]
--AXES--
P      -21                    87 YEAR OLD MAN
QRS    125                    HIS PROBLEMS INCLUDE??                    - ABNORMAL ECG -
```

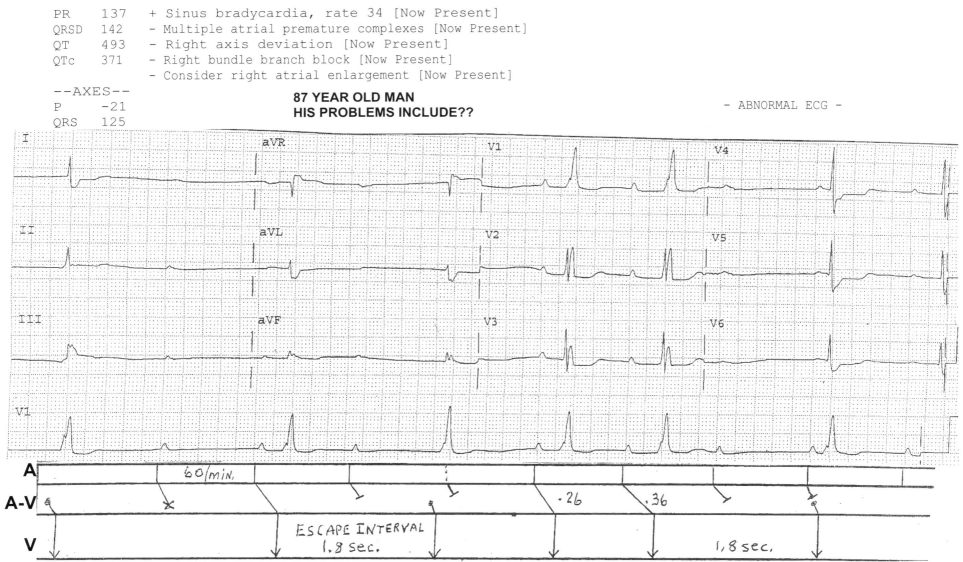

The computer interpretation of the rhythm and axis is incorrect. Right bundle branch block is present, but the "pre-blocked axis" is (+) 10°--not right axis. P waves are regular at 60/min. and are conducted with Wenckebach A-V block. When a "dropped beat" occurs, the resulting lengthy pause allows an _escape_ junctional focus to surface after 1.8 sec. Although there is a P wave preceding the last QRS complex, the shortened PR interval indicates that is not conducted. The problem is not due to impulse _formation_, but to impulse _conduction_ - i.e. - A-V dissociation due to A-V block. Drugs that depress A-V nodal conduction should be considered the possible cause.

77 YEAR OLD MAN
THE "DEGREE" OF AV BLOCK IS??

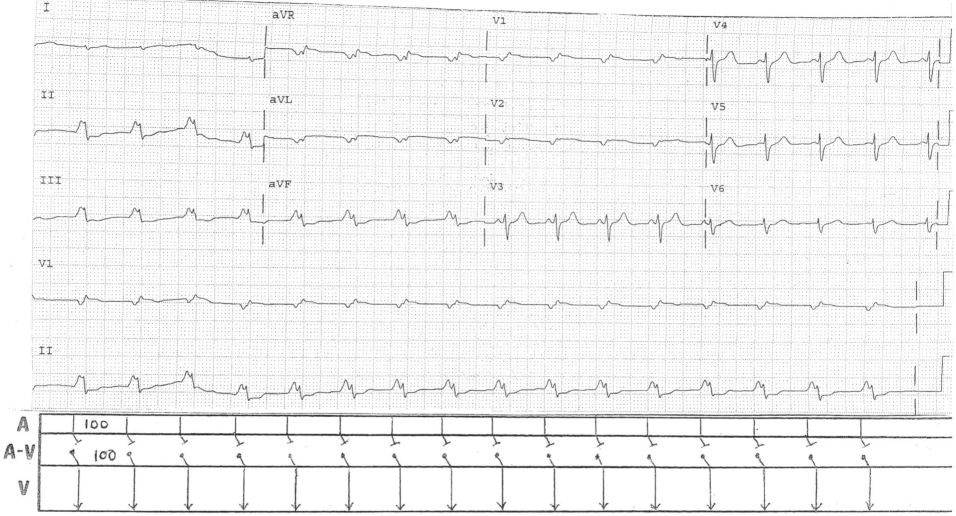

The frontal plane QRS axis is indeterminate, and the voltage is low in both planes. The P-QRS-T are all isoelectric in lead I; that plus the lack of precordial QRS transition and the low-voltage, indicate advanced COPD. The Q waves in leads V1-V2 may indicate a septal M.I. P waves are saddled next to an accelerated junctional focus, both firing at 100/min. This is an example of "isochronic" A-V dissociation, due to the enhanced junctional pacemaker. Although, none of the P waves is conducted, there is likely no A-V block. Despite being partially hidden, the P waves show evidence of biatrial enlargement. Until proven otherwise, this arrhythmia is due to drug excess (digoxin? theophylline? beta-agonist inhaler?).

133

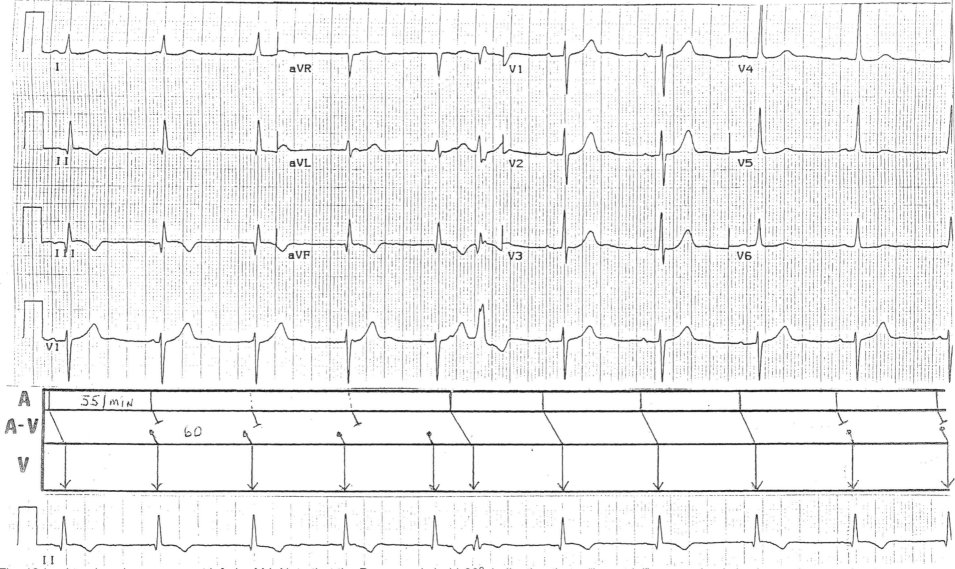

The 12-lead tracing shows a recent inferior M.I. Note that the P wave axis is (-) 30°, indicating that a "low atrial" pacemaker is in charge. Its rate of 55/min is slower than that of an auxiliary junctional focus at 60/min. and A-V dissociation develops, due to the "default" of the atrial impulse. When the sluggish P wave wanders into the relative refractory period of the junctional impulse, it is able to slip across the A-V bridge as an aberrantly-conducted complex and "capture" the ventricle. Its passage extinguishes the junctional site, and the atrial focus resumes control.

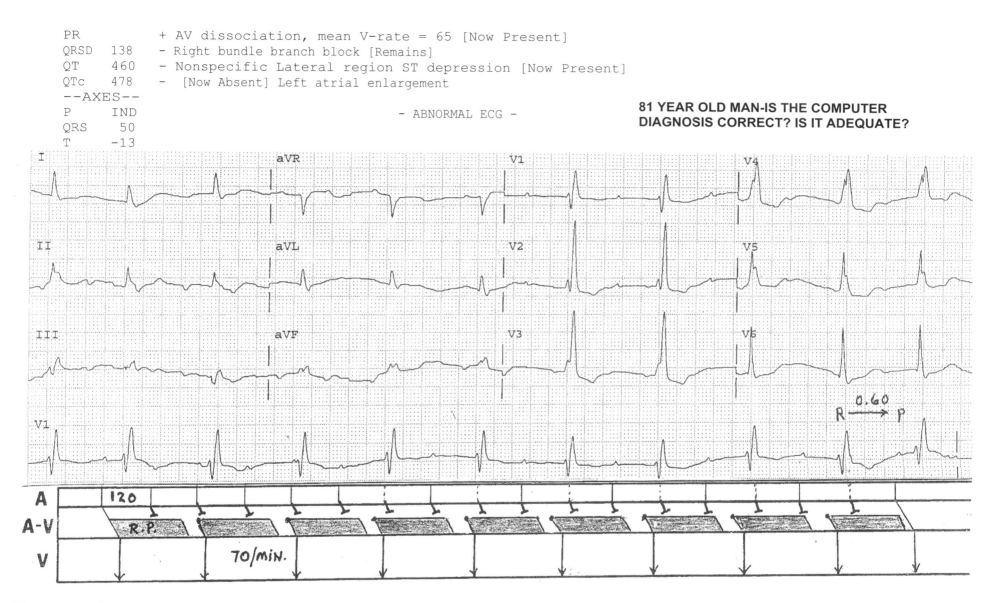

```
PR              + AV dissociation, mean V-rate = 65 [Now Present]
QRSD    138     - Right bundle branch block [Remains]
QT      460     - Nonspecific Lateral region ST depression [Now Present]
QTc     478     -  [Now Absent] Left atrial enlargement
--AXES--
P       IND                          - ABNORMAL ECG -
QRS     50
T       -13
```

81 YEAR OLD MAN-IS THE COMPUTER DIAGNOSIS CORRECT? IS IT ADEQUATE?

The computer interpretation is partially correct, but it has ignored important points. Due to artifact, P waves cannot be identified in the limb leads, but are seen in lead V1. The P waves are regular at 120/min. It is evident that not all the P waves are conducted and, thus, there is "some degree" of A-V block, probably 2:1 transmission. An accelerated junctional focus appears at a rate of 70/min. and remains in command until the end of the tracing. The ladder diagram depicts the problem. When the AV bridge is depolarized, there is a lengthy recovery (refractory period) resulting. The prolonged refractory interlude prevents transmission of the majority of the atrial impulses. However when a P wave is late enough after the QRS complex (R-P interval of 0.60 sec.) conduction occurs. This unusual, but important variety of A-V dissociation has been termed "*block--acceleration dissociation,*" and may be due to digitalis excess.

70 YEAR OLD MAN
ASHD, COPD, CHRONIC RENAL DISEASE
WHAT IS GOING ON??

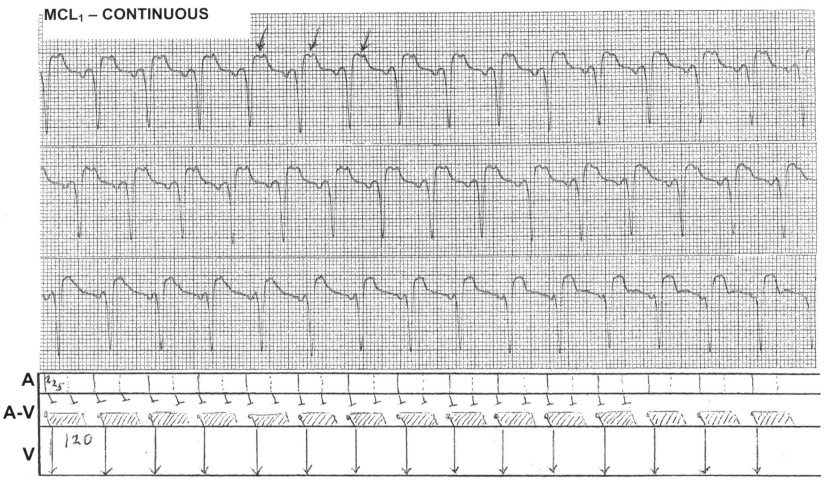

In bygone days, the mainstay of therapy for congestive heart failure was digoxin, and the occurrence of digitalis toxicity was common. Virtually every imaginable arrhythmia could be seen. In this example, the rhythm appears to be sinus tachycardia at 120/min, but look closely. There is another P wave hiding in the ST segment (arrows). Given only the top tracing, this would be an example of atrial tachycardia (? atrial flutter) at 240/min with 2:1 A-V conduction. However, the second and third strips prove that this interpretation is incorrect. The obvious P wave and R-R cycle remain regular, but the "PR interval" gradually shortens. Ultimately, it becomes evident that the P waves are not conducted and that the P waves and QRS complexes are dissociated. An accelerated junctional focus at 120/min is in command. The rhythm represents a combination of some A-V "block," accompanied by a usurping ectopic focus. The status of the A-V bridge cannot be determined because, as diagrammed, the discharge of the junctional focus repetitively sets up a refractory wake that prevents transmission of the atrial stimuli. Digoxin dose in this man was increased because of progressive heart failure. This arrhythmia correlated with a plasma "dig" level of 4.8 ng/ml.

A-V BLOCK

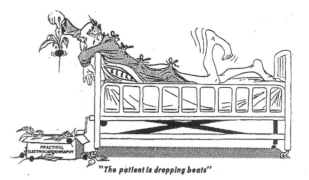

"The patient is dropping beats"

We believe that a major problem with the recognition of AV block stems from the effort to make concepts too simple. The three "degree" of AV block have been a source of confusion and incorrect diagnosis. Although many examples of disturbed AV conduction fit into these categories, many do not!

First-degree A-V block is technically an incorrect term, since there is merely <u>delay</u> and not block of all sinus impulses.
An example is shown below.

PR interval greater than 200ms

FIRST DEGREE AVB

Second-degree A-V block is more complex and the basis of many errors.
Classic type I (Wenckebach) A-V block is due to depressed A-V *nodal* conduction and is recognized by prolonging PR intervals before a "dropped beat." It is frequently due to drugs that depress the A-V node (digitalis, beta-blockers, and calcium channel blockers). Although type I block can occur with inferior wall myocardial infarction, it infrequently requires an electronic pacemaker.

A typical example of Wenckebach block is shown below.

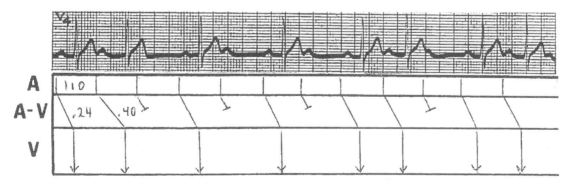

SECOND DEGREE TYPE I AVB (3:2, 2:1)

137

The illustration above depicts the basis of type I AV block. The earlier the P wave is, in the wake of the preceding complex, the longer the PR interval will be. Ultimately, the P wave encounters the absolute refractory period and cannot be conducted.

Diagram illustrating the effect on A-V conduction as successive atrial impulses (1-5) arrive in the A-V junction earlier and earlier in it refractory period. The light stippling = relative refractory period; the dark stippling = absolute refractory period.

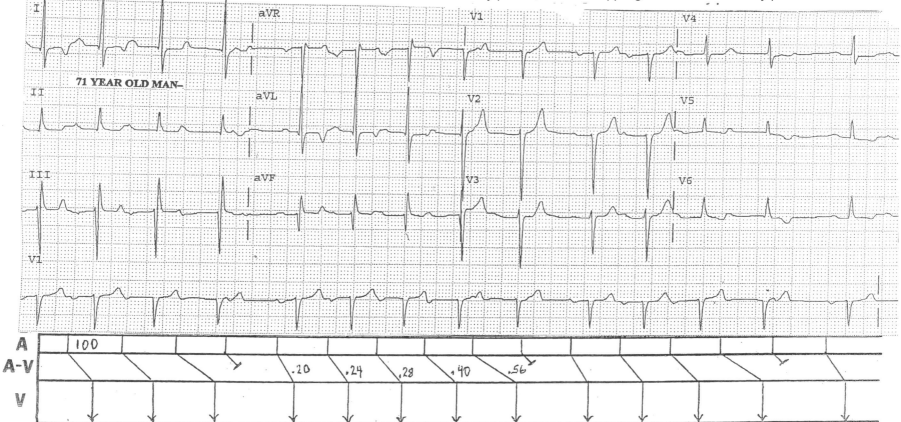

In the tracing above, the prolonging PR intervals and the "dropped beat" indicate Wenckebach A-V block. This example is atypical because of the large increments in the A-V delay.

Type II (Mobitz) A-V block is due to abnormal _infranodal_ conduction, and is usually accompanied by bundle branch block. All conducted impulses share the same PR intervals (usually normal). The "dropped beats" appear without warning and may be sporadic or several in a row. Type II block may be seen with anterior infarction, but is not related drugs in current use. A pacemaker is usually required.

An example of Type II block is shown below.

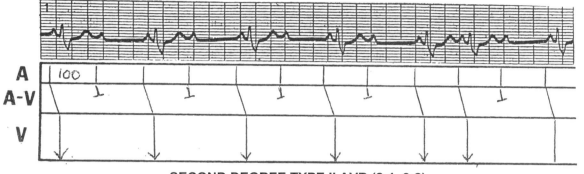

SECOND DEGREE TYPE II AVB (2:1, 3:2)

Second degree A-V block with 2:1 conduction is a particular problem. This ratio of conduction has little meaning unless the _atrial rate_ is provided. For example, in patients with atrial flutter, there are +/- 300 impulses available for A-V transmission. It is evident that if all were conducted, the ventricular rate would be life-threatening. In this circumstance, a conduction ratio of 2:1 is a boon, and represents physiologic refractoriness rather than AV block. Conversely, if the atrial rate is 70/minute, a 2:1 conduction would be a disaster and represent pathologic AV block. 2:1 conduction is often said to represent Type II block. Although this is frequently correct, many cases are due to 2:1 A-V _nodal_ block (Type I). A clue for the latter diagnosis would be the absence of bundle branch block and prolonged PR interval of the conducted P wave.

A number of examples will be presented.

Ladder diagram, illustrating how an increase in atrial rate, without change in the refractory period, can alter the conduction ratio from 1:1 to 2:1. The first two cycles represent a rate of 60/min; the last five cycles, a rate of 78/min. As the rate increases, the alternating P waves encounter the refractory period set up by the prior transmitted impulse and are not conducted. Shaded areas represent an unchanging refractory period.

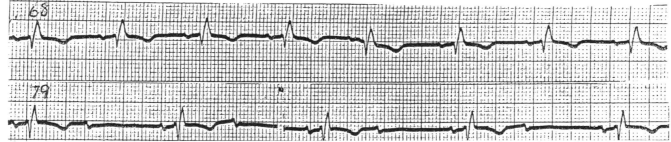

The illustration emphasizes the relationship between a prolonged R-P interval and heart rate. The example above shows that at a rate of 68/min. the A-V conduction is 1:1. When the rate increases only slightly to 79/min. alternating impulses are blocked. This is an example of *rate dependent* A-V block. The presence of bundle branch block would support the conclusion that this is type II infranodal A-V block.

Third-degree (complete A-V block) is a diagnosis to often rendered and too often incorrect. There is a common definition--"if no P waves are conducted, complete AV block is present". This simplistic concept leads to major errors and inappropriate management. It is evident that, to be conducted, an atrial impulse must have an <u>opportunity</u> for conduction. Thus, in order to diagnose complete heart block:

1. P waves should not occur in the absolute refractory period of a preceding activation.

2. P waves should not be in "lockstep" (iso-chronic dissociation) with a competing junctional or ventricular pacemaker.

3. There must be an adequate number of P waves sampling different portions of the cardiac cycle and none are conducted.

4. The rate of an escaping focus should be slow enough (<45/min?) to permit conduction of a dissociated P wave.

5. There should never be an early QRS complex indicating a "capture beat". If one is present, it would require that the A-V bridge be intact.

An example of complete AV block is shown.

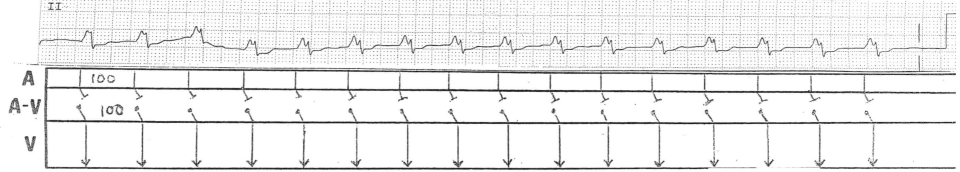

P waves are saddled next to an accelerated junctional focus, both firing at 100/min. This is an example of "iso-chronic" AV dissociation, due to an enhanced junctional pacemaker. Although none of the P waves is conducted, there is no opportunity for conduction because of the short PR interval, and there is likely no AV block.

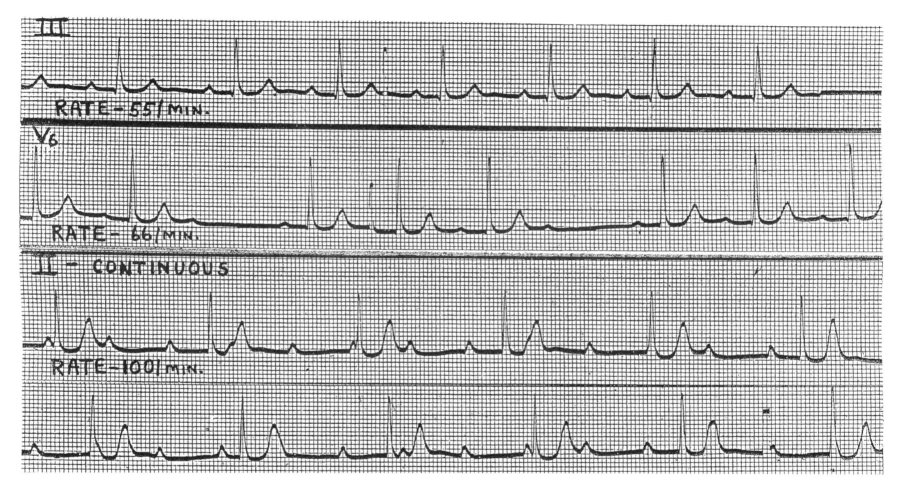

These are segments from a <u>single</u> EKG and are a dramatic example of the effect of changing heart rate when a long refractory period is present. At a rate of 55/min., first-degree A-V block is present. When the rate increases to 66/min., two P waves are blocked-second-degree A-V block. At a rate of 100/min., all P waves arrive in the absolute refractory period of the escape focus, and none are conducted-complete A-V block.

```
PR     254    + Sinus rhythm, rate 81
QRSD    93    - First degree AV block
QT     423    - QT interval long for rate
QTc    491    - Nonspecific Anterior ST depression
--AXES--
P       76                          - ABNORMAL ECG -
QRS     74
T       74
```

70 YEAR OLD WOMAN
MINOR COMPUTER UNDERCALL??

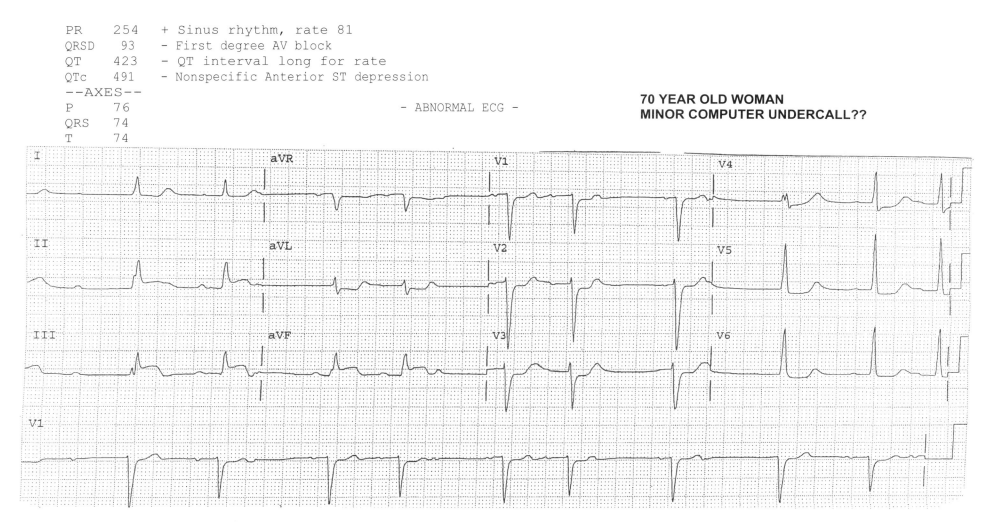

The computer has missed the indicative ST segment elevation in leads II, III, aVF and the accompanying reciprocal depression in leads I and aVL. The ST segment depression in the precordial leads should not be regarded as "nonspecific," but rather as an injury current involving the posterior LV wall. The prolonging PR intervals and "dropped beats" indicate Wenckebach block (type 1) second-degree A-V block. Type 1 A-V block is common with inferior infarction and, if symptomatic, usually responds to atropine.

142

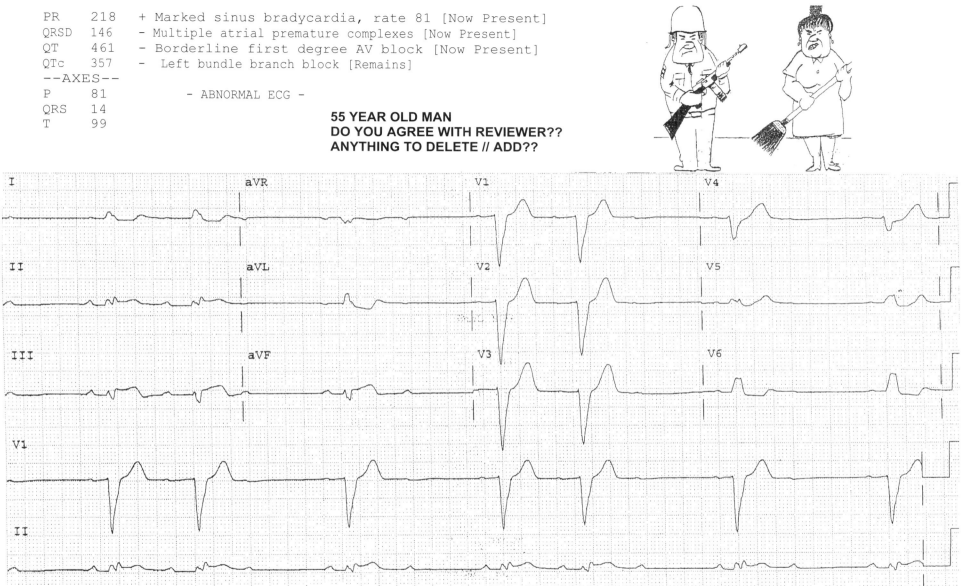

```
PR    218    + Marked sinus bradycardia, rate 81 [Now Present]
QRSD  146    - Multiple atrial premature complexes [Now Present]
QT    461    - Borderline first degree AV block [Now Present]
QTc   357    -  Left bundle branch block [Remains]
--AXES--
P      81              - ABNORMAL ECG -
QRS    14
T      99
```

55 YEAR OLD MAN
DO YOU AGREE WITH REVIEWER??
ANYTHING TO DELETE // ADD??

The cartoon depicts the theme of this tracing—"a minor difference." A minor transposition of letters changes the concept of <u>martial law</u> to <u>*marital law*</u>. (Are they the same in your house?) Some "minor" disagreements with this interpretation:

1. "Marked sinus bradycardia of 36/min." should read sinus rhythm of 75/min.
2. There are no APCs.
3. "Borderline first-degree AB block" is really Wenckebach second-degree AV nodal block.
4. LBBB is correct, but note that there is concordant ST elevation in leads II, III, and aVF indicating an acute inferior MI. Minor differences?

143

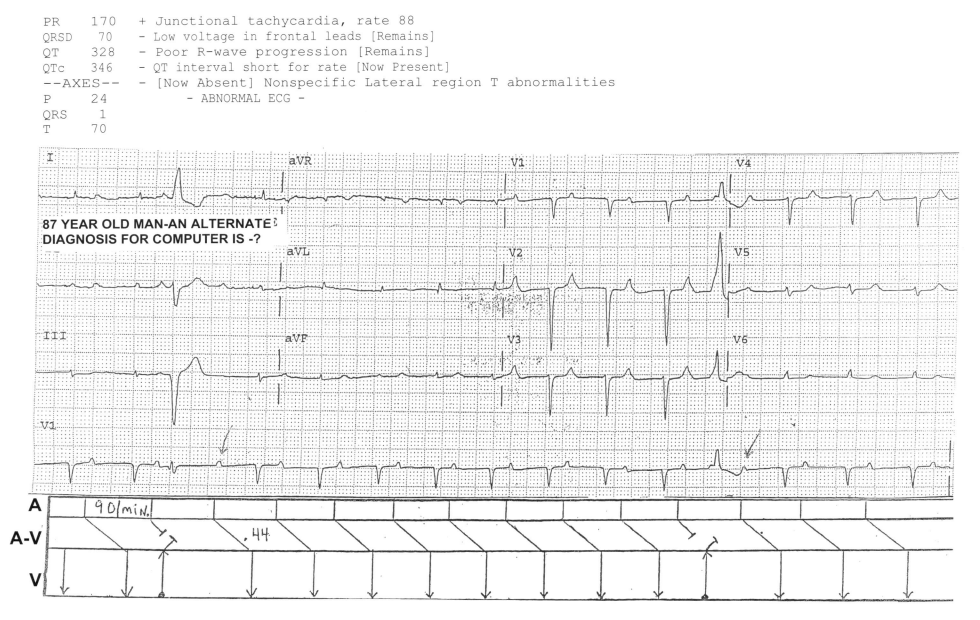

```
PR      170    + Junctional tachycardia, rate 88
QRSD    70     - Low voltage in frontal leads [Remains]
QT      328    - Poor R-wave progression [Remains]
QTc     346    - QT interval short for rate [Now Present]
--AXES--       - [Now Absent] Nonspecific Lateral region T abnormalities
P       24              - ABNORMAL ECG -
QRS     1
T       70
```

87 YEAR OLD MAN-AN ALTERNATE DIAGNOSIS FOR COMPUTER IS -?

The computer has misinterpreted the P waves as T waves, resulting in the incorrect diagnosis of "short QT interval." Importantly, the two VPCs were not recognized and they are the key to the correct diagnosis. Note that during the pause after the VPCs, there are convincing P waves (arrows). The P-P cycle is regular at 90/min. and the P waves bear a constant relationship to the QRS complexes. The PR interval is prolonged to 0.44 seconds--an example of first-degree AV block.

144

```
PR     267    + Sinus rhythm, rate 88
QRSD    84    - Multiple atrial premature complexes
QT     304    - First degree AV block
--AXES--      - Low voltage in frontal leads
P       46    - Nonspecific Inferior T abnormalities
QRS      0              - ABNORMAL ECG -
T      -11
```

76 YEAR OLD WOMAN
DO YOU AGREE WITH THE COMPUTER?

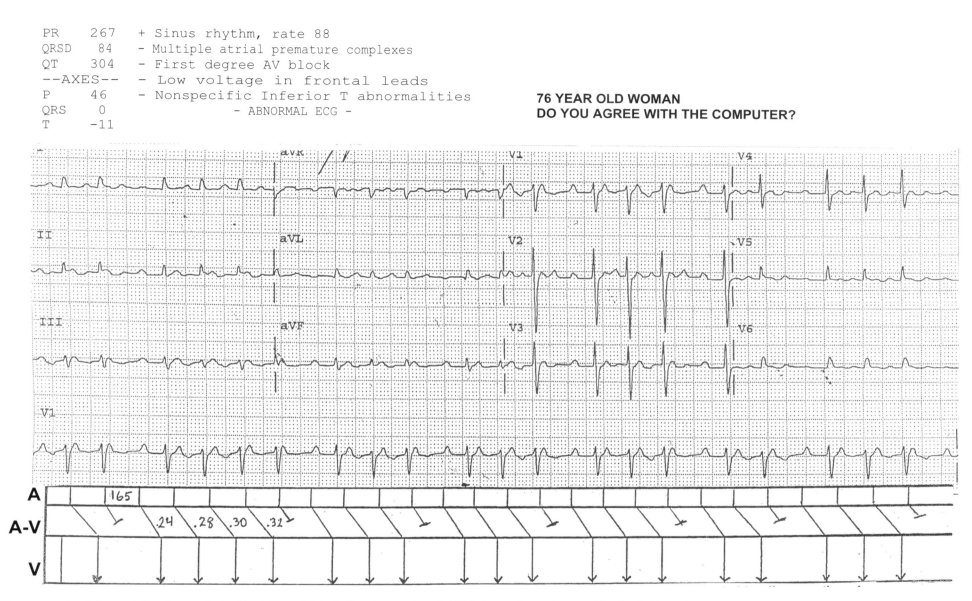

The computer interpretation is sorely lacking! The atrial rhythm is regular at 165/min. and, as depicted in the ladder diagram, there is progressive PR interval prolongation culminating in a dropped beat. This is a classical example of atrial tachycardia with Wenckebach A-V block--representing serious digitalis intoxication.

47 YEAR OLD MAN-6/4
ANY CONDUCTION PROBLEMS??

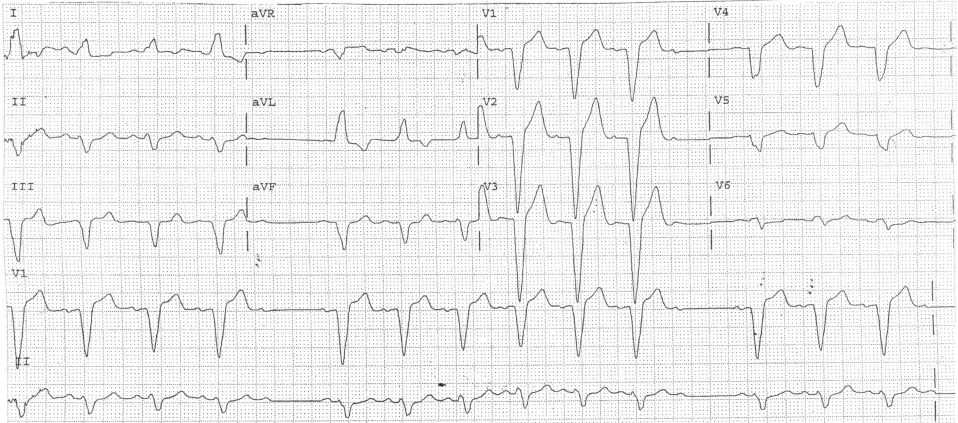

The sinus cycle is regular at 60/min. and PR intervals constant at 0.20 sec. Without warning, P waves are blocked. The presence of left bundle branch block indicates the conduction abnormality is "infra-nodal" type II A-V block. Since the prognosis is uncertain and, if the patient is symptomatic, an electronic pacemaker is warranted.

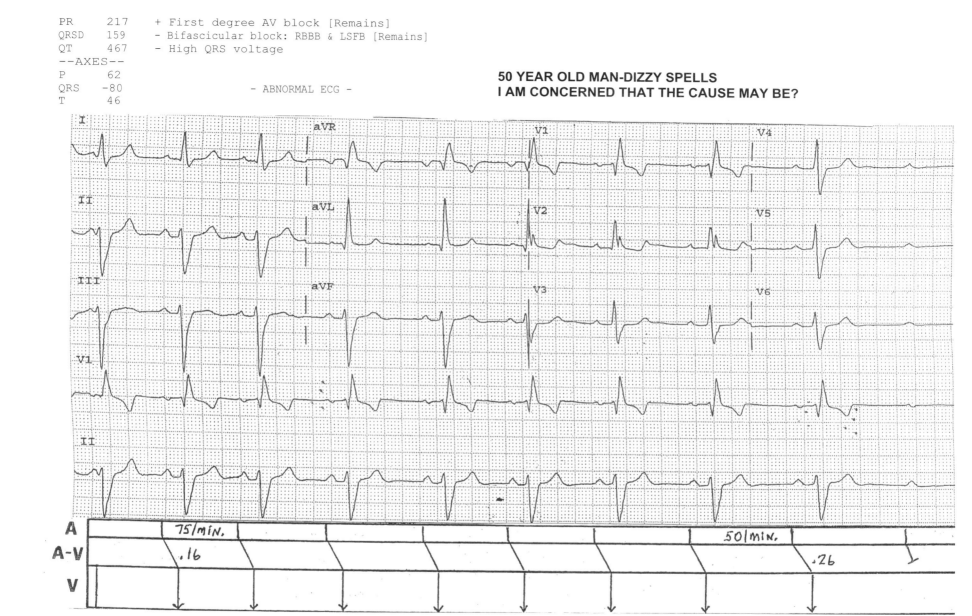

```
PR    217   + First degree AV block [Remains]
QRSD  159   - Bifascicular block: RBBB & LSFB [Remains]
QT    467   - High QRS voltage
--AXES--
P      62                                    50 YEAR OLD MAN-DIZZY SPELLS
QRS   -80        - ABNORMAL ECG -            I AM CONCERNED THAT THE CAUSE MAY BE?
T      46
```

I   aVR   V1   V4

II   aVL   V2   V5

III   aVF   V3   V6

V1

II

A   75/min.   50/min.
A-V   .16   .26
V

The interpretation is correct, but incomplete. A significant omission is that the final P wave is not conducted. This is an unusual example of AV "block." Note that the rhythm begins at 75/min. with a PR interval of 0.16. The rate gradually slows to the 50/min. and the PR interval prolongs to 0.26 seconds. This phenomenon can be seen during a marked vagatonic state--resulting in both sinus node depression and increased AV node refractoriness. It is possible that the last P wave is not conducted because of the markedly prolonged recovery time of the AV node? However, the patient's symptoms are concerning and the bifascicular block and non-conducted P wave may be due to type 2 infranodal block.

6/6-HIS PROBLEM NOW IS ---?

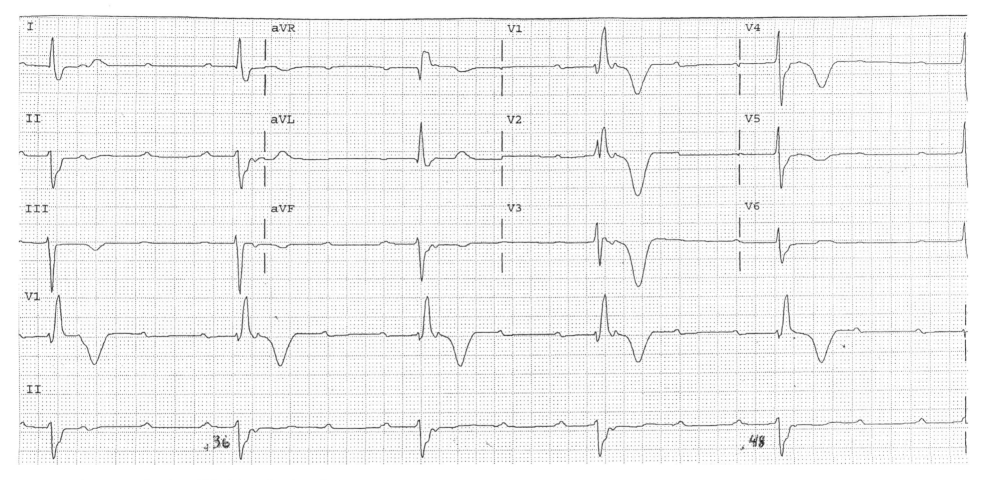

Two days later, complete heart block has developed.
A simple exercise to help clarify the relationship of the P wave and QRS complexes is to ask a series of three questions:
1. Is the P-P cycle regular?
2. Is the R-R cycle regular?
3. Is the PR interval constant? If the answer to all three questions is "yes," the atrial and ventricular events are related as cause and effect. However, if the P-P and R-R cycles are regular, but the PR interval is not constant, the P waves and the QRS complexes are dissociated. In this example, dissociation is present and is due to third-degree A-V block. Now this young man really needs a pacemaker.

= Atrial fibrillation with V. response of 75
= Left bundle branch block [Remains]
-ABNORMAL ECG-

80 YEAR OL WOMAN 6/30
HOW MANY OBSERVATIONS??

Significant errors are present in the computer interpretation. P waves are evident at 100/min. and the rhythm is not atrial fibrillation. Atrial impulses are conducted with prolonging PR intervals until one is not conducted-type I AV block. The conduction ratios vary-3:2 and 4:3. The diagnosis of left bundle branch block is correct, but there is an important omission. Note that there is ST segment elevation greater than 1mm in leads II, III, and aVF, which by the "GUSTO" criteria indicate an acute inferior wall infarction.

149

```
PR     207    + Regular rhythm, undetermined origin, rate 87
QRSD    96
QT     350
QTc    421
--AXES--
P      IND
QRS     79              - BORDERLINE ECG -
T       30
```

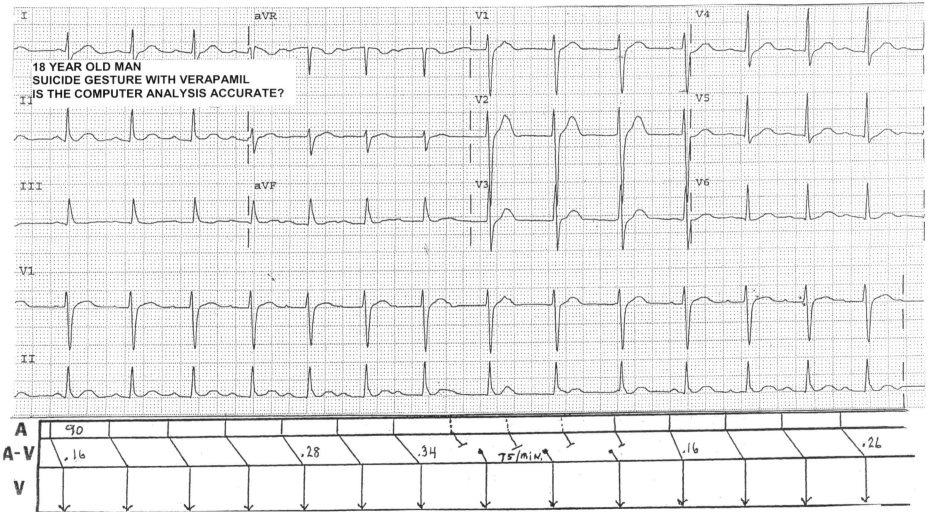

18 YEAR OLD MAN
SUICIDE GESTURE WITH VERAPAMIL
IS THE COMPUTER ANALYSIS ACCURATE?

This unhappy young man took a large dose of calcium channel blocker which resulted in a lengthened refractory period of the A-V node. The prolonging PR intervals and dropped beat indicate type 1 A-V block. This tracing shows a common finding that makes the example "atypical." Note that when the Wenckebach pause occurs, and before the next atrial impulses can be conducted, an accelerated junctional focus appears at 75/min. and discharges three times in sequence.

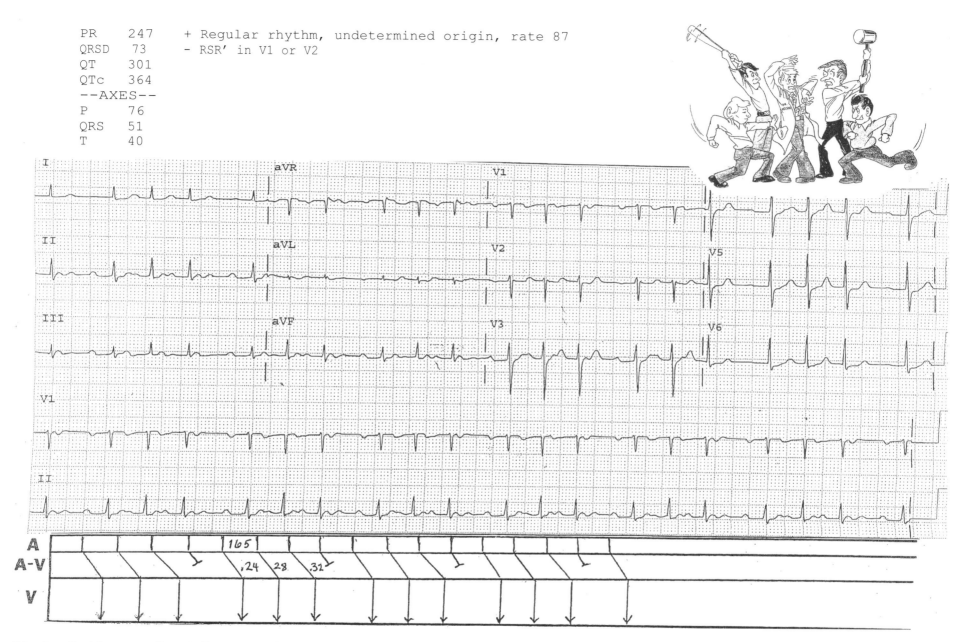

```
PR     247      + Regular rhythm, undetermined origin, rate 87
QRSD    73      - RSR' in V1 or V2
QT     301
QTc    364
--AXES--
P       76
QRS     51
T       40
```

It is clear that there are discrete P waves and that the rhythm is not atrial fibrillation. This tracing is a typical example of atrial tachycardia at 165/min, with type 1 A-V block. The conduction ratio is repetitively 4:3, resulting in a pattern of three QRS complexes separated by pauses. The term applied for this is suggested by the cartoon-"group beating." This is another example in which digitalis toxicity should be considered.

```
PR     218    + Marked sinus bradycardia, rate 36 [Now Present]
QRSD   146    - Multiple atrial premature complexes [Now Present]
QT     461    - Borderline first degree AV block [Now Present]
QTc    357    - Left bundle branch block [Remains]
--AXES--                  -ABNORMAL ECG-
P      81
QRS    14
T      99
```

55 YEAR OLD MAN
DO YOU AGREE
ANYTHING TO DELETE//ADD??

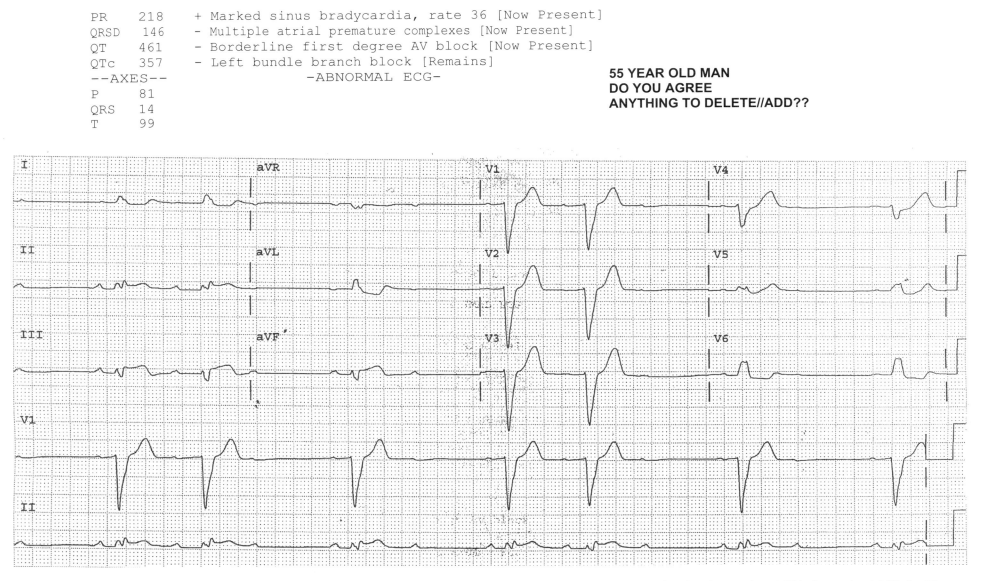

If we acknowledge correct diagnosis, let's give the computer one point for recognizing LBBB, but the sinus mechanism is regular at 72/min. and not 36/min. There are no APCs. The sinus impulses are conducted with Wenckebach A-V nodal block, with variable 3:2 and 2:1 transmission. The concordant elevation of the ST segment in lead II lead raises concern about an acute inferior wall myocardial infarction. Therapy with atropine should be considered.

70 YEAR OLD MAN
WHAT IS BILATERAL BUNDLE BRANCH BLOCK?

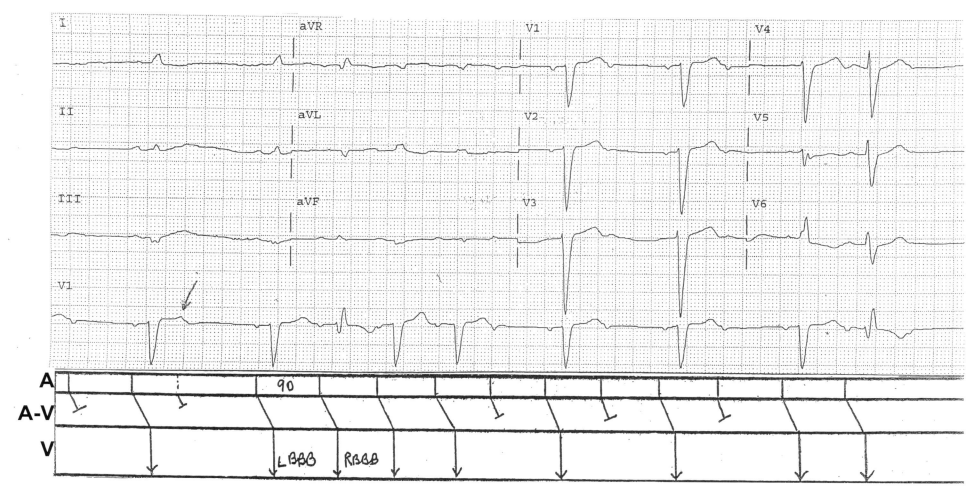

A single APC (arrow) disturbs an otherwise regular sinus rhythm at 90/min. Subsequently, the atrial impulses are transmitted in peculiar fashion. Some are not conducted; some are conducted with LBBB morphology; and some with RBBB. The varying bundle branch conduction has been termed "bilateral bundle branch block," and signals the imminent demise of the intraventricular pathways, and justifies the insertion of an electronic pacemaker.

```
PR              + 3RD degree AV block, Ventricular rate = 44 [Now Present]
QRSD    90      - Vertical axis, unusual for age [Now Present]
QT      443     - Diffuse ST-T abnormalities, [Now Present]
QTc     379     - [Now Absent] Junctional rhythm, rate 43
--AXES--        - [Now Absent] LVH with ST-T abnormalities
P                              -ABNORMAL ECG-
QRS     81
T       100
```

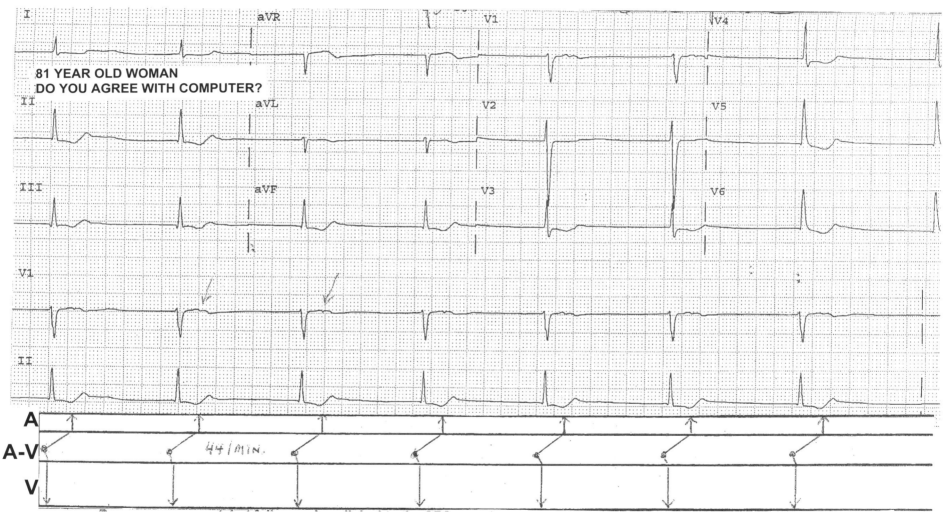

81 YEAR OLD WOMAN
DO YOU AGREE WITH COMPUTER?

P waves are present, but follow and are linked to the QRS complexes. The rhythm is due to a slow, escaping junctional focus with a retrograde atrial activation (arrows). No P waves are available for anterograde conduction and therefore no judgment can be made about "AV block."

```
PR          + Junctional tachycardia, rate 125 [Remains]
QRSD   141  - Long R-R interval measured
QT     301  - Right axis deviation [Remains]
QTc    434  - Nonspecific intraventricular conduction delay [Now Present]
--AXES--    - RVH with ST-T abnormalities [Now Present]
P           - Consider Inferior infarct [Now Present]
QRS    126      -ABNORMAL ECG-
```

61 YEAR OLD MAN
DO YOU AGREE WITH THE COMPUTER?

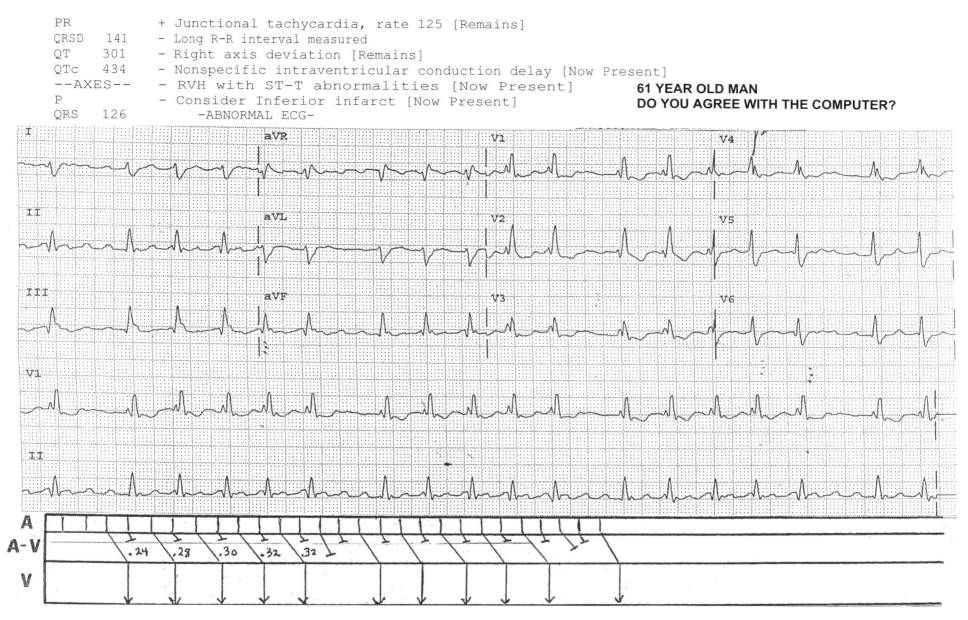

The computer is mostly wrong! The rhythm is atrial flutter. There is right bundle branch block, and, although there is a right axis of the "pre-blocked forces," there is no evidence of RVH. This rhythm is a common finding in patients with atrial flutter. Obviously, it would be foolhardy to conduct 300 stimuli/min. The physiologic refractoriness of the AV node blocks alternating impulses and the patient usually presents with 2:1 AV conduction, and an effective rate of 150/min. Two possibilities exist: all of the *conductible* stimuli may be transmitted, or they may be transmitted with gradual prolongation (Wenckebach AV block). This phenomenon has been termed "bi-level AV block"- i.e.-2:1 block at an upper level of the AV Junction, and Wenckebach block at a lower level. Hopefully, the ladder diagram should make this concept evident.

```
PR     206    + Bradycardia with wide rate variation Mean V-rate = 49, range form 38 to 64
QRSD   127    - Right bundle branch block [Remains]
QT     483    - [Now Absent] 2^{nd} degree Av block (A-rate= 63, V-rate = 47)
QTc    436
--AXES--
P      IND
QRS    3                 -ABNORMAL ECG-
T      12
```

73 YEAR OLD MAN
AGREE WITH THE COMPUTER?
AGREE WITH "NOW ABSENT"?

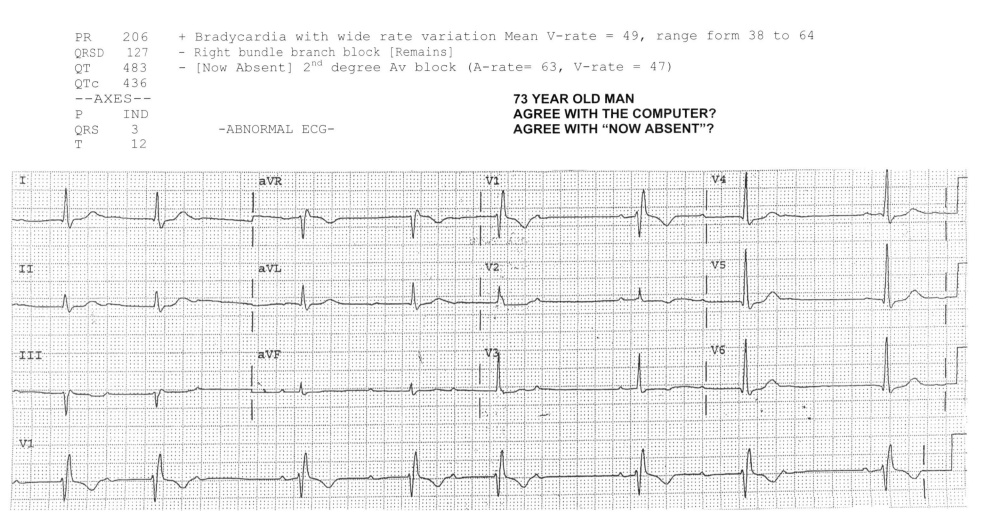

The computer recognized right bundle branch block, but missed the sinus rate of 65/min. Prolonging PR intervals of type 1 A-V block are obvious. Of interest, the computer has previously interpreted "second-degree A-V block," but regards it as "now absent." It is difficult to understand why!

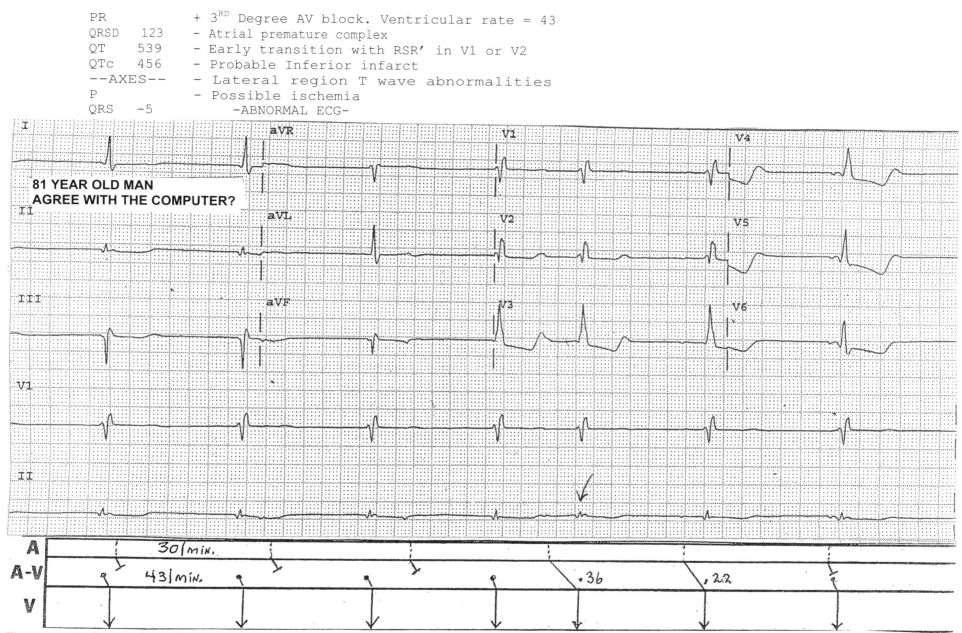

PR   + 3RD Degree AV block. Ventricular rate = 43
QRSD   123   - Atrial premature complex
QT   539   - Early transition with RSR' in V1 or V2
QTc   456   - Probable Inferior infarct
--AXES--   - Lateral region T wave abnormalities
P   - Possible ischemia
QRS   -5   -ABNORMAL ECG-

**81 YEAR OLD MAN
AGREE WITH THE COMPUTER?**

A   30/min.
A-V 43/min.   .36   .22
V

The computer frequently confuses A-V dissociation and A-V block. In this example, there is marked sinus bradycardia at 30/min. An "escape" junctional focus assume command at 43/min. It is conducted with RBBB and Q waves of inferior wall infarction. The dissociated P waves gradually occur later and later after the QRS complexes. When the refractory period from the junctional discharge lessens, the impulse is conducted and "captures" the ventricles (arrow). The next atrial impulse is conducted with only a slight PR prolongation. The capture beat proves that the A-V bridge is intact and denies "third-degree A-V block." The problem is due to the default of the sinus node, rather than A-V block.

72 YEAR OLD MAN. WHAT IS "BLOCK-ACCELERATION DISSOCIATION"?

```
COMPLETE HEART BLOCK ATRIAL RATE 110, WITH
ACCLERATED JUNCTIONAL RHYTHM (NO P-WAVES FOUND)
VENTICULAR RATE 85
RIGHTWARD AXIS
CANNOT RULE OUT INFERIOR INFARCT AGE UNDETERMINED
ABNORMAL ECG
```

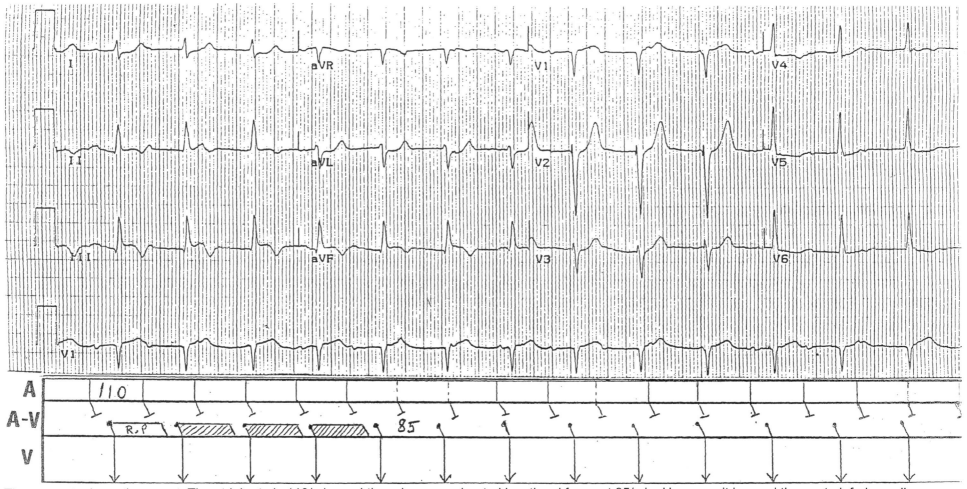

The computer is partly correct. The atrial rate is 110/min. and there is an accelerated junctional focus at 85/min. However, it ignored the acute inferior wall infraction, and concluded that the dissociation of the P waves and QRS complexes was due to complete heart block. It is agreed that there must be "some degree" of AV block, or the atrial rate of 110 would be in command of ventricular activation. The ladder diagram depicts the solution. The repetitive discharge of the accelerated junctional focus and the resulting refractory period (R.P.) prevents transmission of all atrial stimuli. The dissociated P waves "leap frog" over the QRS-ST-T of the accelerated junctional pacemaker, but are unable to find a "window" that would permit A-V passage. Thus, there is a combination of A-V block (probably minor) and an enhanced junctional pacemaker. A descriptive term for this is "block-acceleration dissociation."

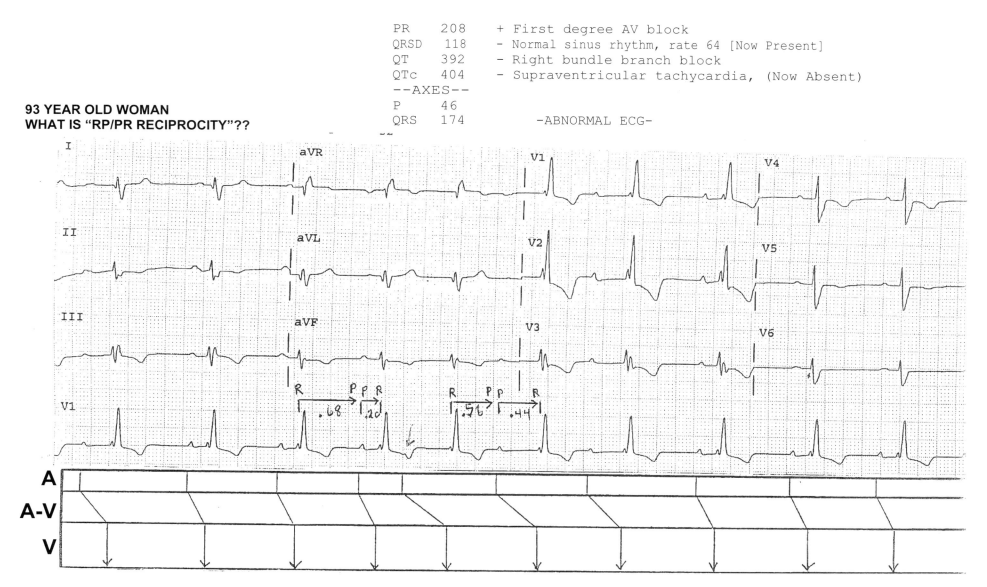

```
PR     208     + First degree AV block
QRSD   118     - Normal sinus rhythm, rate 64 [Now Present]
QT     392     - Right bundle branch block
QTc    404     - Supraventricular tachycardia, (Now Absent)
--AXES--
P      46
QRS    174        -ABNORMAL ECG-
```

93 YEAR OLD WOMAN
WHAT IS "RP/PR RECIPROCITY"??

When an atrial (or ventricular) stimulus enters the A-V junction, it establishes a zone of refractoriness. If the next impulse attempts passage, it may encounter this zone and be conducted with delay, or not al all. In the example above, an APC discharge arrives in the relative refractory period of the preceding beat and its A-V transmission is prolonged. Note the measurement: if the R-P is long (0.68 sec) the subsequent P-R is short (0.20 sec) if the R-P is shorter (0.56 sec), the P-R interval is longer (0.44 sec). This relationship carries the elegant term, "R-P/P-R reciprocity."

159

ELECTROLYTE DERANGEMENTS

The seriously ill patient frequently prompts a request for "STAT" laboratory studies. Usually, the abbreviation STAT should be replaced by "SAWLI" (sit and wait for lab information) because the requested results often are unavailable for 30 minutes (or more). If the patient has a threatening electrolyte derangement, EKG features frequently show characteristic abnormalities and are <u>immediately available</u>. Thus, the clinical relevance is evident, and all physicians should be familiar with EKG changes indicating an electrolyte disturbance which is causative, or contributing, to the patient's illness. The identification of an electrolyte abnormality is relatively straightforward from the characteristic EKG "patterns" that result. However, it is important for clinical correlation to understand the underlying electrophysiological events that result in the EKG changes.

NORMAL ACTIVITY

Despite the fact that Dr. Nernst won the Nobel Prize for his work in cellular electrophysiology, none of us frequently reflect on the "Nernst equation," and we need not worry about it! Nonetheless, it is important to emphasize his conclusions; the level of resting *membrane potential* (RMP) of the cellular action potential is related to the gradient of (K^+) across the cell membrane. Normally, the concentration of <u>intracellular</u> potassium (K^+)i = 160 meq. and <u>extracellular</u> potassium (K^+)o = 4.5 meq. The potassium <u>ratio</u> across the semipermeable cell wall = 35 to 1, and this transcellular concentration difference results in a resting membrane potential of (-) 90 millivolts. This is displayed in the illustration. In the "working" myocardial cell the *threshold potential* (TP) for stimulation is (-) 60 mv. The difference between the RMP and the TP is normally 30 mv. This is the "excitability" requirement.

If the myocardial cell receives the required 30 mv. stimulus, it reaches the threshold potential and there is an inrush of (Na) ions and the cell rapidly depolarizes. This is phase zero of the action potential and corresponds to the "QRS" of the surface EKG. Repolarization begins with a brief phase 1, followed by a longer, and more important phase 2. The dotted line in the diagram depicts the "slow calcium current," which is a major cause of the "plateau" during this phase. (The ST segment on the surface EKG). The major portion of recovery is in phase 3--reflecting potassium movement across the cell membrane (the surface T wave). Phase 4 is the reestablishment of the resting membrane potential.

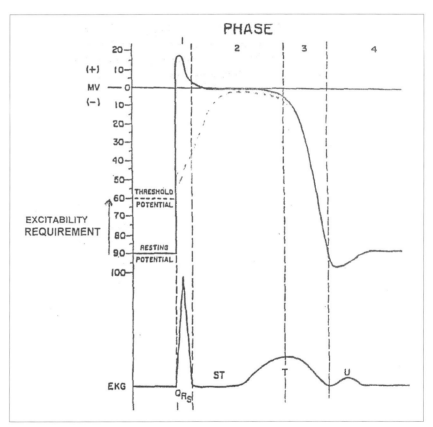

HYPERKALEMIA

Hyperkalemia is a common and life-threatening condition. Causes include renal failure, diabetic acidosis, muscle injury, and medications. The most evident and early EKG feature of hyper (K^+) is due to change in the repolarization phase 3. This becomes steeper, resulting in a T wave that is taller than normal, peaked, and narrow at the base...a "tented" T wave. The result of the increase in extracellular (K^+) is also a <u>decrease</u> in the intra and extracellular potassium ratio. For example, a marked increase in extracellular (K^+)--let's say to 9 meq.--will result in *hypopolarization* of the RMP--let's say to 70 mV. The membrane now requires only a 10 mV. stimulus to reach the threshold level and is, thus, *hyperexcitable*. In addition, when the exciting stimulus reaches the threshold level, it has a diminished "running start" and the depolarization upstroke velocity (phase 0) is decreased, resulting in an increase in the QRS duration. The T wave morphology identifies the problem, and, in general, the QRS duration indicates the severity. Obviously, the rapidity of the (K^+) increase will determine the clinical impact. The example shown was from a woman with diabetic acidosis and a serum potassium of 6.8 meq.

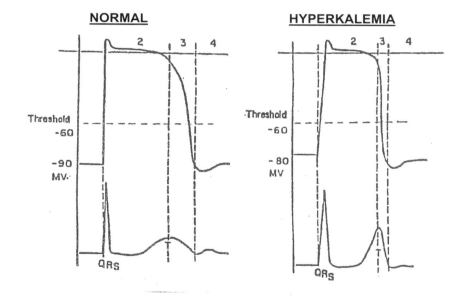

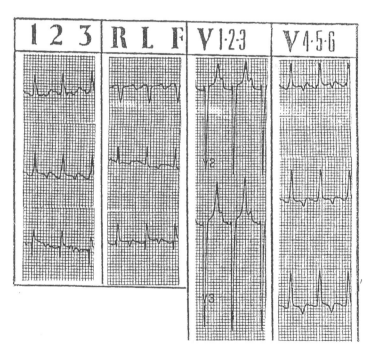

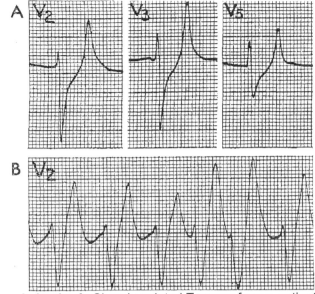

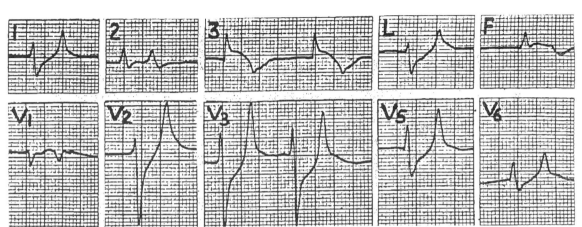

Hyperkalemia. **A**. Sharply pointed T waves from a patient with diabetic acidosis and a serum potassium of 8 mEq/L. **B**. Note the widening QRS and the almost straight line from the nadir of QRS to the apex of disproportionately tall T wave.

Hyperkalemia in a 77-year-old man with diabetic acidosis and a potassium level of 7.7 mEq/L, simulating the pattern of acute inferior injury (with ST elevation in leads III and aVF and depression in other leads). The ST-T configuration in the mid-precordial leads is classical for potassium toxicity.

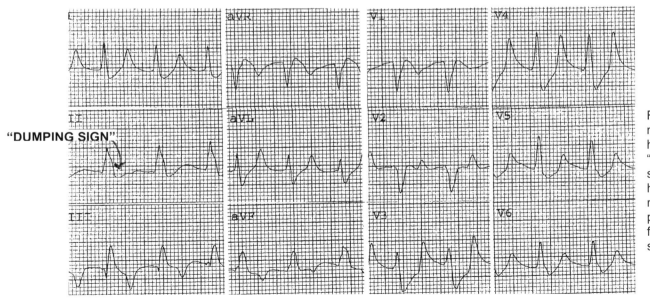

"DUMPING SIGN"

From a patient in renal failure with a potassium of 8.1 mEq/L. Occasionally, the pattern of significant hyperkalemia includes what may be called the "dumping sign." The morphology appears as though some rotund body has been dumped into the hammock of the ST segment. This has the effect of making the ST segment sag horizontally and of pushing the proximal limb of the T wave further away from the QRS, so that the upstroke of the T wave is steeper than its downstroke.

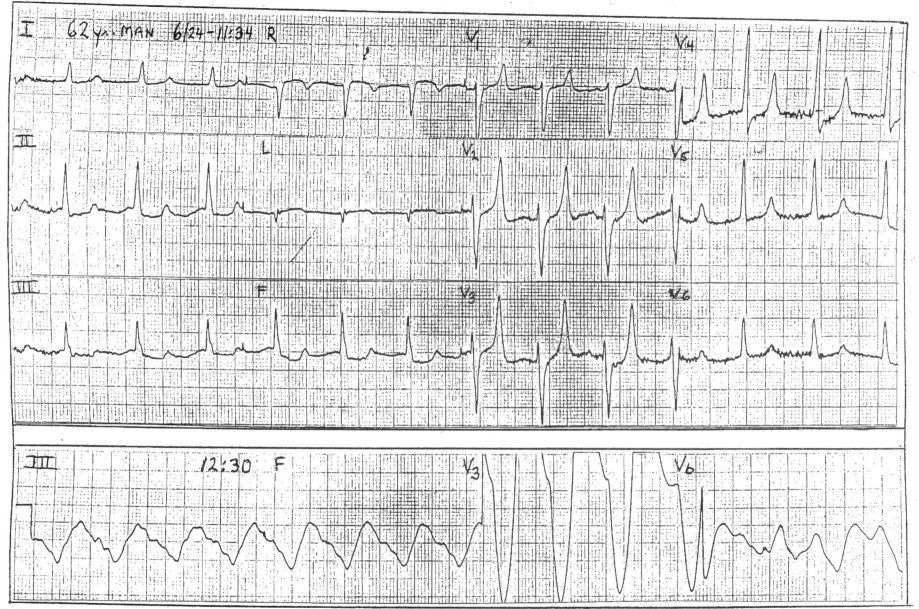

This man had chronic renal failure requiring dialysis. On this day, he presented to the renal clinic and announced that he was leaving the dialysis program. His potassium in the upper tracing was 9.0 mEq/L Note the lack of P waves and the tall and narrow T waves. Efforts to dissuade him were unsuccessful. An hour later, while waiting for his ride home, he collapsed. A segment of his final EKG is shown. The waveforms in leads II and aVF spill together with little indication of what is depolarization and repolarization. This pattern is the end-stage of hyperkalemia and has been termed "sine wave pattern." It signals imminent death.

HYPOKALEMIA

Potassium deficits occur with gastrointestinal or renal losses and are much too frequently due to excessive diuretic therapy. When the serum (K^+) decreases--let's say from 4.5 mEq to 2.0 mEq-- the _ratio_ of potassium concentration across the cell membrane increases and the resting membrane potential is _hyperpolarized_ (let's say from (-) 90mV to (-) 110mV). With a normal threshold potential of (-) 60mV, the usual "excitability" requirement to reach the TP is 30mV, but is now increased to 50mV. The membrane may become so hyperpolarized that it is difficult, or impossible, to reach the threshold level, and the patient is weak, or paralyzed. The phase 3 of the action potential--dependent on (K^+) movement across the cell--becomes longer and slower and encroaches on phase 2. The result on the surface EKG is that the ST segment is depressed, the T-wave is smaller, and a secondary repolarization event-the U wave-increases.

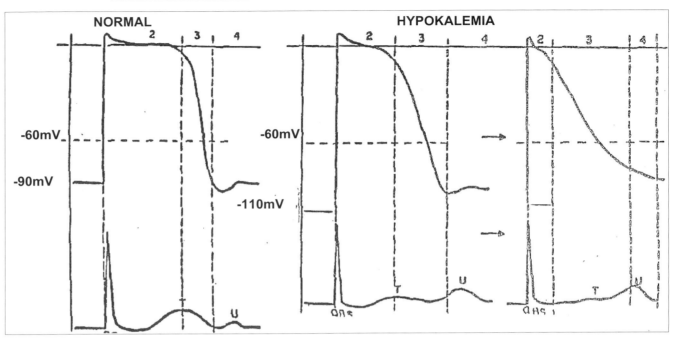

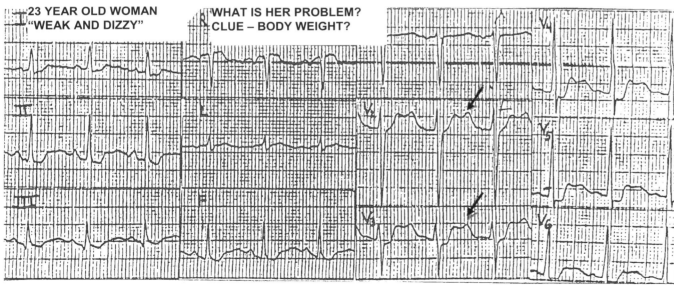

23 YEAR OLD WOMAN "WEAK AND DIZZY"

WHAT IS HER PROBLEM? CLUE – BODY WEIGHT?

The example was obtained from a young woman with "anorexia nervosa" who, in addition to starving herself, had taken emetics, laxatives, and a diuretic drug. Her body weight of 80 lbs. was accompanied by a (K^+) of 1.8 mEq. Note the depressed ST segments, the flattened T-waves and the large U waves (arrows). The morphology of the T-U in V2-V4 is a "camel-hump" effect.

From a patient with a serum potassium of 2.6 mEq/L. As the extracellular potassium concentration declines, a "seesaw" develops between the T wave and the U wave. As the U wave gets taller, the T wave shrinks. When the serum level is somewhere between 2.5 and 3.0 mEq./L their height is usually about equal, and the two rounded peaks may produce a "camel-hump" effect. At lower levels, the U wave may tower over the T-wave. In many patients the T and U waves, instead of retaining their individual identity, unite to form a single upward bulge. This can produce the contour of a rather tame "roller coaster." The blend of T and U wave may result in the U wave being included in the measurement of the QT interval--a mistake that has led to the erroneous belief that the QT interval is prolonged in hypokalemia.

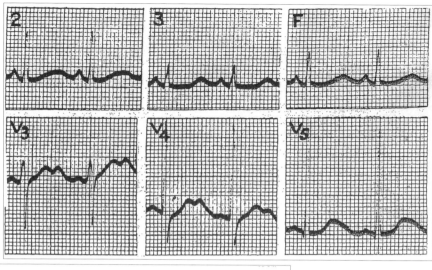

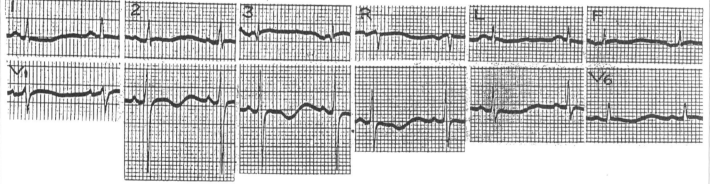

The "roller coaster" pattern in a patient with a K$^+$ of 2.3 mEq/L.

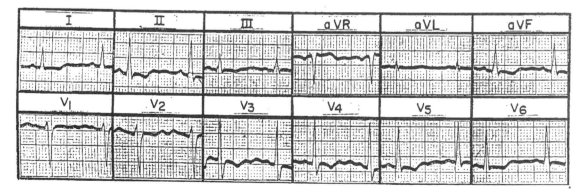

A 39-year-old woman with primary hyperaldosteronism resulting in a potassium level of 2.4 mEq/L. The undulations of the ST-T-U produce a pattern characteristic of hypokalemia.

HYPERCALEMIA

Hypercalcemia is seen in hyperparathyroidism, numerous malignancies, prolonged immobilization, sarcoidosis, and excess vitamin D and calcium intake. As mentioned previously, the slow (Ca^{++}) current influences phase 2 of the cellular action potential (the ST segment of the EKG). With an increase in (Ca^{++}) ions, the phase 2 is _shortened_, causing the T-wave to be closer to the end of the QRS complex. The surface EKG shows a decreased interval between the beginning of the QRS complex and the _onset_ of the T wave (Q<u>o</u>T interval); the _apex_ of the T wave (Q<u>a</u>T interval); and the _end_ of the T-wave (QT interval). Thus, the T-wave reaches an early peak and the upstroke is steeper than the ensuing down stroke. An important additional effect of hypercalcemia is to alter the level of the threshold potential--<u>raising</u> it from (-) 60 mV. to--let's say (-) 50 mV. The difference between the resting membrane potential and the threshold potential is increased, requiring a 40 mV. stimulus to reach the membrane "take off" point. The importance of this effect will be seen shortly.

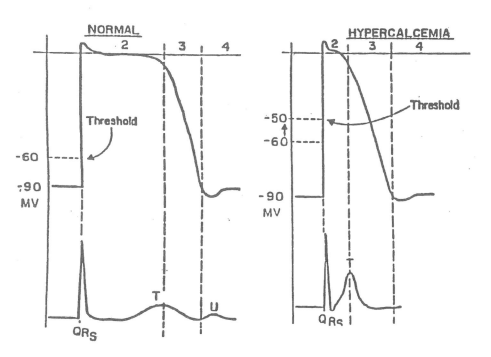

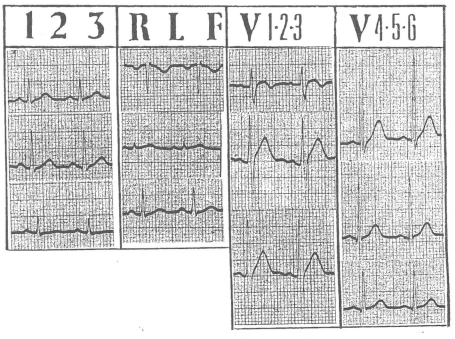

This 19-year-old man had a hematologic malignancy with bone destruction. His (Ca^{++}) level was 14--increased from the normal level of +/- 10.
Note in leads V2-4 that the T wave begins immediately at the end of the QRS complex ("short Q to onset of T"). The measured onset of the QRS to the _apex_ of the T wave, corrected for rate, (QaTc) is 0.26 sec. (normal = 0.34 sec.).

166

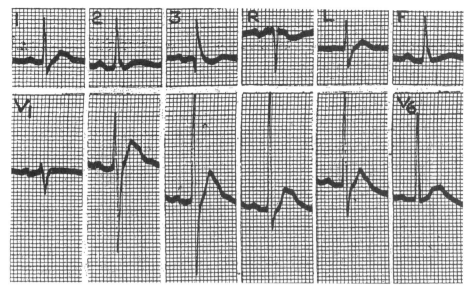

Hypercalcemia. Note the steep upstroke of the T-wave with more gradual return to the baseline. From a patient with hyperparathyroidism and a serum calcium of 15 mg/100 ml.

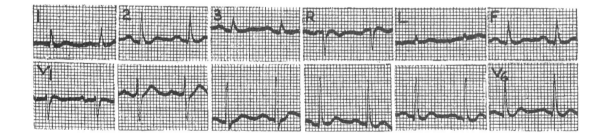

An example of hypercalcemia secondary to bronchogenic carcinoma. Subtle evidence of the early T wave apex is best seen in lead V2; serum calcium was 12.9 mg%.

HYPOCALCEMIA

Causes of hypocalcemia include hypoparathyroidism, malabsorption syndromes, vitamin D deficiency, acute pancreatitis, and some cases of renal insufficiency. Just as hypercalcemia shortens phase 2 of the action potential, hypocalcemia prolongs it. The T-wave is delayed and all components of the QT interval are prolonged. The figure depicts the delay in the onset (QoT), apex (QaT) and end of phase 3 (QT interval). Since the time for repolarization depends on the heart rate, the measurements must be corrected for the cycle length. The correction formula and the limits for the corrected intervals are shown. The alteration in phase 2 is not the only effect of hypocalcemia. It also results in a change in the threshold level, which *decreases* from (-) 60 mV. to--let's say (-) 70 mV. The stimulus required to pass from the resting membrane level of (-) 90 mV. to the threshold level is less--now 20 mV. and the membrane is "hyperexcitable." All neuromuscular structures participate in this increased responsiveness and skeletal muscle spasm may signal the abnormality. Cardiac arrhythmias can be promoted by this electrolyte derangement.

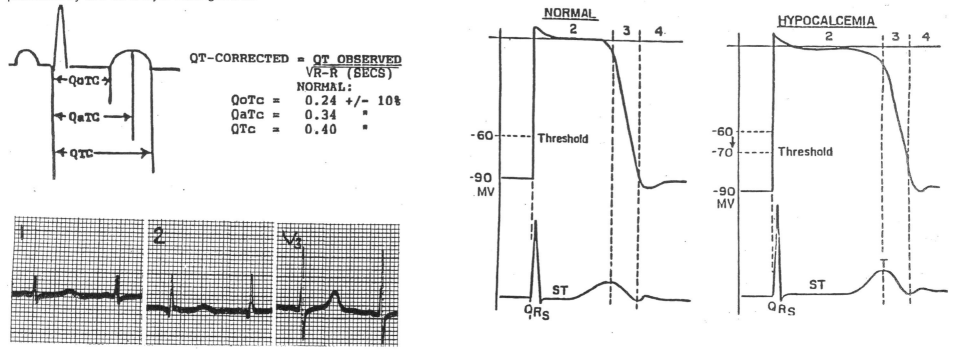

$$QT\text{-}CORRECTED = \frac{QT\ OBSERVED}{\sqrt{R\text{-}R}\ (SECS)}$$

NORMAL:

QoTc = 0.24 +/- 10%
QaTc = 0.34 "
QTc = 0.40 "

Hypocalcemia. A, Long Q-T interval because of prolonged ST segment; from a patient with serum calcium of 7 mg/100ml

168

KINDLY MAKE AN OBSERVATION ON THIS CONTINUOUS RECORDING OF LEAD III.

WHAT IV MEDICATION IS BEING ADMINISTERED?

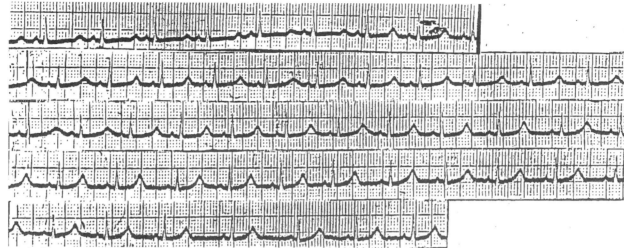

This 14 year-old girl has congenital hypoparathyroidism. Her calcium metabolism had been controlled with vitamin D and calcium supplement. Upon reaching the age or reason (?) she refused to take her medications. She presented with a seizure, a serum (Ca^{++}) of 4 mg% and this EKG. I.V. calcium gluconate was administered, with the striking response show in this continuous tracing. The first complex shows a marked prolongation of the Q to onset of T (0.36 sec.) The measurement quickly shortens and at the end of the recording is normal.

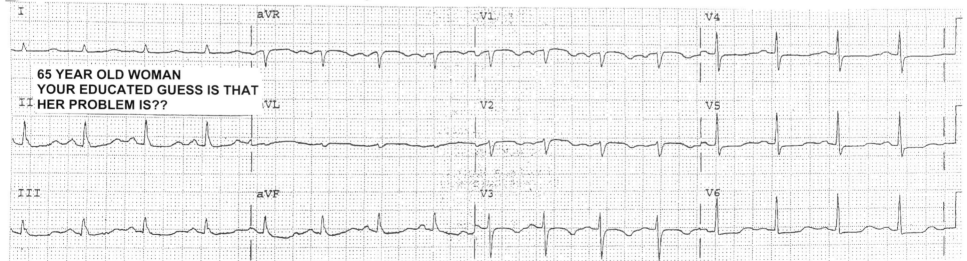

65 YEAR OLD WOMAN
YOUR EDUCATED GUESS IS THAT HER PROBLEM IS??

The tracing shows a prolonged Q to the onset of T, characteristic of hypocalcemia. An interesting and unusual explanation: this woman had used a "Fleets enema" nightly, providing herself with a large dose of sodium phosphate. On admission, her phosphate level was 19 mg% and her calcium was 5.0 mg%. Recall the principle of physiology that nature desires the Ca x PO4 product ± 40, so if the phosphate increases, the calcium decreases. A rather bizarre but true story.

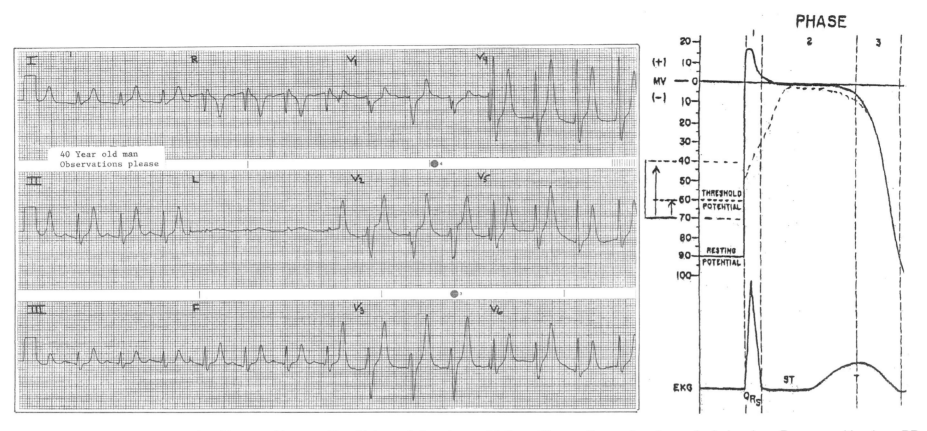

An E.D tracing from a hypotensive 40-year-old man with a history of chronic renal failure. Observations, at a glance, include: sinus P waves with a long PR interval, broad QRS complexes and gigantic T waves with a relatively narrow base. The immediate reaction should be-marked hyperkalemia (measured at 8.7 mEq/L). The most specific and immediate therapy should be calcium gluconate. Why? The illustration provides an answer. As previously discussed, hyperkalemia results in "hypopolarization" of the membrane, and the resting membrane potential is decreased from (-) 90 mV to, let's say, (-70) mV. With a normal threshold potential of (-) 60 mV, now only a 10 millivolt stimulus is required for depolarization and the cell is "hyperexcitable." When calcium is administered, the threshold potential is shifted form (-) 60 to, let's say (-) 40 mV and normal excitability is restored. The QRS duration and PR interval are normalized and the T wave changes regress. Calcium is the only treatment that directly alters the electrophysiology of the cell.

Other therapies are certainly worthwhile and work but not as quickly or specifically. They depend on either excretion of the potassium excess or transfer of the cation into the cell to normalize the transcellular ratio.

Affecting "excretion"	**Affecting "transfer"**
Diruretics	Glucose & Insulin
Binding Resins	Na bicarbonate
Dialysis	Beta agonists
	Hyperventilation

82 YEAR OLD MAN – PROBLEM??
CLUE: THEM BONES, THEM BONES

```
PR              + Atrial fibrillation with V. response of 55
QRSD    99      - Borderline low voltage in frontal leads
QT     449      - Nonspecific Anterior ST elevation
QTc    429
--AXES--
P
QRS     25         -ABNORMAL ECG-
T        6
```

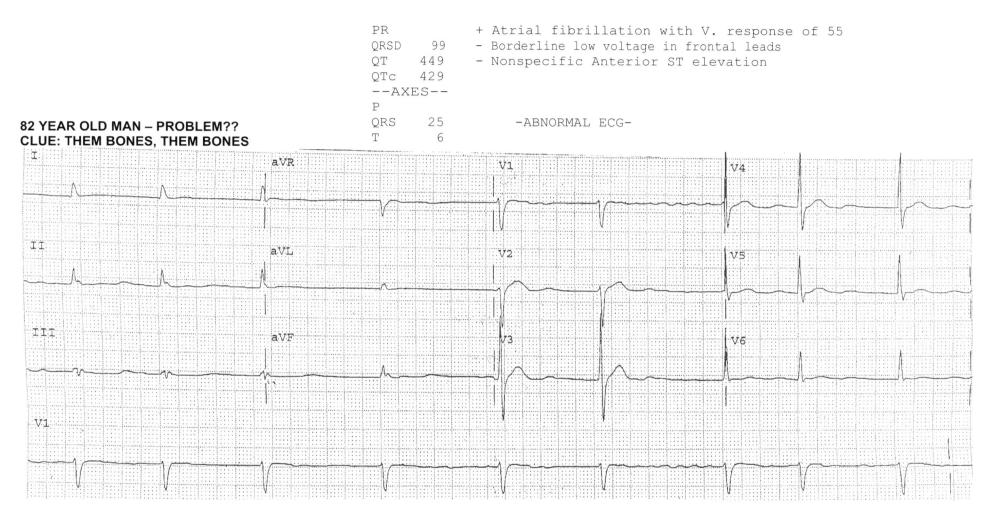

The generous clue should suggest that the patient's problem relates to calcium metabolism. Aside from atrial fibrillation, the noteworthy EKG observation is the markedly short interval between the end of the QRS complex and the onset of the T wave, indicating hypercalcemia. This man was prescribed HCTZ and calciferol to "help preserve his bones" and presented with a serum (Ca^{++}) of 14.8 mg%--bad therapy don't you think?

47 YEAR OLD MAN
"I COULDN'T MOVE THIS MORNING"

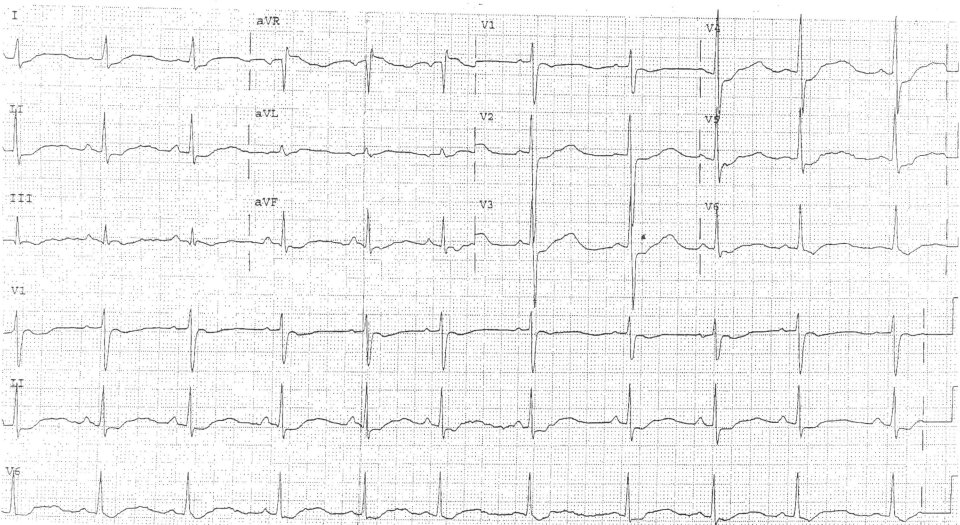

The long Q-T-U interval is evident with large U wave in V2-V5 and the ST segment depression consistent with hypokalemia. This young man has had numerous episodes of profound weakness due to "familial hypokalemic paralysis." His potassium level in the Emergency Department was 1.5mEq/L. Advice: Don't marry into this family!

172

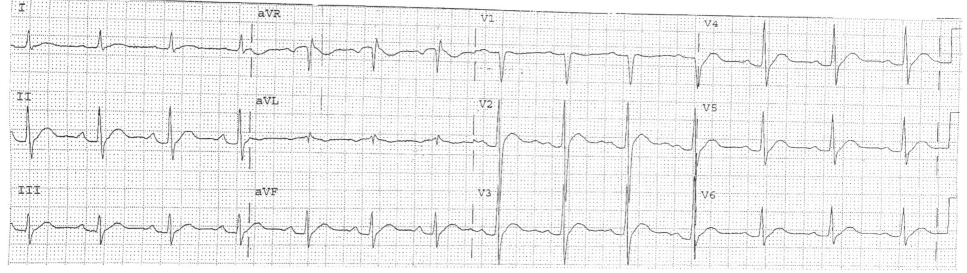

Nicely shown in lead V2-V3 is a short Q to the onset of T, indicating hypercalcemia. Her calcium level was 16.4 mg%, due to hyperparathyroidism. The small U wave in lead V2 correlated with a potassium of 2.5 mEq/L.

173

86 YEAR OLD WOMAN
VOMITING FOR 4 DAYS
KINDLY FILL IN THE BLANKS

Na=_____   Cl=_____

K=_____ CO_2=___

```
PR     136    + Sinus rhythm, rat 74
QRSD   101    - Atrial premature complex
QT     409    - Inferior Q waves noted
QTc    454    - Diffuse ST-T abnormalities
--AXES--
              -ABNORMAL ECG-
```

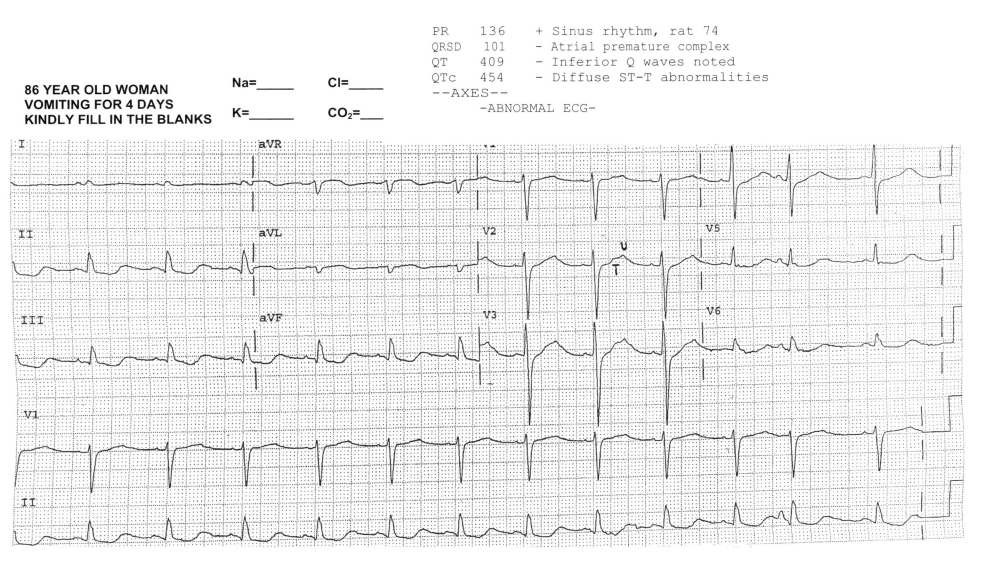

The computer analysis is correct, but not informative. A blend of T wave and large U wave is seen in V2-V4. The sagging and depressed ST segments are a result of hypokalemia secondary to vomiting and diarrhea. Labs values: (Na^+) = 128 mEq/L (K^+) = 2.3 mEq/L ($HCO3^-$) = 30 mEq/L (Cl^-) = 80 mEq/L

74 YEAR OLD WOMAN
C/O MARKED WEAKNESS
ION SUFFICIENCY?? –DEFICIENCY??
EFFECT ON EXCITABILITY??

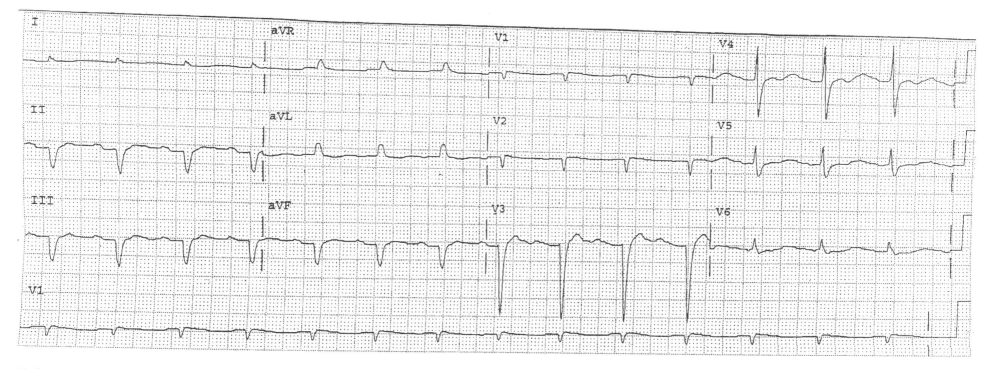

Unfortunately, this was single EKG from the emergency department and there is no clinical correlation available. Noteworthy observations are the short Q to the onset and apex of the T wave and the very prominent U waves, the combination consistent with hypercalcemia and hypokalemia. Recall that cellular "excitability" reflects the difference between the resting membrane potential = (-) 90 mV and the threshold potential = (-) 60 mV. Thus, normal excitability is ± 30 mV. Hypokalemia increases the resting membrane potential (let's say to 100 mV), and hypercalcemia decreases theresold level (let's say to -50 mV.) With the combined electrolyte derangement, the stimulus now required to reach the threshold is 50 mV, with resultant profound weakness.

47 YEAR OLD WOMAN WITH ACUTE PANCREATITIS
PELASE PROVID HER LAB VALUES:

K^+=_____ Ca^{++}=_____

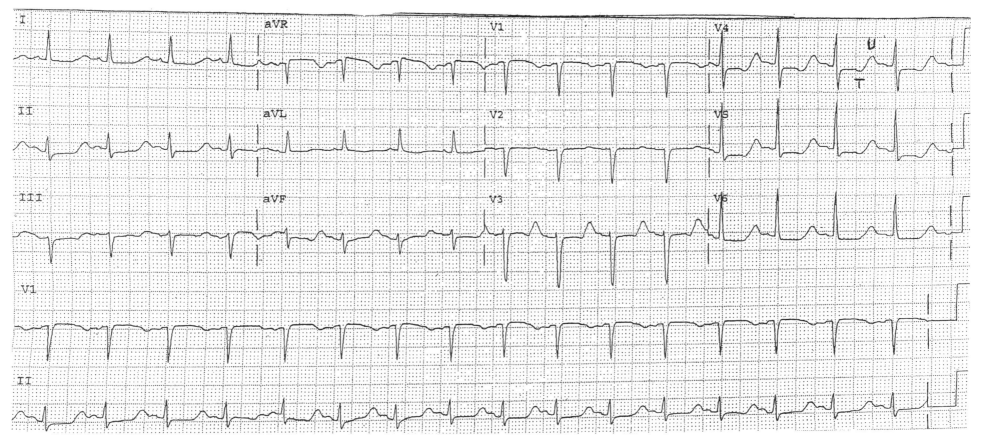

The T waves are almost invisible, and the large deflection is a prominent U wave (note lead V4). Although it is difficult to measure, there is a long interval between the QRS and T wave, consistent with hypocalcemia (Ca^{++} = 7.0 mg%). This was due to the release of pancreatic lipase resulting in increase in free fatty acids (which are saponified by calcium). Repetitive vomiting caused potassium loss with resulting hypokalemia. The large U wave reflected a potassium of 2.7 mEq/L. The Q waves indicating inferior and anterior MI provide additional concern to the electrolyte derangement.

77 YEAR OLD WOMAN
HER PROBLEMS INCLUDE:
1. **DIABETES**
2. **CHRONIC RENAL FAILURE**
3. **PANCREATITIS**

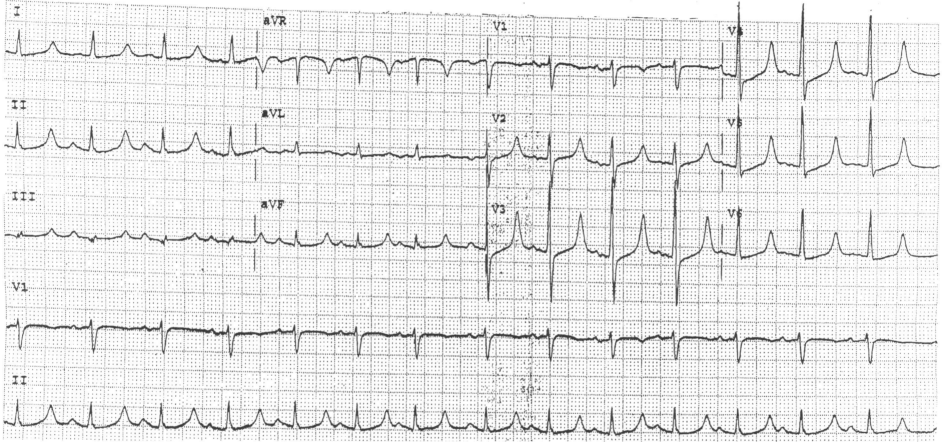

The prolonged Q to the onset of the T wave indicates hypocalcemia, and tall, narrow based T waves, hyperkalemia. All three of the suggested problems are present. The patient's pancreatitis caused the release of amylase and lipase, and the resulting free fatty acids were "saponified" by calcium, resulting in a decreased calcium level of 7.2 mg%. Her diabetic ketoacidosis and chronic renal failure combined to increase the potassium to 8.2 mEq/L.

ATRIAL & JUNCTIONAL RHYTHMS

Before launching into a discussion of supraventricular <u>tachycardias</u>, let's review other supraventricular arrhythmias.

In the normal individual, the sinoatrial node, in the roof of the right atrium, is in command of cardiac activation because it has the fastest inherent rate. Right and left atrial depolarization then continues from above-down and, thus, the normal P wave axis is (+) in leads I and aVF. (The first quadrant).

Varieties of atrial rhythm include
Atrial premature complexes--conducted or not
Ectopic atrial rhythm
Sinus arrhythmia
Sinoatrial exit block
Atrial parasystole
"Sick sinus syndrome"--"Tachy-brady syndrome"

Varieties of junctional rhythm include
Wandering atrial pacemaker
Junctional "escape" rhythm
Reciprocal rhythm
Accelerated junctional rhythm

All of us have seen and have had episodes of sinus bradycardia (rate <60/min.) and sinus tachycardia (rate >100/min.). Examples are so familiar that none need to be shown.

ATRIAL PREMATURE COMPLEXES

Atrial premature complexes occur during the refractory period of the conducting system. If the occurrence is sufficiently early (0.48 sec.), the AV bridge has not recovered and the APC is not conducted. If later (0.56 sec.), the APC may achieve AV nodal transmission, but find that the right bundle branch has not recovered, and is conducted with RBBB aberration. When late enough (0.60 sec.) the APC is normally conducted.

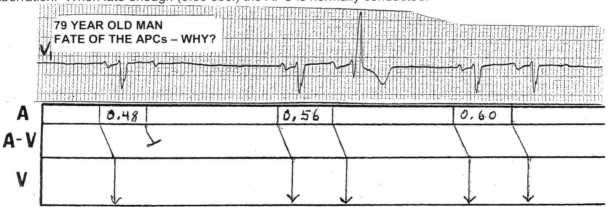

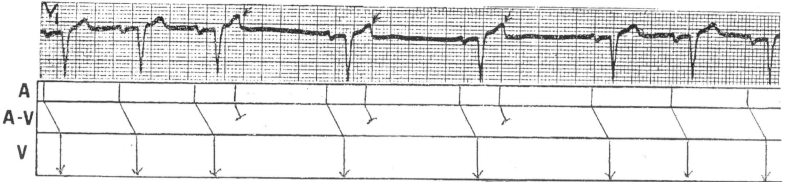

A devious patient might attempt to fool an interpreter into saying "intermittent sinus bradycardia." In reality, note that the morphology of the 3rd, 4th, and 5th T waves is different than all others. The subtle change indicates that there is a premature P wave which is hiding in the T wave. The stimulus is sufficiently early that it encounters junctional refractoriness and is not conducted.

ECTOPIC ATRIAL RHYTHM

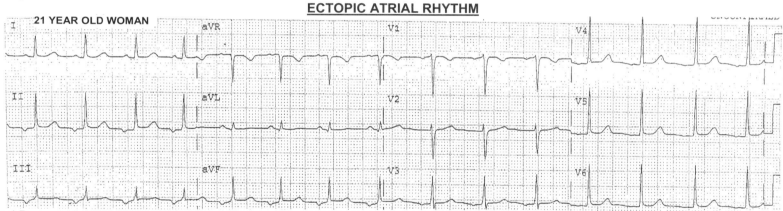

21 YEAR OLD WOMAN

Note the inverted P waves in leads II, III, and aVF (P wave axis = (-) 60°). Beta agonist therapy for asthma has awakened an ectopic atrial pacemaker, firing at 88/min. The tracing is otherwise normal. When this site slows or the SA node accelerates, the rhythm will return to normal.

SINUS ARRHYTHMIA

Sinus arrhythmia is a normal phenomenon indicating changes in sinus rate with respiration. With inspiration, and the resulting increase in venous return, the rate increases, and decreases with expiration. When long rhythm strips are recorded, the variation in rate correlates with the respiratory cycle.

38 YEAR OLD MAN-WHERE DID THIS MAN EXPIRE??   **A NICE EXAMPLE OF RATHER MARKED RESPIRATORY SINUS ARRHYTHMIA**
HE INSPIRED HERE----------AND EXPIRED HERE

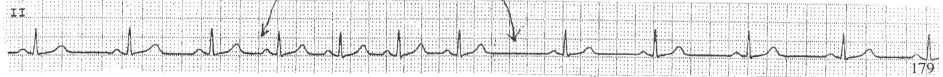

SINOATRIAL "EXIT BLOCK"

When the sinus node continues to fire, but its stimulus does not leave the sinus node "island", and there is a "missing" P wave, the term "exit block" is applied. Analogous to <u>AV nodal</u> block, the disturbed transmission may be considered "type 1 block" or "type 2 block." Examples are shown below. Sinoatrial exit block is frequently due to waning sinoatrial node "strength" (sick sinus syndrome) but can be due to drugs that depress the sinus node (digitalis excess, beta-blockers, or calcium channel blockers) or to vagatonic depression related to inferior wall myocardial infarction.

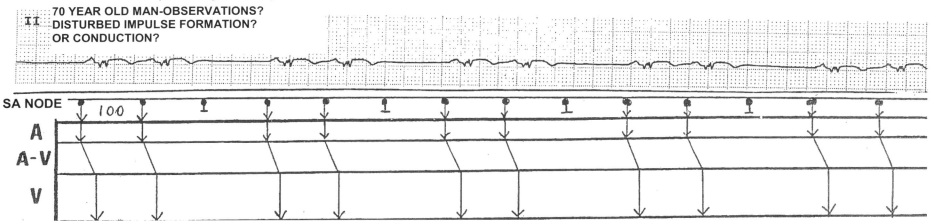

The evident "group beating" could be simply atrial bigemini, with a lengthy post extra systolic pause. An alternate solution is diagrammed, indicating that there is 3:2 type 2 *sinoatrial exit block* which results in the missing P wave. This is occurring during acute inferior myocardial infarction.

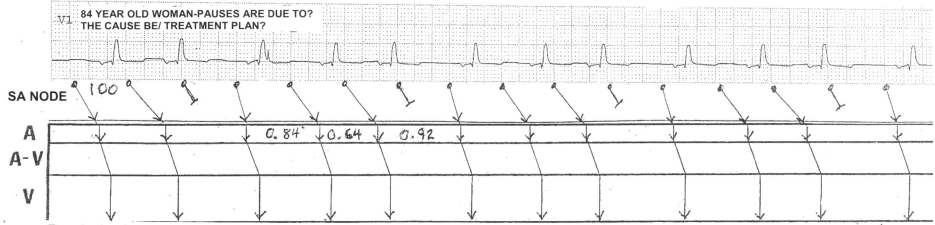

Even in the rhythm strip, you can recognize that the sinus impulses are conducted with the right bundle branch block. But what about the pauses? The rhythm is an example of *type 1 sinoatrial exit block*. The repetitive QRS pattern and the "missing" P waves serve as an alert to the problem. The simple math to determine the true rate of the sinus node and explain the ladder diagram is shown. The sum of the sinus cycles, including the dropped beat, is 2.40 sec. (0.84 + 0.64 + 0.92 = 2.40 sec.) Since this represents 4 sinus node discharges, the sinus interval = 0.60 second-rate = 100/minute. In this woman, digitalis excess was the culprit, and the exit block disappeared when it was discontinued.

ATRIAL PARASYSTOLE

Atrial parasystole is an interesting and unusual arrhythmia. It represents the coexistence of two atrial pacemakers functioning independently of each other. The criteria for diagnosis are as follows: The ectopic focus has an inconstant relationship to the sinus node cycle ("non-fixed coupling"). It is not depolarized by the sinus node discharge ("entrance block"). Its rate remains *reasonably* constant ("interectopic interval"). If the ectopic focus attempts to fire when the sinus node has just discharged, it will be unsuccessful ("exit block"). When the timing of the two pacemakers, by accident, coincide, an atrial fusion complex results.

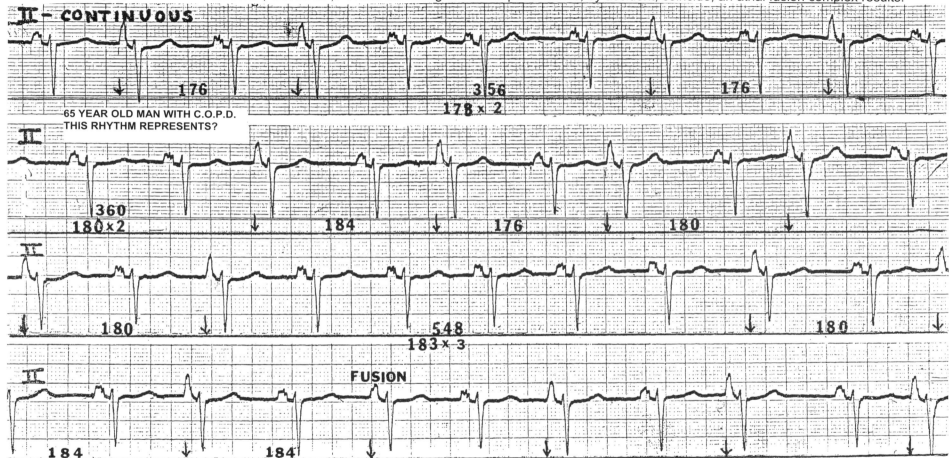

The example shows that a long rhythm strip and careful measurements are required to establish the diagnosis of atrial parasystole. The measured intervals between discharges of the slow ectopic focus indicate that its rate is 32-34/min. There is a minor variation in the ectopic discharges from 176 to 184 hundredths of a second ("centiseconds"). Multiples of this basic interectopic interval are seen when exit block occurs. And atrial fusion complex is identified in the bottom strip.

"SICK SINUS SYNDROME" & "TACHYCARDIA-BRADYCARDIA SYNDROME"

Sick sinus syndrome is a common problem and can be due to the abnormality of sinoatrial node impulse <u>formation</u> or <u>conduction</u>. With advancing age, or drug excess, the activity of the nodal pacemaker cells ("P cells") may decrease. They may no longer "fire", or the signal may not be enough to depolarize the surrounding tissue (sinoatrial exit block). The resulting slow rate permits junctional "escape beats" to occur, and frequently allows <u>ectopic</u> atrial pacemakers to surface. All premature atrial stimuli will depolarize the sinoatrial node and the "insult" can result in marked delay in its recovery (termed "post extra-systolic sinus node suppression"). Conversely, a premature ectopic discharge may trigger episodes of tachycardia (atrial fibrillation or atrial flutter). The end result is that the episodes of bradycardia are blended with bursts of supraventricular tachycardia.

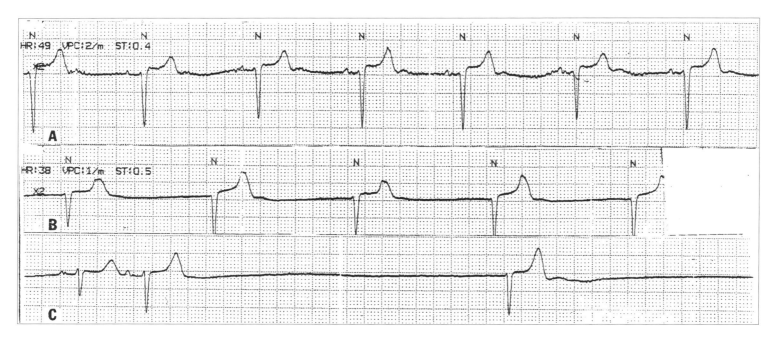

This 60-year-old woman presented with recurring "dizzy spells." Holter monitoring revealed the cause. Her basic rhythm (**A**) was sinus bradycardia at 49/min. Later (**B**) sinus node activity is no longer present and an escape junctional focus activates the heart at 38/minute. Segment (**C**) shows her real problem. A sinus beat is followed by an APC which is conducted, but results in a striking depression of sinus node activity. A sluggish junctional focus finally awakens after a 4 second pause, and after its discharge neither pacing site returns.

A dramatic and instructive example of the "sick sinus--tachy-brady syndrome." The patient was a 78-year-old man with recurrent syncope. The continuous and lengthy monitor lead was obtained in the ICU, and during its recording he was aware only of "palpitations."

Strip #1- shows coarse atrial fibrillation with a ventricular response averaging 100/min.

Strip #2-shows atrial fibrillation which converts to atrial flutter.

Strip #3-shows atrial flutter, which abruptly stops and a 3.2 second pause is recorded before a slower junctional focus surfaces at 35/min.

Strip #4-an alarm signals the patient's arrhythmia and the slower junctional rhythm persists.

Strip #5-sinus rhythm returns at 60/minute.

Strip #6-aberrrantly conducted APCs accompany the sinus beats.

Strip #7-sinus beats are present, until an APC triggers a return to atrial fibrillation.

Strip #8-the atrial irregularity of atrial fibrillation converts to atrial flutter with a 2:1 conduction ratio in strip #9.

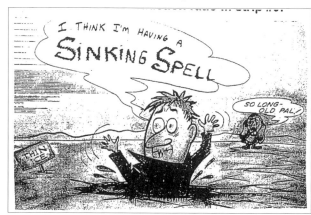

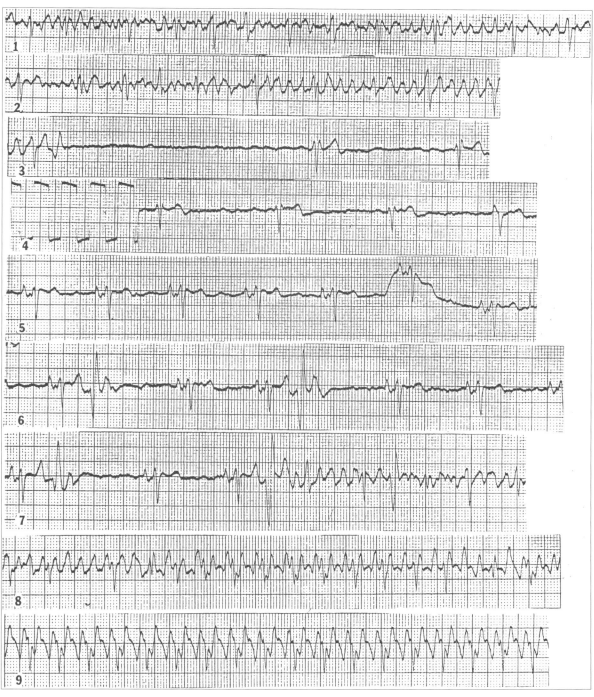

JUNCTIONAL RHYTHMS

Previous terminology was "nodal rhythm," but studies indicated that the AV node lacks pacemaker cells, and the less specific term "junctional rhythm" was substituted. It is generally believed that most pacemaker cells in the AV junction are in the perinodal cells or in the His bundle. A junctional focus may surface if the sinus node falters or fails, the auxiliary focus functioning as an "escape" pacemaker. (rate of 60/min. or less). Conversely, the junctional rate may increase inappropriately (> 60/min.) and assume command of cardiac activation ("usurpation" by an accelerated junctional site). The junctional discharge will activate the ventricle and has the *opportunity* to conduct retrograde to the atria. Accelerated junctional rhythms should always raise suspicion of digitalis toxicity or, in its absence, myocardial ischemia. If the junctional stimulus does conduct retrograde, the location of the retrograde P wave will depend on the relative velocity of conduction of the anterograde and retrograde impulses.

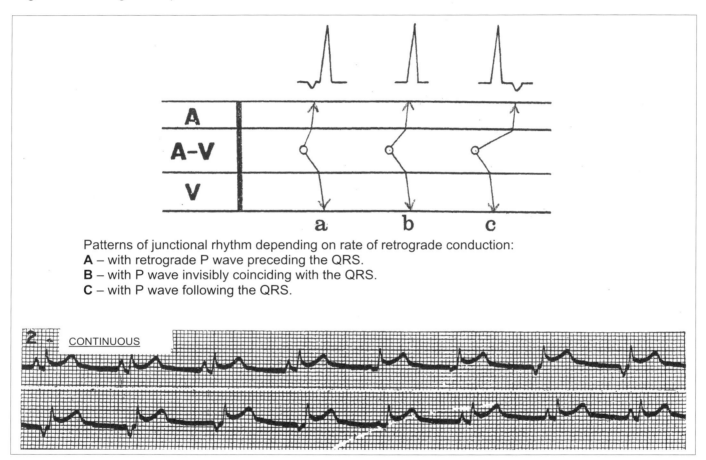

Patterns of junctional rhythm depending on rate of retrograde conduction:
A – with retrograde P wave preceding the QRS.
B – with P wave invisibly coinciding with the QRS.
C – with P wave following the QRS.

Sometimes the pacemaker controlling the heart may shuffle back and forth between sinus node and A-V junction, and then the term *shifting* or *wandering* pacemaker applies. The top strip begins with sinus rhythm; by the end of this strip, the rhythm has changed with junctional retrograde P waves preceding the QRS; by the end of the bottom strip, the sinus has resumed control. The 5th and 6th P waves in the top strip, and the 3rd, 4th, and 5th in the bottom strip are atrial fusion beats.

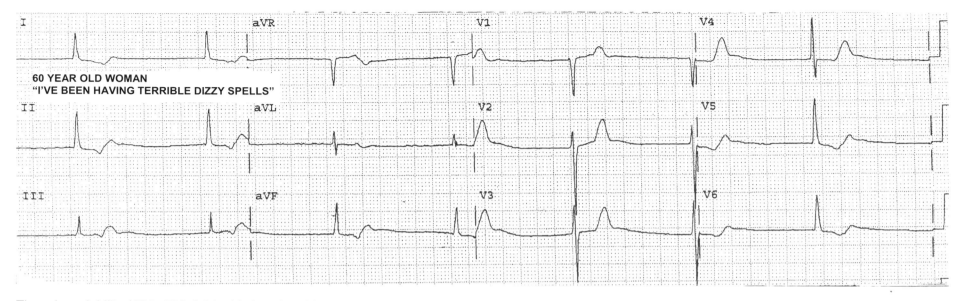

**60 YEAR OLD WOMAN
"I'VE BEEN HAVING TERRIBLE DIZZY SPELLS"**

There is variability (42 to 50/min) in this junctional focus. The slow rate may explain the patient's symptoms, but more likely, they are the result of retrograde atrial conduction. The inappropriate location of the P wave removes any atrial contribution to ventricular filling. Atrial contraction now occurs *during ventricular systole* and the atrial blood flow is sent into the vena cava ("Cannon A waves") and the pulmonary venous circuit. Additionally, the retrograde atrial conduction depolarizes and resets the sinus node. If the sinus impulse is tardy in its recovery, the junctional focus will remain in charge, and the hemodynamic abnormality will persist.

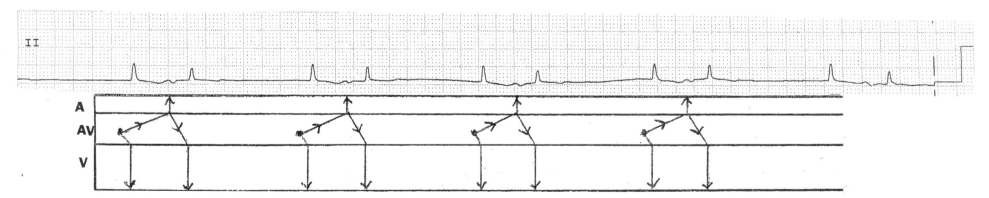

A slow junctional focus is in command, with an unusual twist. They doublets of ventricular complexes, with a P wave sandwiched in between, are termed "reciprocal rhythm." As diagrammed, the junctional stimulus is conducted slowly to the atria and finds a "reflection point," turns around, and returns to ventricle. Although the retrograde impulse discharges the sinoatrial node, it must be seriously depressed to permit the arrhythmias to continue.

185

LEAD II - CONTINUOUS

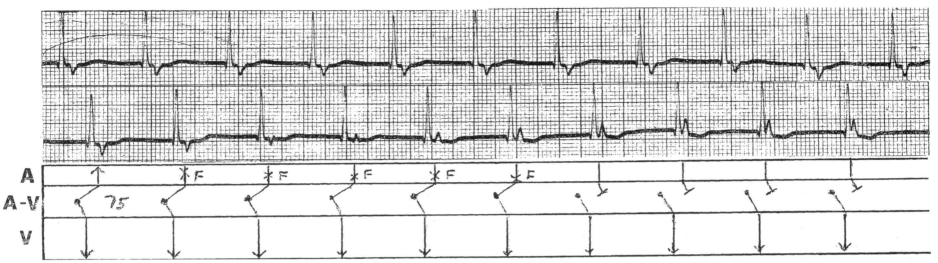

In the top strip, the ventricular rhythm is due to an accelerated junctional focus at 75/min, with 1:1 retrograde conduction to the atria. The lower strip is more interesting. Contrast the first and last complexes. The first shows a retrograde P wave and the last shows return of an upright sinus P wave, living at the end of the junctional QRS complex. There are five atrial fusion complexes (F) occurring when the retrograde and sinus P waves share in atrial activation. The P wave morphology of fusion beats changes when there is more of the sinus impulse contributing.

68 YEAR OLD MAN-DIGOXIN 0.25MG/DAY

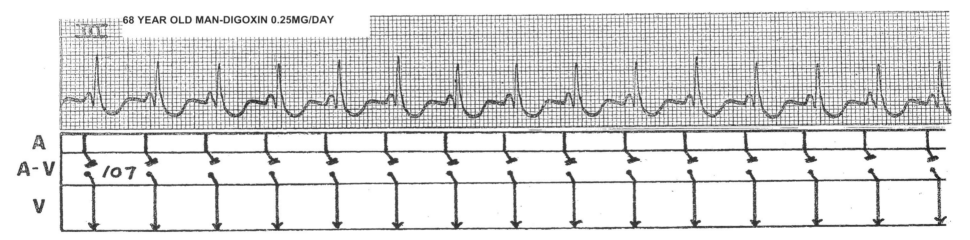

Although the P wave is living in front of the QRS complexes, the short PR interval indicates that it cannot result in ventricular activation. Sinus P waves and an accelerated junctional focus coexist at a rate of 107/min. The coincidental relationship of the two represents what is termed "isochronic dissociation." The junctional pacemaker has been enhanced in rate due to digitalis access.

186

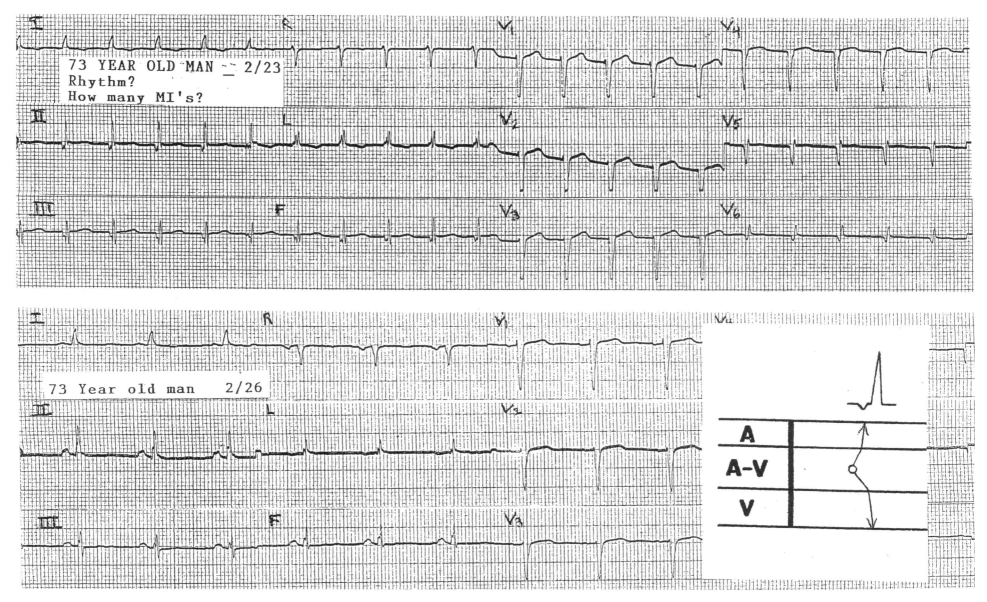

73 YEAR OLD MAN -- 2/23
Rhythm?
How many MI's?

73 Year old man   2/26

Some junctional misbehavior! The "Q waves" evident in leads II, III, and aVF in the upper tracing are not due to inferior wall infarction. They represent retrograde conduction from an accelerated junctional focus, which is inscribing negative P waves at the beginning of the QRS complexes. The features of extensive anterolateral infarction are not altered by the junctional tachycardia. In the lower tracing, after resumption of sinus rhythm, the evidence of inferior wall MI has disappeared. The correct diagnosis could not be made without serial tracings.

SUPRAVENTRICULAR TACHYCARDIAS

Supraventricular tachycardia (SVT) is a common problem plaguing the clinician, particularly the Emergency Department physician. In bygone days, every SVT that was not atrial fibrillation or atrial flutter, was termed "paroxysmal atrial tachycardia" ("PAT"). It is now recognized that the arrhythmia boasts many varieties, and that they may be difficult to differentiate from each other. Currently, atrial tachycardias can be catalogued as due to:
  Disturbed impulse formation (i.e. a rapidly firing focus due to an enhanced automaticity)
      Examples include ectopic atrial tachycardia (uniform or multiform) and accelerated junctional rhythm.
  Disturbed impulse conduction (reentry, reciprocation). Intracardiac recording techniques provide compelling evidence
    that the great majority of SVTs are due to reentry, and not to enhanced impulse formation. Included are: atrial fibrillation, atrial flutter, sinoatrial reentrant tachycardia, AV nodal reentrant tachycardia, and atrioventricular tachycardia utilizing an accessory pathway. By far, the commonest *regular* reentrant SVT is AV nodal reentrant tachycardia.

1. A POTENTIAL CIRCULAR PATHWAY
2. A ZONE OF DEPRESSED CONDUCTION
3. AN AREA OF UNIDIRECTIONAL BLOCK

The features of a reentrant circuit are depicted. Like an auto raceway, only a single *direction* of impulse passage can be permitted. One limb of the circuit must prevent *anterograde* conduction, but permit *retrograde* transmission. There must be an area in which the speed of passages is slowed, to permit recovery of the other limb.

Hemodynamic Considerations

It is important to keep in mind that it is not so much the origin of the tachycardia which determines its seriousness, as it is a number of other variables.
> **1**. Absolute ventricular rate.
> **2**. Relationship between atrial and ventricular contraction.
> **3**. Size of the heart.
> **4**. Presence of additional abnormalities.

Ventricular rate: As rate increases, the time available for diastolic ventricular filling is decreased, compromising stroke volume. At a rate of 60/min., there is approximately 0.6 sec available for diastolic flow into the ventricle; at a rate of 180/min. the time available will be a fraction of that required and may be intolerable, even with a normal heart.

A-V relationships: Atrial contribution to ventricular filling does not occur if there is an inappropriate relationship of P and QRS. Thus, if the P wave follows the QRS, the AV valves are closed, and atrial "kick" is lost because atrial contraction is frustrated by the barrier of unopened AV valves. The pressure generated is reflected into the jugular veins, producing characteristic "cannon A" waves. Loss of atrial contribution is particularly important in patients with a non-compliant ventricle.

Heart size: An enlarged ventricular chamber requires both effective atrial contribution and sufficient time for filling. A tachycardia with dissociated P waves may be disastrous in a patient with ventricular dilatation.

Additional abnormalities: If the tachycardia occurs in the presence of hypovolemia, sepsis, ventricular hypertrophy or acute myocardial infarction tolerance may be sharply reduced.

188

DISTURBED IMPULSE FORMATION

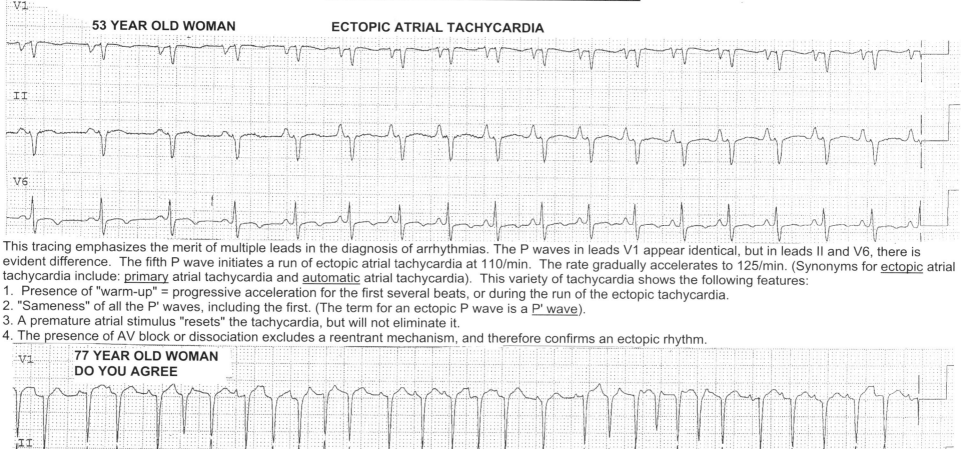

53 YEAR OLD WOMAN   ECTOPIC ATRIAL TACHYCARDIA

This tracing emphasizes the merit of multiple leads in the diagnosis of arrhythmias. The P waves in leads V1 appear identical, but in leads II and V6, there is evident difference. The fifth P wave initiates a run of ectopic atrial tachycardia at 110/min. The rate gradually accelerates to 125/min. (Synonyms for ectopic atrial tachycardia include: primary atrial tachycardia and automatic atrial tachycardia). This variety of tachycardia shows the following features:

1. Presence of "warm-up" = progressive acceleration for the first several beats, or during the run of the ectopic tachycardia.
2. "Sameness" of all the P' waves, including the first. (The term for an ectopic P wave is a P' wave).
3. A premature atrial stimulus "resets" the tachycardia, but will not eliminate it.
4. The presence of AV block or dissociation excludes a reentrant mechanism, and therefore confirms an ectopic rhythm.

77 YEAR OLD WOMAN
DO YOU AGREE

The rhythm strips show multiple, multiform, and irregular P waves, characteristic of multifocal atrial tachycardia. In the "good old days" this warranted the term "chaotic atrial rhythm." There are at least three P wave morphologies and most of the P waves are conducted. The rhythm is most often encountered in patients with serious chronic pulmonary disease. Calcium channel blocker therapy can suppress the ectopic foci.

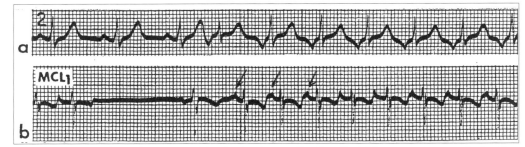

Ectopic atrial tachycardia. In these two examples of supraventricular tachycardia, the first P' wave appears to be the same as the subsequent P' waves, indicating an ectopic, automatic mechanism. In **a**, the first few P'-P' intervals show progressive shortening ("warm-up"). In **b**, the arrows indicate the first few ectopic P' waves.

Atrial tachycardia with block--the block excludes a reentrant mechanism.
A) atrial tachycardia with 2:1 A-V block.
B) atrial tachycardia with mostly 2:1 but varying A-V block.

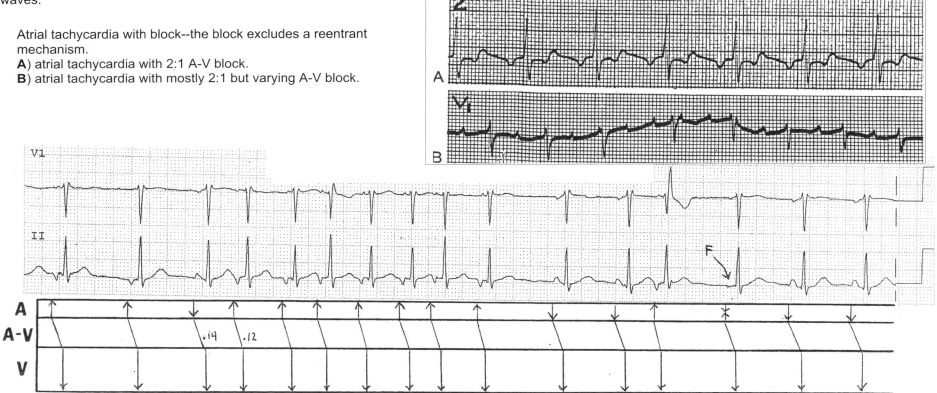

Ectopic atrial stimuli may be single discharge or can "stack up" into bursts of tachycardia. The P' waves frequently lack regularity but their morphology remains constant indicating origin in the same ectopic site. In this example, there are single ectopic beats and a run of an irregular ectopic atrial tachycardia. One premature stimulus is aberrantly conducted with RBBB morphology; another occurs at the same time as the sinus impulse resulting in an atrial fusion complex (**F**). The few sinus beats that are present have a PR interval of 0.14 sec. The ectopic atrial beats have a shorter PR interval because of their proximity to the A-V bridge.

190

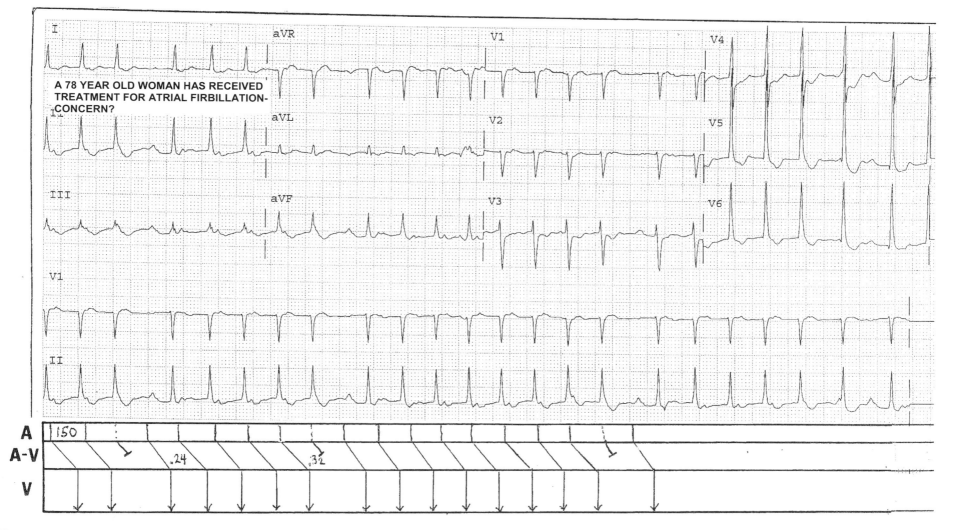

A 78 YEAR OLD WOMAN HAS RECEIVED TREATMENT FOR ATRIAL FIRBILLATION- CONCERN?

The computer interpretation is obviously incorrect, however the previous day she did have atrial fibrillation. She received digitalis to achieve rate control. This tracing shows an atrial tachycardia of 150/min. conducted to the ventricle with variable Wenckebach AV block. For many years it has been known that, with digitalis excess, atrial fibrillation frequently converts to an ectopic atrial tachycardia, often somewhat irregular (such as this example). The suppressive effect of digitalis on the AV node usually results in accompanying AV block. The phenomenon has led to the axiom, "atrial tachycardia with block should be considered due to digitalis toxicity until proven otherwise."

87 YEAR OLD WOMAN
DO YOU ARGREE WITH THE REVIEWER?

NORMAL SINUS RHYTHM FIRST DEGREE BLOCK
LEFT ATRIAL ENLARGEMENT
LEDT AXIS DEVIATION
NON-SPECIFIC INTRA-VENTRICULAR CONDUCTION DELAY
ST&T WAVE ABNORMALITY, CONSIDER LATERAL ISCHEMIA
ABNORMAL ECG
WHEN COMPARED WITH ECG OF 01-AUG 10:04
SINUS RHYTHM HAS REPLACED ATRIAL FIBRILLATION
VENT. RAT HAS INCREASED BY 34 BPM

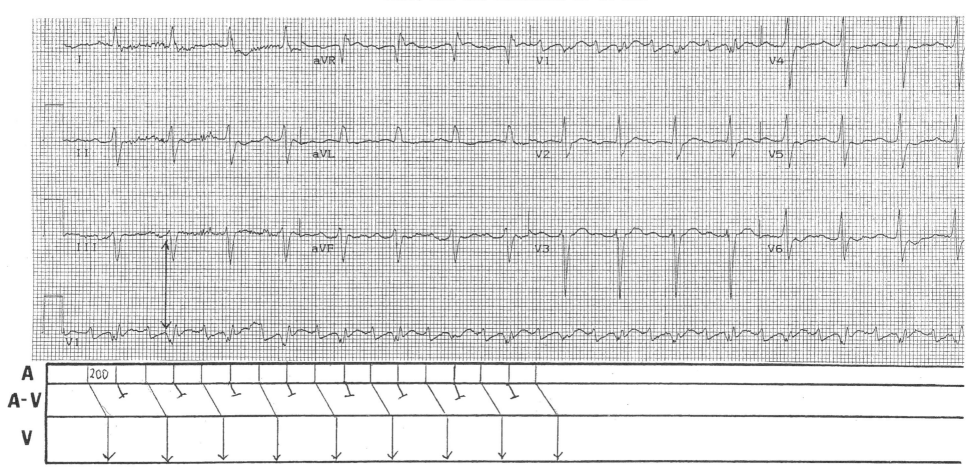

Another example of atrial tachycardia (200/min.) with 2:1 AV conduction due to digitalis excess. Perhaps understandably, the computer has mistaken the rhythm as "normal sinus." The truth is available in the rhythm strip of lead V1. Compare the timing of the QRS onset in lead III and V1 (arrow). Not that the diphasic event are the P waves and the troughs are the QRS complexes. When digitalis was withheld, this threatening arrhythmia disappeared.

192

15 YEAR OLD BOY
"MY HEART RUNS AWAY WHEN I EXERCISE"
MECHANISM OF THE TACHYCARDIA?

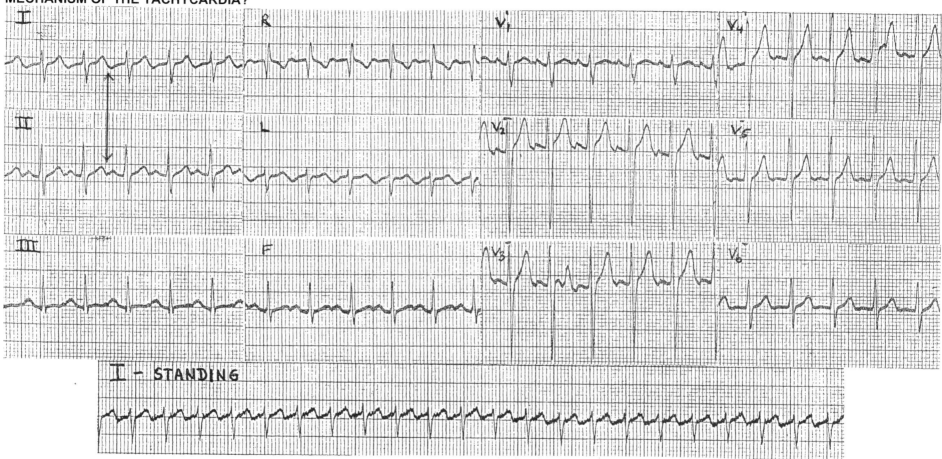

This young lad could not participate in any sport activities because of "heart racing." The P wave in lead II suggests that the rhythm is merely sinus tachycardia at 140/min. However, the negative P waves in lead I provide an alert to his problem. The P wave axis is (+) 120° indicating that the stimulus does not arise in the SA node, but is an ectopic source of impulse formation. Merely standing accelerates the focus to 170/min. Referral to an electro physiologist for possible ablation of the ectopic site would be appropriate.

```
PR      189   +   Possible arrhythmia; review (A-rate = 214, V-rate = 107
QRSD     88   -   Rightward axis
QT      303   -   Nonspecific Lateral region T wave abnormalities [Remains]
QTc     404   -   Probable Inferior injury [Now Present]
--AXES--      -   [Now Absent] Atrial fibrillation with V. response of 73
P        86   -   [Now Absent] Right axis deviation
QRS      97         -ABNORMAL ECG-
```

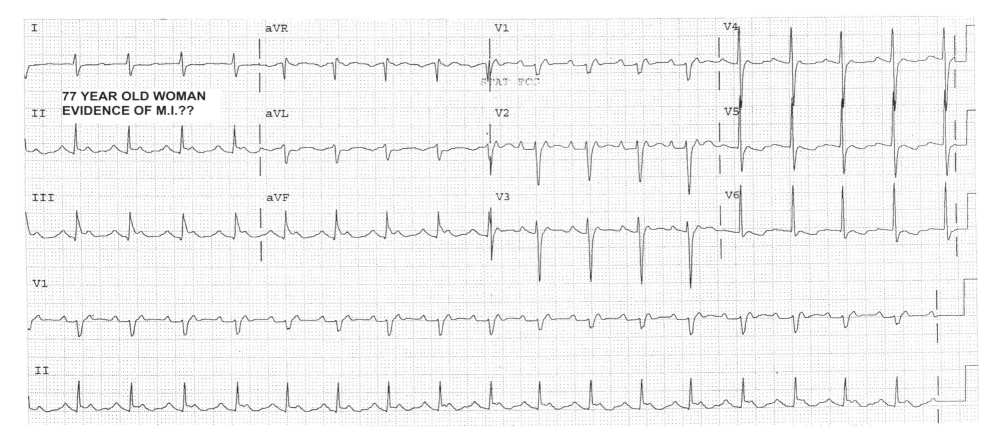

**77 YEAR OLD WOMAN
EVIDENCE OF M.I.??**

The computer makes a half-hearted attempt to diagnose the rhythm, but prompt forgets its observation! There are P waves at 214/min conducted with a 2:1 ratio.
The non-conducted P wave is saddled at the end of the QRS complex and simulates ST segment elevation. The computer misinterprets this as "inferior injury."
This is another example of atrial tachycardia with block due to digitalis excess.

54 YEAR OLD WOMAN -9/91

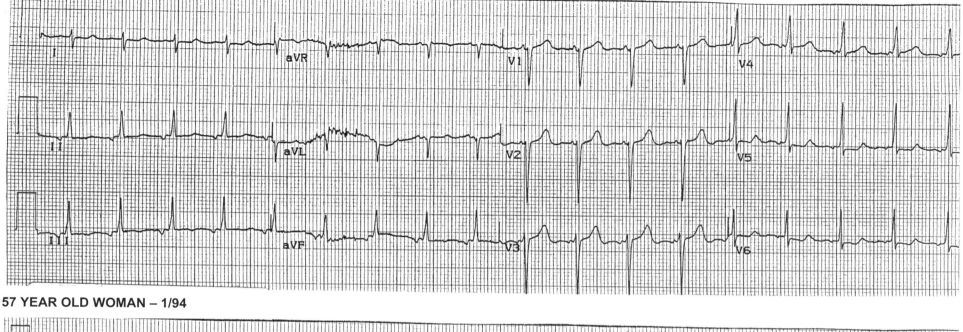

57 YEAR OLD WOMAN – 1/94

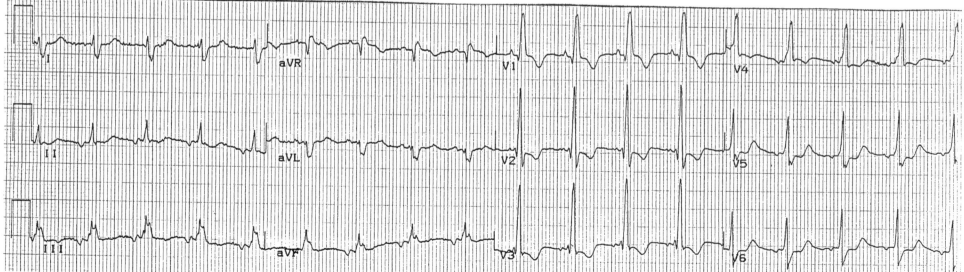

An example of the perils of chronic ectopic tachycardia. In both tracings, the P wave vector is (-) 75°, indicating an abnormal site of atrial (or junctional?) impulse formation at 110/min. The upper tracing is abnormal showing right axis deviation of 100°, probably due to left posterior fascicular block, and widespread repolarization abnormality. Three years later, she presented with congestive heart failure and bifascicular block (RBBB plus LPFB). Although the cardiac rate burden was "only 110/min," the impact of the tachycardia 24 hours a day may lead to "tachycardia-induced cardiomyopathy."

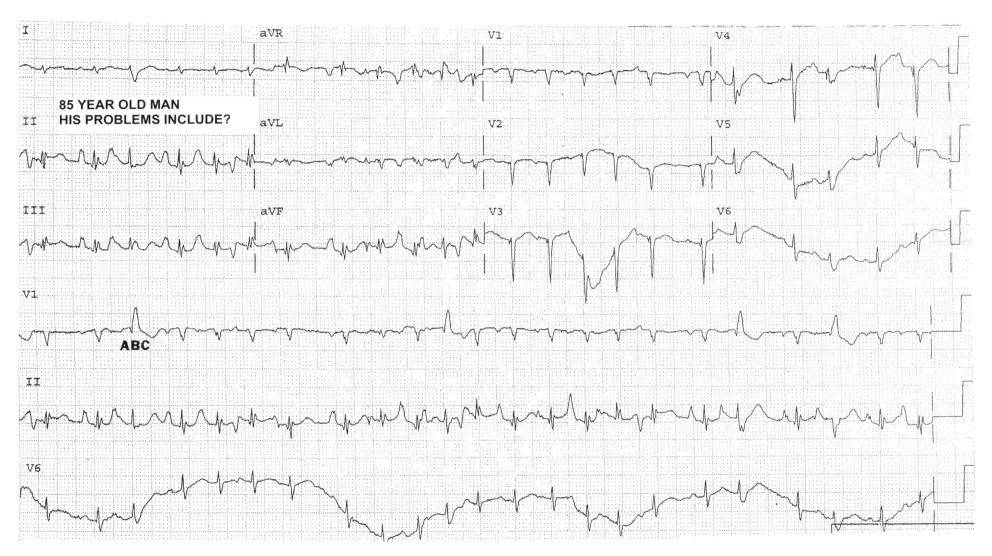

I   aVR   V1   V4

85 YEAR OLD MAN
HIS PROBLEMS INCLUDE?

II   aVL   V2   V5

III   aVF   V3   V6

V1

ABC

II

V6

The tracing is from an elderly man with advanced chronic obstructive pulmonary disease. The respiratory variation ("dyspnea pattern") in the rhythm strip of V6 identifies the patient's discomfort. The frontal plane axis is (+) 90°--right axis deviation for age 85. The lack of R waves in V1-3 may indicate an anterior M.I., but could be due to cardiac displacement with the depressed diaphragms. The multiple morphologies of the P waves and the irregularity of the R-R cycle indicate that the rhythm is *multifocal atrial tachycardia*. Four of APCs are aberrantly conducted with a pattern of right bundle branch block. The arrhythmia reflects the marked changes present with serious lung disease (hypoxia, hypercarbia, and atrial wall stretch) and medications in use (beta agonists and theophylline).

DISTURBED IMPULSE CONDUCTION

ATRIAL FIBRILLATION

Atrial fibrillation (AF) was originally called "delirium of the heart" (*delirium cordis*) because the atrial behavior was erratic. It is the commonest of the atrial tachycardias in adults and goes hand-in-hand with congestive heart failure. AF is recognized in the EKG by the absence of regularly formed P waves, the uneven rippling baseline due to fibrillatory waves ("**ff**"), and chaotic irregularity of the ventricular response. For descriptive purposes, the fibrillation can be characterized as coarse, medium, or fine. The number of stimuli present in the AF is impossible to define, but most often exceeds 400/min. It is often precipitated by a critically timed premature atrial stimulus, as shown in the example below.

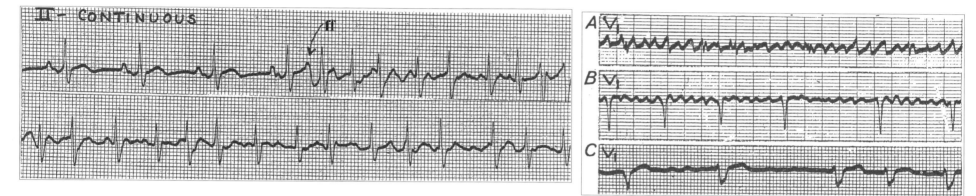

Just as the ventricles have a "vulnerable period," there is a point in the atrial cycle in which an APC is likely to precipitate an atrial tachycardia. Dr. Thomas Killip has formulated the situation as follows: if a P-P' interval (i.e. the interval from the preceding P wave to the premature P' wave) is <u>less than one half</u> the preceding P-P interval, it is likely to land in the atrial vulnerable period and initiate atrial fibrillation.

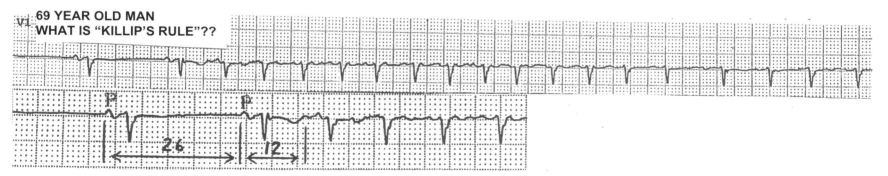

In the enlarged segment, the sinus cycle (P-P) measures 26 mm. The rhythm is interrupted by an APC occurring at less than half this cycle (12 mm), and atrial fibrillation results.

The initiating APC may arise in either atrium. Interestingly, evidence indicates that in many patients, the precipitating stimulus arises in one of the pulmonary veins at the left atrial junction. The mechanism of atrial fibrillation appears to be a myriad of "microreentry" circuits in the atrium. Ventricular transmission of the numerous fibrillatory impulses is modulated by the AV node and, obviously, can range from many to few. The faster the ventricular rate, the less easy it is to recognize the QRS irregularity, and the less the opportunity to identify the typical baseline oscillations. The ventricular response to atrial fibrillation is variable. If the AV junction is normal and unhampered by digitalis, beta-blocker, or calcium antagonist, rates of 200/min. frequently develop. On the other hand, if the AV node is diseased or suppressed by drugs, the ventricular response may be markedly reduced.

Atrial fibrillation from 4 different patients.
A) With rapid ventricular response
(rate about 180 beats/min.)
B) With moderate ventricular response
(rate about 70 beats/min.)
C) With slow ventricular response
(rate about 50 beats/min.)
D) With regular, independent escape
pacemaker at 43/min.

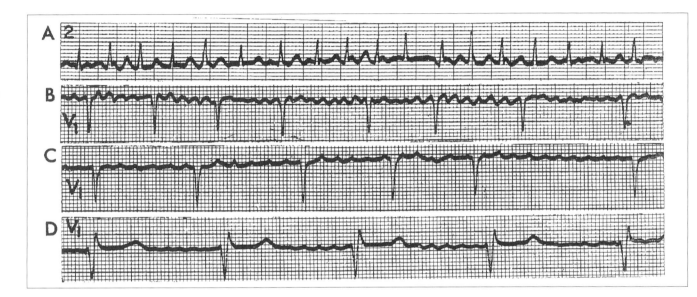

The irregularity of the ventricular response to atrial fibrillation is the result of incomplete transmission ("concealed conduction") of some of the innumerable atrial impulses. Although not conducted to the ventricle, these impulses establish a refractory wake in the AV junction. This wake results in blocking of one or more of subsequent stimuli and insures irregular delivery.

If there is characteristic fibrillatory baseline in the presence of a regular ventricular rhythm, it is proof that the ventricles are responding to an independent pacemaker, and not to the fibrillating atrium. This combination of findings should always prompt suspicion of digitalis intoxication.

198

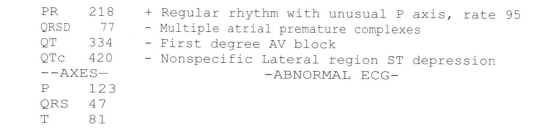

```
PR    218    + Regular rhythm with unusual P axis, rate 95
QRSD   77    - Multiple atrial premature complexes
QT    334    - First degree AV block
QTc   420    - Nonspecific Lateral region ST depression
--AXES—              -ABNORMAL ECG-
P     123
QRS    47
T      81
```

85 YEAR OLD WOMAN
COMPUTER CRAZINESS??

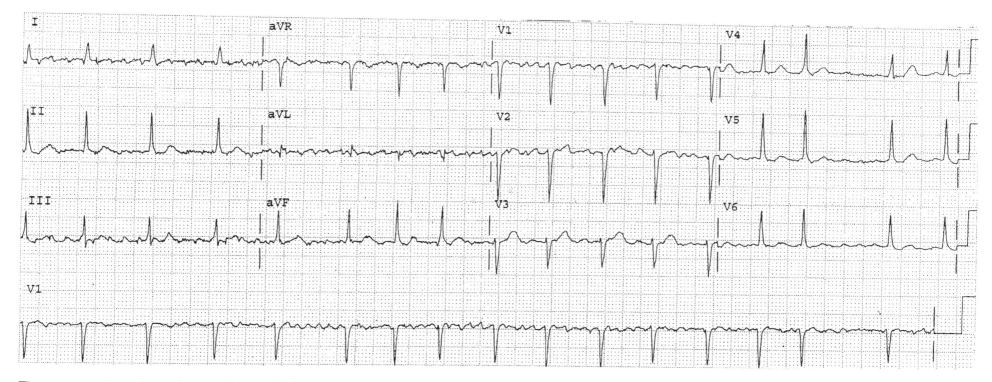

The computer has missed the baseline and R-R cycle irregularity characteristic of atrial fibrillation, and its analysis of the rhythm is way off base!

ATRIAL FLUTTER

Atrial flutter trails behind atrial fibrillation in the frequency of occurrence. Like AF, the arrhythmic mechanism is <u>reentry</u>, but instead of "micro-reentry" it involves a "*macro reentry*" circuit in the right atrium. (Figure). The size of this raceway permits generation of 300 atrial stimuli/min. (usual cited range = 250 to 350/min.). Obviously, it would be imprudent to conduct all of these impulses and a frequent presentation is a transmitted ratio of 2:1. The observation of a regular tachycardia at or near 150/min. has led to the "150 rule," which states: if the ventricular rate is regular at, or near, 150/min. <u>consider</u> atrial flutter with 2:1 conduction. If the patient has associated AV block or after drug treatment, the ratio can be usually 4:1, resulting in a normal ventricular rate of 75/minute.

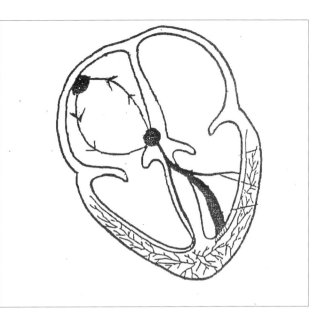

The diagnosis of atrial flutter may be obvious at a glance if typical flutter ("FF") waves are visible. They have a "saw- tooth" appearance in leads II, III, and aVF; but in the precordial leads they have the appearance of "P-like" waves. The difficulty of recognizing 2:1 atrial flutter stems from the fact that, at an AV conduction ratio of 2:1, every alternate atrial wave is inevitably entangled with or distorted by some part of the ventricular events, and may be obscured thereby. It is important to scrutinize all 12 leads, because 2:1 atrial activity may be obvious in only one lead and be obscured in all the others.

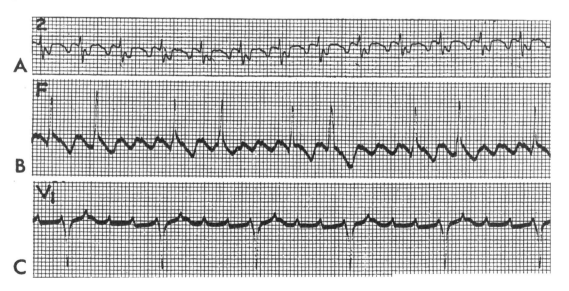

Atrial flutter from 3 different patients, with atrial rates between 250 and 290 beats/minute. **A**: with 2:1 AV conduction. **B**: with alternating 2:1 and 4:1 conduction. **C**: with 4:1 conduction.

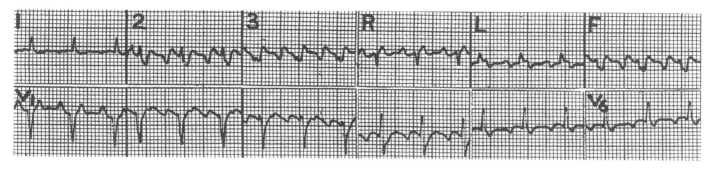

A 12 lead display of atrial flutter with 2:1 AV conduction; the atrial rate is about 275 beats/min. Note the P-like waves in the chest leads, positive V1, negative in V6; and the absence of diagnostic atrial activity in lead I. Usually, the best leads for diagnosing atrial flutter are the "inferior leads" II, III, and aVF.

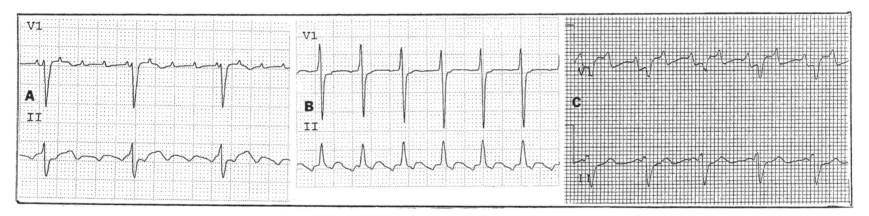

A contrast of simultaneous leads V1 and II to establish "which one is the best" in the diagnosis of atrial flutter.
A = A 76 year old woman. Flutter waves are evident in both leads.
B = A 63 year-old man. The "saw teeth" flutter waves in lead II are not seen in lead V1.
C = An 89 year-old woman with "slow flutter" at 200/min. present in V1 but missing in lead II.
The point is obvious. An arrhythmia may be identified in some leads and not appear in others. _Single "rhythm strips" often do not permit the correct conclusion regarding an arrhythmia_.

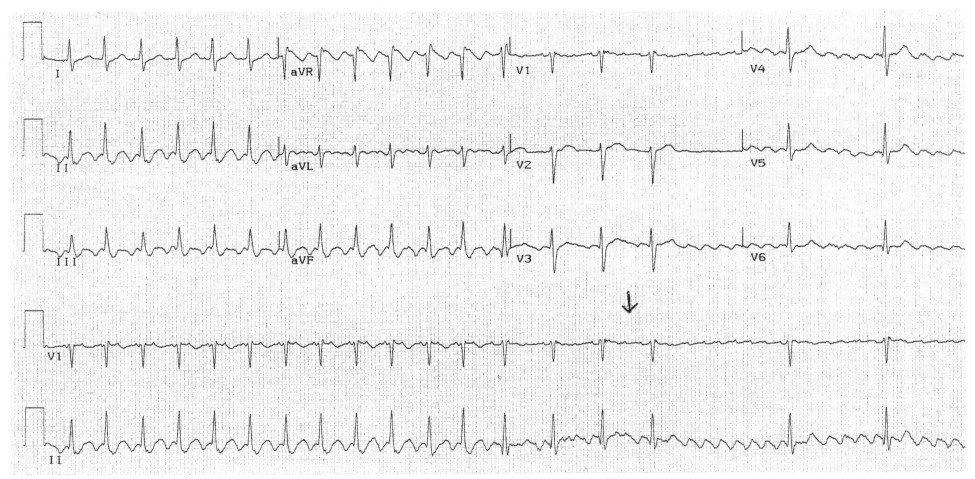

The rhythm strips of leads V1 and II show fairly convincing evidence of atrial flutter with 2:1 A-V conduction. To prove the issue, carotid sinus massage was performed at the arrow. The vagatonic influence on the AV node "blocked" numerous flutter waves, revealing the typical "saw tooth" pattern of the atrial arrhythmia.

- Supraventricular bygeminy. Mean V-rate = 89
- First degree AV block
- Left axis deviation
- Borderline intraventricular conduction delay
- Consider left atrial enlargement
- Poor R-wave progression   -ABNORMAL ECG-

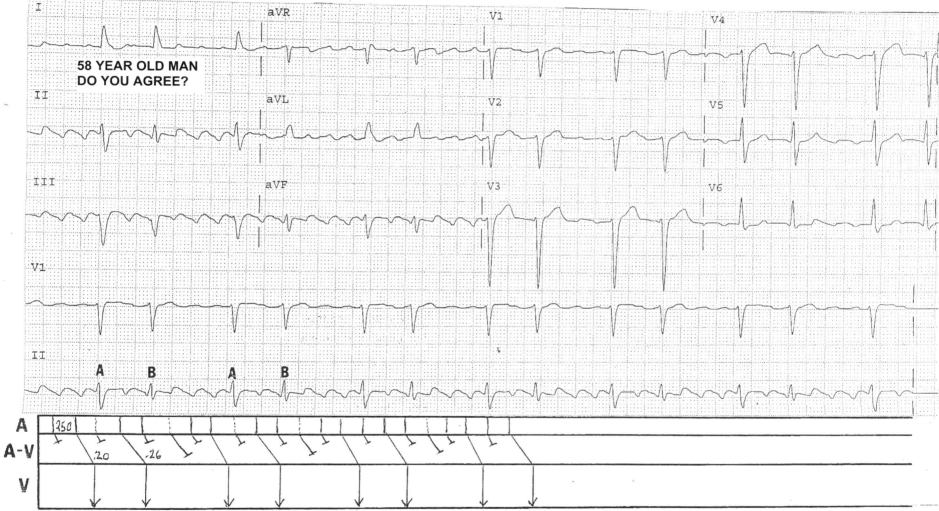

**58 YEAR OLD MAN
DO YOU AGREE?**

Another example of atrial flutter with variable A-V conduction. Alternate F waves are "blocked" and the conductible ones are transmitted with prolonging A-V nodal delay (Wenckebach block). The conduction ratio is usually termed 2:1, 4:1, 2:1, etc. The changing relationship of the flutter waves to the ventricular depolarization can result in interesting changes in QRS morphology. If the trough of a flutter wave coincides with the QRS complex, it can increase the apparent depth of the S wave. Contrast morphology A vs. B and the apparent "alternation." The increased "S waves" in complex A is due to superimposed negative flutter waves at the end of the QRS complex.

203

**83 YEAR OLD MAN-12/5
HOW MANY
OBSERVATIONS??
WHAT IS "BIX'S RULE?"**

PR		+	Tachycardia, ? origin, rate 139
QRSD	142	-	Left anterior fascicular block and nonspecific intraventricular conduction delay
QT	345	-	Prominent anterior forces with ST-T negative (?RVH or old posterior MI)
Tc	525	-	Anterolateral region infarct, age indeterminate
--AXES--		-	Inferior ST elevation
P			- ABNORMAL ECG -
QRS	-74	*	Supraventricular Tachycardia

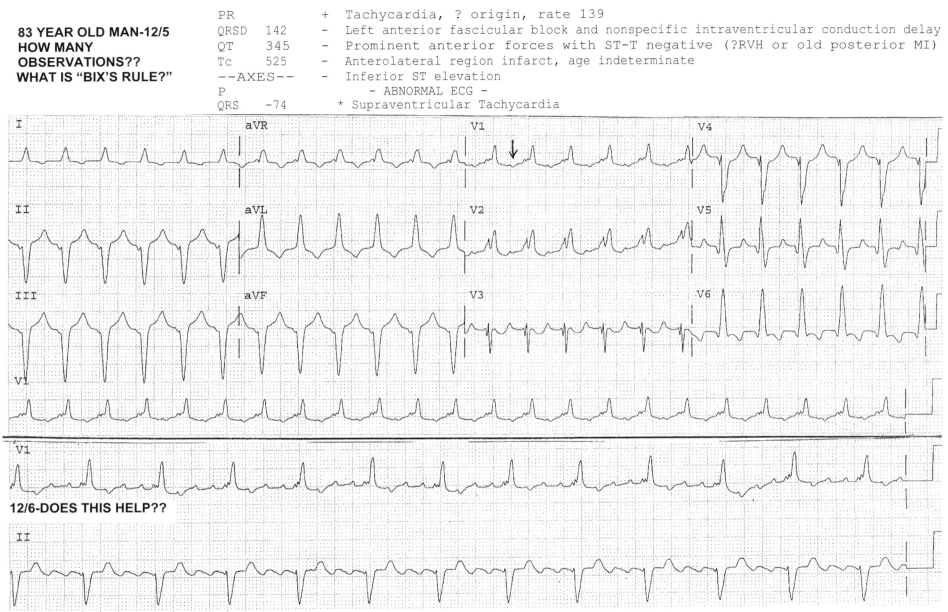

12/6-DOES THIS HELP??

The QRS duration is increased consistent with RBBB. The pre-block axis is (-) 75°, with Q waves in leads II, III, and aVF consistent with inferior MI of uncertain age (? acute). The Q waves in V3-V6 indicate lateral wall involvement in the infarction. The repolarization time -QT interval- is significantly prolonged. Dr. Harold Bix made the observation that an apparent P wave saddled halfway between the QRS complexes (arrow) often signals the presence of another hiding P wave. The ventricular rate of 150/min. suggests that the atrial mechanism is flutter with 2:1 conduction. The bottom strips show evident flutter and prove that Bix's observation was correct.

204

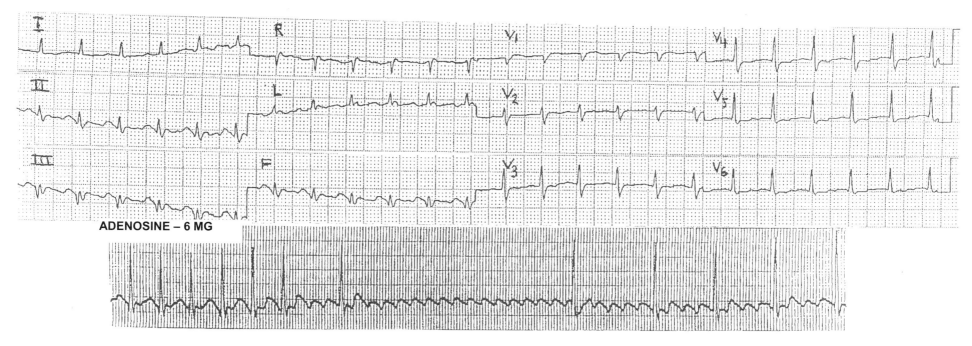

ADENOSINE – 6 MG

This instructive tracing will either tickle your fancy, or fire your ire. This 77-year-old man had sustained an inferior wall infarction in the past. He presented with ischemic infarction of the bowel, necessitating surgery, and made difficult because of his morbid obesity (340 lbs.). Postoperatively, he developed sepsis and this EKG was obtained looking for a cardiac cause for hypotension. The rhythm appears to be sinus tachycardia at 140/minute. There is low QRS voltage, evidence of prior inferior infarction, and intraventricular conduction delay. Because the heart rate had persisted *unchanged at 140* for several hours and was unresponsive to carotid sinus massage, it was thought that it might represent other than "simple sinus tachycardia." IV adenosine was given and the result provided proof that the rhythm was atrial flutter with 2:1 conduction. He was cardioverted and his blood-pressure normalized. EMPHASIS: *Sinus tachycardia does not remain unchanged for lengthy periods. When a rate appears "locked in" consider an underlying arrhythmia.*

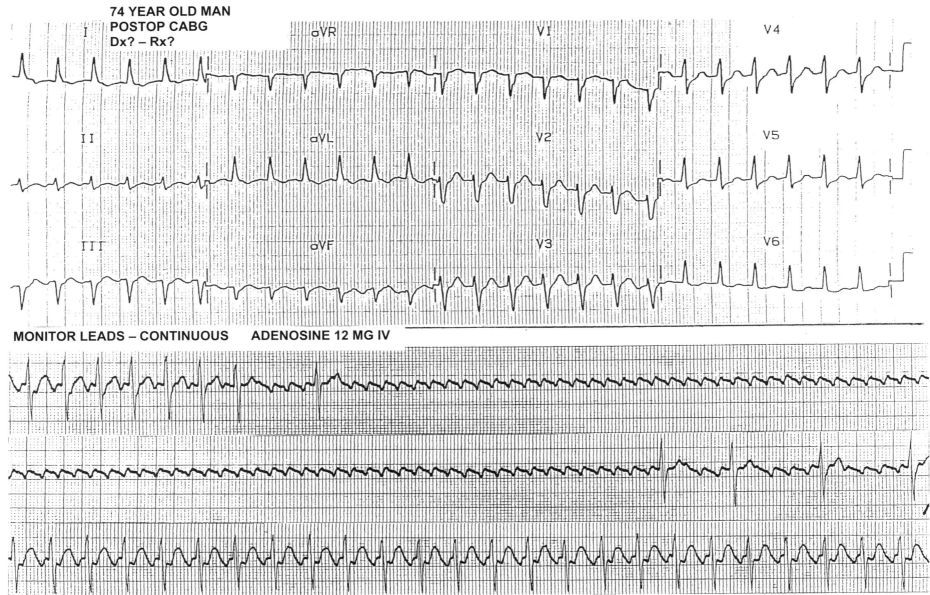

74 YEAR OLD MAN
POSTOP CABG
Dx? – Rx?

I aVR V1 V4

II aVL V2 V5

III aVF V3 V6

MONITOR LEADS – CONTINUOUS   ADENOSINE 12 MG IV

Postoperative tachycardia, persisting at 150/min., raised concern that the rhythm was atrial flutter with 2:1 conduction. Since the diagnosis was not conclusive, an A-V nodal blocking drug--adenosine--was given. The result is obvious, but undesirable. Atrial flutter was proven, but the blocking effect of the drug continued for a remarkably long interval. The result was ventricular asystole for 13.5 sec. and syncope. Message: Adenosine is a very effective drug, but the older patient often is intolerant of large doses. Small IV doses are frequently effective and, when needed, incremental amounts can be given to prevent this "therapeutic misadventure."

A-V NODAL REENTRANT TACHYCARDIA

AV nodal reentrant tachycardia (AVNRT) is third in frequency of occurrence, well behind atrial fibrillation and atrial flutter. However, emergency departments are visited by many symptomatic patients yearly with this arrhythmia. Unlike individual with the more common arrhythmias, often, these patients have no underlying heart disease. Early electrophysiologic studies demonstrated that many individuals have "dual AV nodal pathways"--electrically, but not anatomically definable. The presumption was that the pathways resided in the AV node, hence the name of the arrhythmia. Evidence now indicates that the "dual pathways" are usually *extranodal*. However, let's use the diagram below to describe the circuitry of this very common variety of SVT. It has been established that the pathways have different electrical properties. One has a more rapid <u>conduction velocity</u> (termed the "beta pathway"); the other a slower transmission (the "alpha pathway"). Interestingly and importantly, the fast (beta) path has a longer <u>refractory period</u> than the slow alpha limb.

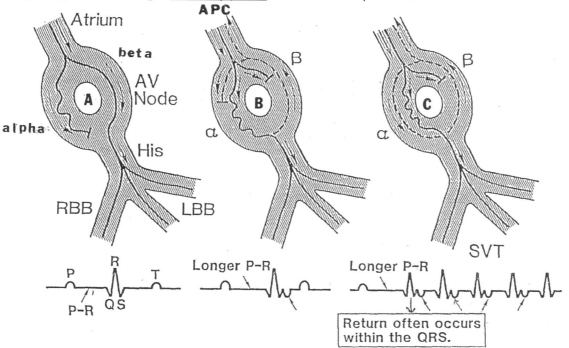

In the illustration, the slow (alpha) and fast (beta) limbs of the "dual AV nodal pathways" are depicted.

In **segment (A):** a sinus node impulse finds the beta path available and is conducted rapidly to the ventricle, with a normal PR interval and a single ventricular response. Impulse transmission over the alpha limb is slower and it arrives at the His bundle to find it refractory.

In **segment (B):** because of its longer refractory period, a premature atrial impulse (APC) blocks in the fast path. It conducts over the slow pathway, with a long PR interval resulting. Since the beta limb was not "used" it is available for retrograde conduction to the atrium. This results in a negative P wave which is either buried in the QRS complex or appears in its shadow (arrow).

In **segment (C):** the reentrant tachycardia becomes established, with the antegrade limb the slow path, and the retrograde limb the fast. Thus, typical AVNRT is "slow--fast" in its conduction. The retrograde P waves may be lost in the QRS complex, but often they appear as a late contribution to the QRS--as so-called "pseudo s waves."

The ladder diagram depicts the onset and circuitry of A-V nodal reentrant tachycardia. Despite the availability of "dual AV nodal pathways," an atrial premature complex (APC), to initiate the tachycardia, must occur at the proper time. This is termed the "echo-zone" (EZ). When the APC occurs later (**A**), it will conduct with a single of ventricular response. When earlier (**C**), it will encounter A-V nodal refractoriness and be blocked. When the APC lands in the EZ, it will encounter the differing refractory periods of the dual pathways and begin the reentrant circuit. The result is cycling anterograde slow, retrograde fast--typical AVNRT.

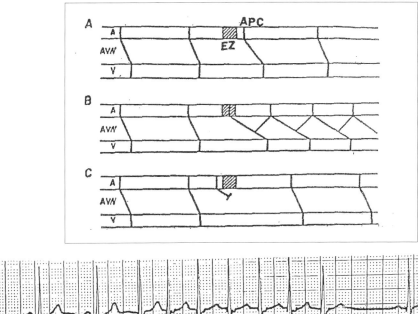

26 YEAR OLD WOMAN-"PALPITATIONS"
WHY DO THE SALVOS OF SVT START AND STOP?

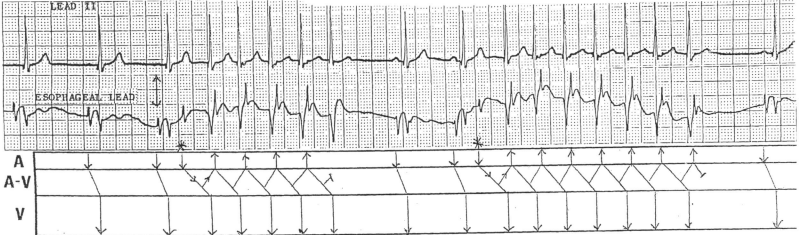

In bygone days, puzzling arrhythmias were often studied utilizing an "esophageal lead." An electrode was advanced, like a nasogastric tube, and placed in the mid-esophagus behind the left atrium. In this position, it could record atrial potential. The P waves in the E-lead were often evident, and not seen in the standard EKG leads. The top tracing of lead II would be frustrating and probably not permit a complete analysis. The E-lead, however, clarifies the rhythm. The salvos of SVT are due to AV nodal reentrant tachycardia. After three sinus beats, an APC (*) is conducted over the slow pathway and initiates an anterograde slow-retrograde fast tachycardia as diagrammed. The burst stops when the impulse blocks in the <u>retrograde</u> path. After a pause, there are two sinus beats, followed by another APC and another run of "slow--fast" tachycardia. This time, the circuit is interrupted when the signal blocks in the <u>anterograde</u> limb. An evident conclusion is that both slow and fast pathways are vulnerable. If an impulse blocks in either one the tachycardia will cease.

For any circulating wave to perpetuate itself, the advancing head (arrow) must not catch up with refractory tail. Thus, there must always be an "excitable gap" of non-refractory tissue between the head and tail of the reentrant wave. If an extraneous impulse such as a premature systole manages to find the excitable gap between the head and tail, it will render it refractory and the circulating wave will be halted. Similarly, if the refractory wake can be prolonged (vagatonic effect or drugs), the head of the advancing circuit will encounter the refractory zone and it will be extinguished.

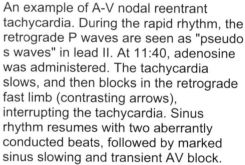

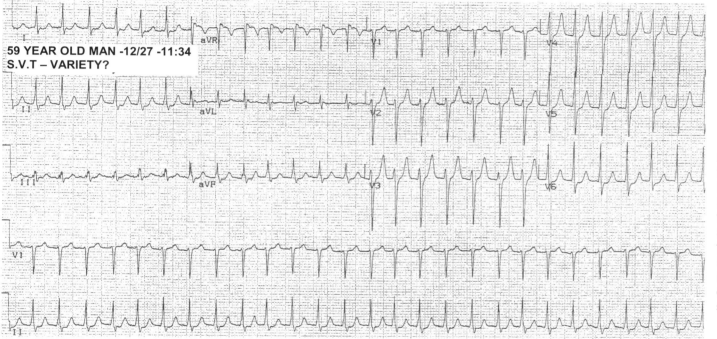

59 YEAR OLD MAN -12/27 -11:34
S.V.T – VARIETY?

An example of A-V nodal reentrant tachycardia. During the rapid rhythm, the retrograde P waves are seen as "pseudo s waves" in lead II. At 11:40, adenosine was administered. The tachycardia slows, and then blocks in the retrograde fast limb (contrasting arrows), interrupting the tachycardia. Sinus rhythm resumes with two aberrantly conducted beats, followed by marked sinus slowing and transient AV block.

12/27 – 11:40

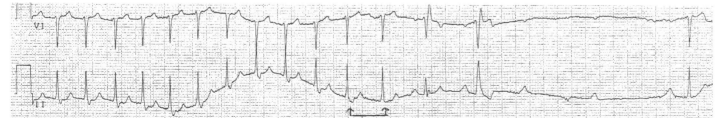

209

77 YEAR OLD MAN -1/14 – 01:02
S.V.T – WHAT VARIETY??
BAD TIME TO HAVE S.V.T??

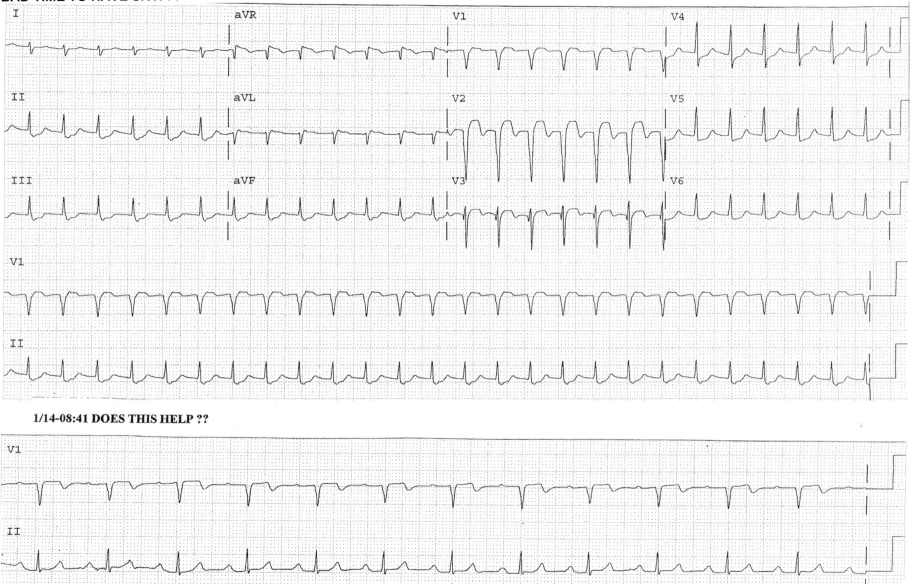

1/14-08:41 DOES THIS HELP ??

The timing of this typical AV nodal reentrant tachycardia of 160/min. is unfortunate since it is occurring in the throes of acute anterior myocardial infarction. The post-conversion tracing confirms the AVNRT, with loss of the "pseudo s" in lead II and the "pseudo r'" in lead V1, reflecting the retrograde P waves present during the tachycardia and due to the retrograde P waves.

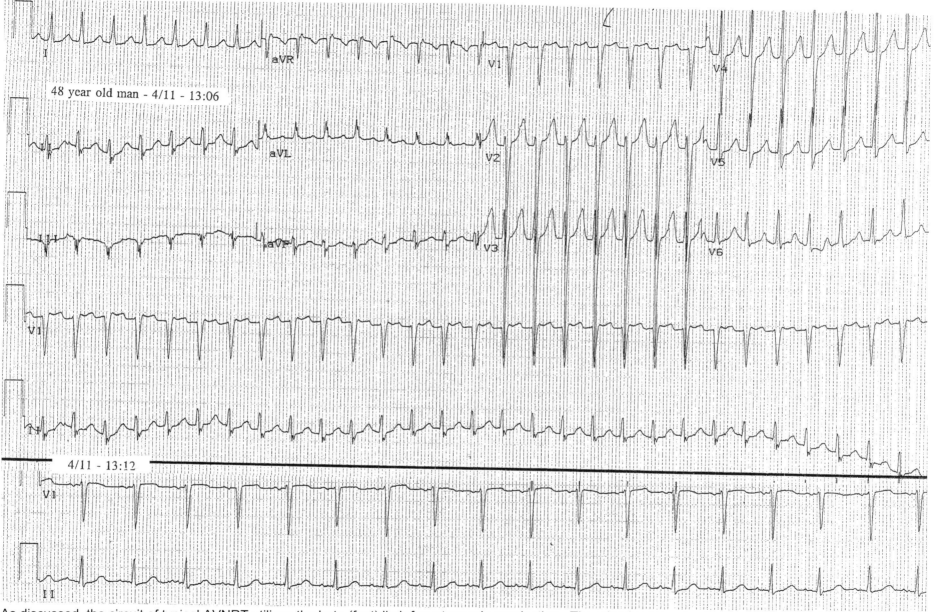

As discussed, the circuit of typical AVNRT utilizes the beta (fast) limb for retrograde conduction. The stimulus returning to the atria is often inscribed as a retrograde P' wave at the end of the QRS complex in the frontal plane. It is seen as a "pseudo s wave" in leads II, III, and aVF. In the horizontal plane, the retrograde P' has an anterior tilt and can be recorded as a terminal <u>positive</u> wave in V1 and seen as a terminal r'. In this example, contrast the QRS of leads II and V1 during the SVT and after conversion. The pseudo s wave in lead II and pseudo r' in V1 which are present during the tachycardia disappear during sinus rhythm, establishing the diagnosis as AVNRT.

Observations include: SVT of 150/min., low-voltage QRS complexes in the limb leads, and inferior and anterior myocardial infarctions, likely acute. The most common causes of R' morphology in lead V1 include delayed RV activation (incomplete RBBB) and excess right ventricular forces (RVH). Neither is the cause in this EKG. The rhythm turned out to be AV nodal reentrant tachycardia and the prominent terminal R' is the retrograde P. Note the V1 morphology after conversion--a real fooler!

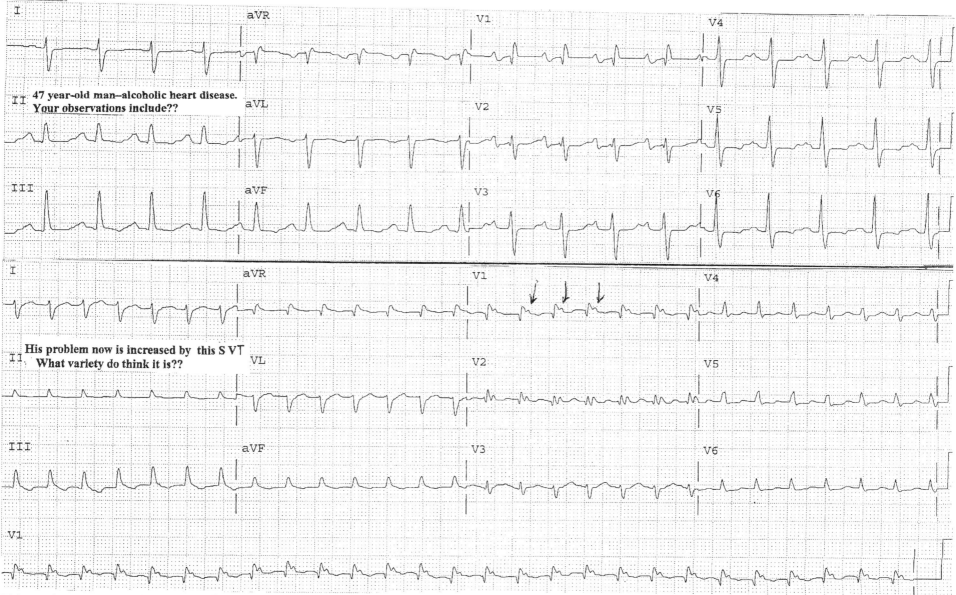

I aVR V1 V4

47 year-old man--alcoholic heart disease.
II **Your observations include??** aVL V2 V5

III aVF V3 V6

I aVR V1 V4

His problem now is increased by this S VT
II **What variety do think it is??** VL V2 V5

III aVF V3 V6

V1

This tragic young man drank himself into an alcoholic cardiomyopathy with profound right and left ventricular "failure." The top tracing displays: biatrial abnormality, increased PR interval, right axis deviation, prominent R' in V1--consistent with RVH (vs. incomplete RBBB + LPFB), and a markedly long QT interval. In the bottom tracing, some months later, the tachycardia is due to an AV nodal reentrant circuit. Note the retrograde P waves in lead V1 (arrows). Imagine the impact of this rhythm on a heart already severely damaged! The significant decrease in QRS voltage is probably due to progressive loss of myocytes before he died.

213

79 YEAR OLD MAN
THIS SVT IS AN EXAMPLE OF --?

```
PR     70     +  Tachycardia of undetermined origin, rate 133
QRSD   104    -  Extensive Anterior infarct, age indeterminate
QT     285    -ABNORMAL ECG-
QTc    424
```

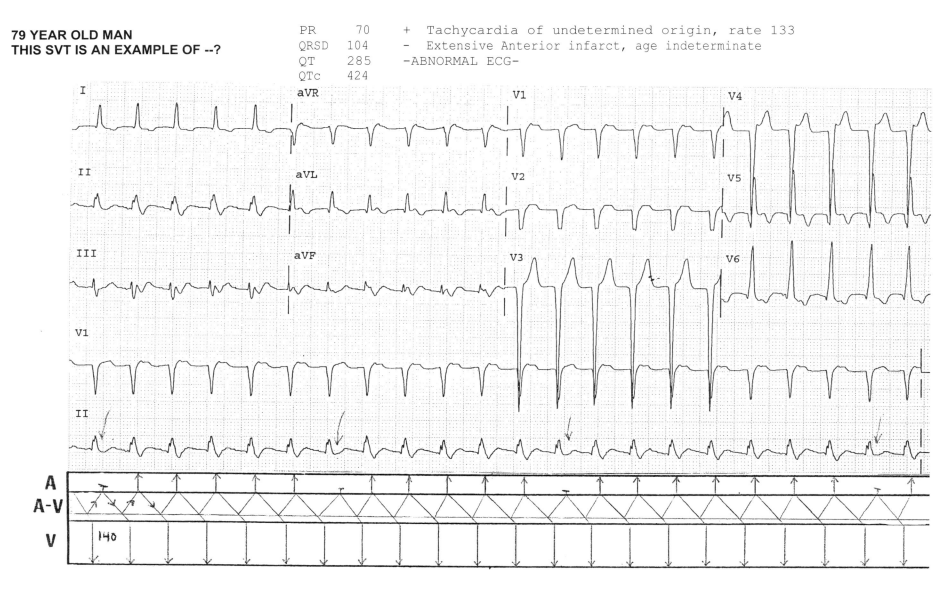

Note the morphology difference in the QRS complexes in the rhythm strip--therein lies the key to the answer. Note that some (arrows) do not show the wide terminal troughs seen in the rest, indicating that this portion of the QRS is really a retrograde P wave. The ladder diagram depicts that reentrant circuit responsible for this SVT. Since the tachycardia is able to continue without consistent atrial participation, it <u>cannot</u> be due to an ectopic (automatic) atrial focus. Similarly, it cannot be reentry utilizing an accessory pathway (A-V reentry) since this requires participation by both atrium and ventricle to continue. Thus, this must be SVT due to *AV nodal reentry*. The 12 lead tracing shows that this arrhythmia is occurring during an acute anterolateral myocardial infarction, which is not the best time to have a heart rate of 140/min.!

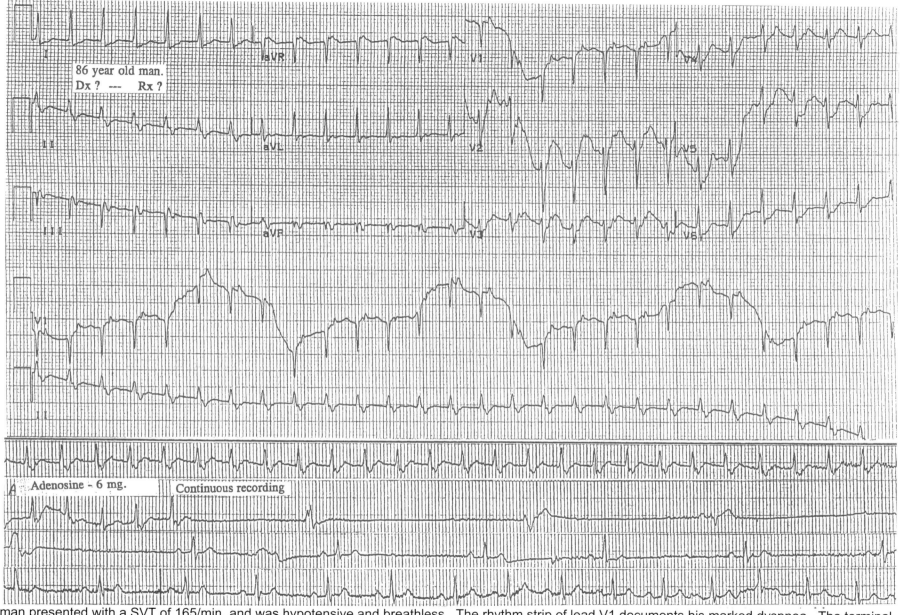

86 year old man.
Dx ? --- Rx ?

Adenosine - 6 mg.

Continuous recording

This man presented with a SVT of 165/min. and was hypotensive and breathless. The rhythm strip of lead V1 documents his marked dyspnea. The terminal negative deflection in leads II, III, and aVF. and the r' in V1 indicates that the arrhythmia is probably AVNRT. In treatment, 6 mg of adenosine was given IV. The rhythm promptly converts, but there is lengthy atrial "standstill" requiring a ventricular escape focus to surface. Gradually, sinus node activity resumes. The QRS morphology in the bottom strip shows that the "pseudo s" and "pseudo r' " waves are no longer present, proving the diagnosis. Although the recommended dose of adenosine is 6 mg, it clearly was too much for this elderly man.

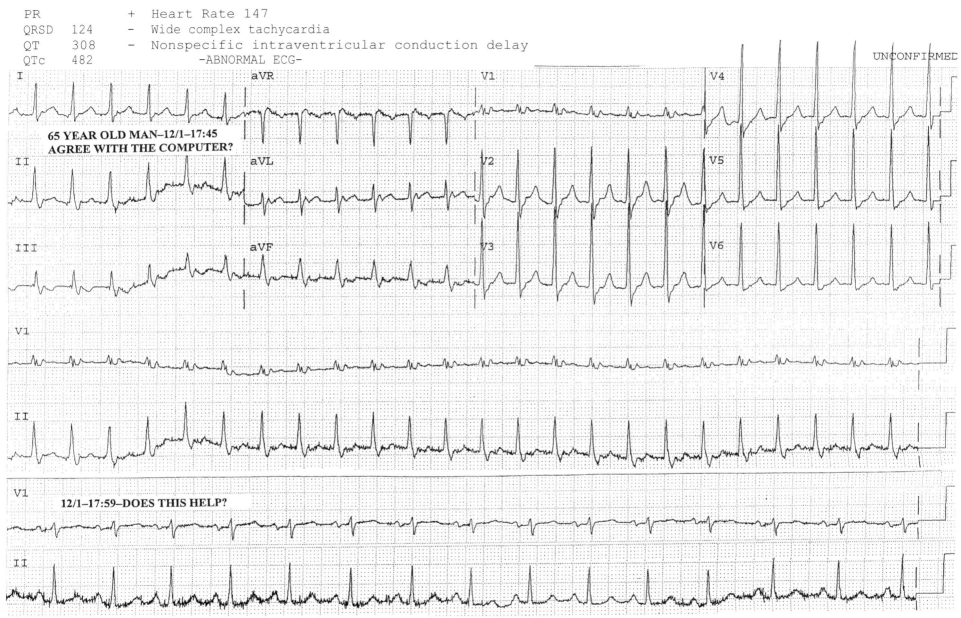

PR   +   Heart Rate 147
QRSD   124   -   Wide complex tachycardia
QT   308   -   Nonspecific intraventricular conduction delay
QTc   482   -ABNORMAL ECG-   UNCONFIRMED

I   aVR   V1   V4

**65 YEAR OLD MAN–12/1–17:45
AGREE WITH THE COMPUTER?**

II   aVL   V2   V5

III   aVF   V3   V6

V1

II

V1

12/1–17:59–DOES THIS HELP?

II

The tachycardia is due to a typical AV nodal reentrant mechanism. Note the prominent "pseudo-s waves" in leads II, III and aVF; and the "pseudo-r wave" in V1. The bottom strips show that these are absent during sinus rhythm. The computer has misinterpreted the combination of the initial R + the pseudo-r' as a "wide complex," but assigns the causes to a "nonspecific IVCD." The early transition and broad R waves in V1-V3 point to a posterior infarct-age uncertain.

216

81 YEAR OLD WOMAN –YOUR CHOICE
1. TYPICAL A.V.N.R.T?
2. ATYPICAL A.V.N.R.T?
3. PRIMARY ATRIAL TACHYCARDIA?
4. A.V.R.T?

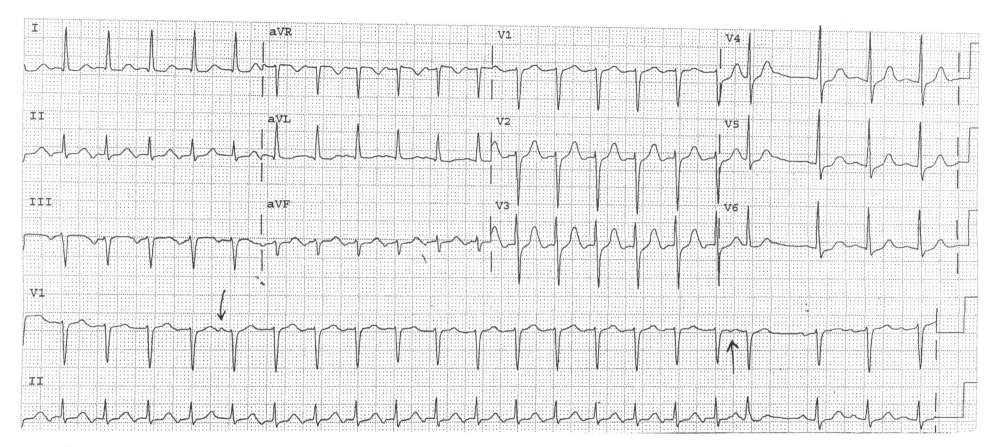

It is evident that the inverted P wave in front of the QRS is responsible for this supraventricular tachycardia. It is interrupted by an APC (lower arrow) indicating it is a reentrant mechanism. That would be evidence against primary artrial tachycardia. The earlier APC (upper arrow) does not alter the tachycardia and, therefore, it would be unlikely that the mechanism is AVRT using an accessory pathway. The timing of the negative P wave eliminates typical AVNRT. Voila, the best choice is atypical AVNRT. Do you agree?

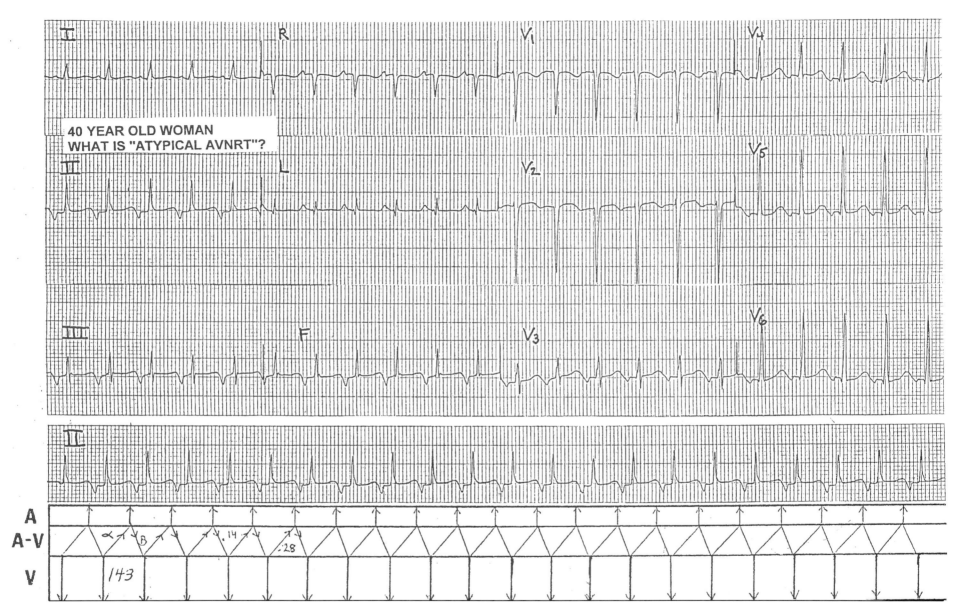

40 YEAR OLD WOMAN
WHAT IS "ATYPICAL AVNRT"?

The retrograde P' wave can follow the QRS to which it 'belongs" and at a considerable distance, so that the R-P' is longer than the P-R interval. This can mean that the circulating impulse is using the slow (alpha) pathway for the *retrograde* passage and the fast (beta) limb for *anterograde* conduction. This "fast--slow" circuit is an *atypical* variety of AVNRT and is infrequent compared to the typical.

81 YEAR OLD MAN – DIFFERENTIAL Dx OF THE RHYTHM??

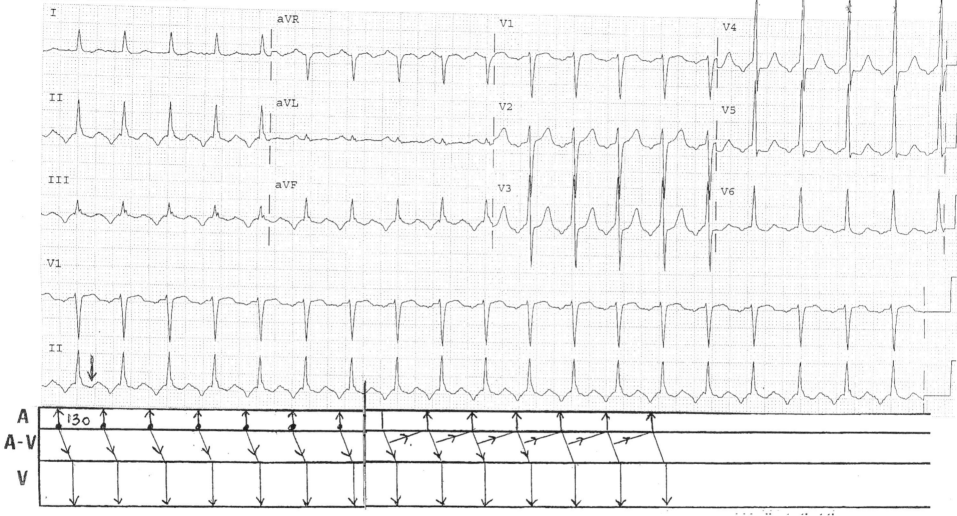

Two possible solutions for the rhythm are provided in the ladder-diagram. In the first, the negative P waves could indicate that the rhythm is an ectopic atrial tachycardia at 130/min. In the second, the mechanism is diagrammed to indicate atypical AV nodal reentrant tachycardia. The conduction in that circuit is such that the anterograde limb conducts fast and the retrograde limb slow. Absence of an atrial wave at the arrow indicates this is not atrial flutter with 2:1 conduction.

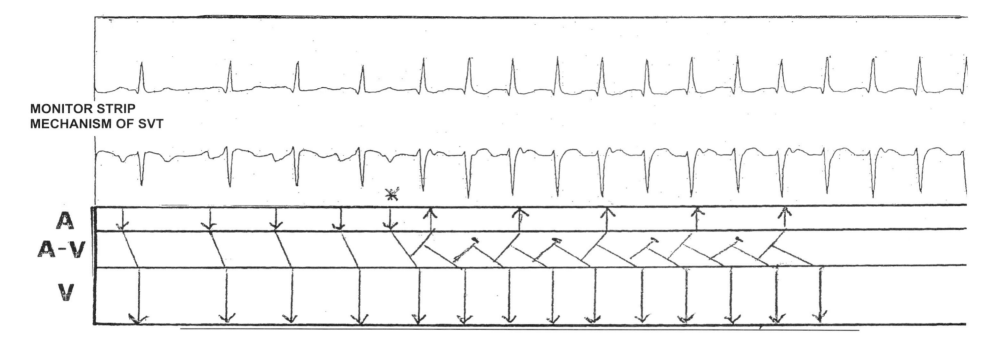

MONITOR STRIP
MECHANISM OF SVT

An interesting example of AV nodal reentrant tachycardia. The Holter monitor strip reveals what is happening. The APC (*) is conducted anterograde over the slow pathway and returns to the atrium with a "pseudo r' " resulting, and initiating a burst of AVNRT. Note that the circuit conducts to the atria only in <u>alternate</u> passes, since the pseudo r' is only present in every other QRS complex. This represents *retrograde 2:1 conduction*. Such observations proved to early observers that the atria were not a <u>necessary</u> link in the reentrant circuit.

ATRIOVENTRICULAR REENTRANT TACHYCARDIA

SINUS RHYTHM

If instead of the abnormality of dual AV nodal pathways, one is born with an accessory pathway (AP), there are two routes for impulses into the ventricle. With sinus rhythm, the atrial stimulus has an option. The impulse may cross over the AV bridge and activate the ventricles normally (the dotted lines in the EKG illustration). However, it may be transmitted over the accessory pathway and result in abnormal ventricular activation and repolarization. When the AP is used, the familiar Wolff- Parkinson-White complex is recorded. Features include a short PR interval, "slur" at the beginning of the QRS complex (delta wave), and QRS widening (depicted as the solid lines in the illustration).

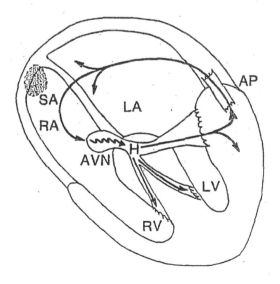

The two anatomic pathways into the ventricles provide a perfect reentrant circuit.

The illustration shows the impulse passage during <u>A-V reentrant tachycardia</u>. An atrial stimulus crosses the bridge, activates the ventricles, and finds the accessory pathway available for retrograde connection to the atria--and the chase is on! A term for this variety in the SVT is "orthodromic tachycardia," meaning the anterograde conduction is over the normal bridge, with the retrograde ventriculo-atrial conduction via the accessory pathway. Since the reentrant impulse enters the ventricles normally, the QRS morphology is normal, unless there is pre-existing bundle branch block.

ATRIOVENTRICULAR REENTRY

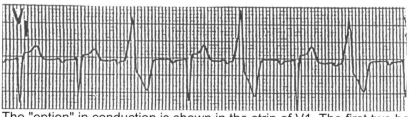

The "option" in conduction is shown in the strip of V1. The first two beats are normal, the third is conducted over the accessory pathway (W. P. W. complex) and the next four alternate between the AV bridge and the AP. Much more regarding "W. P. W." will be presented in a subsequent chapter.

30 YEAR OLD MAN -7/13 – 18:01 SVT – WHAT IS "WELLENS' SIGN"?

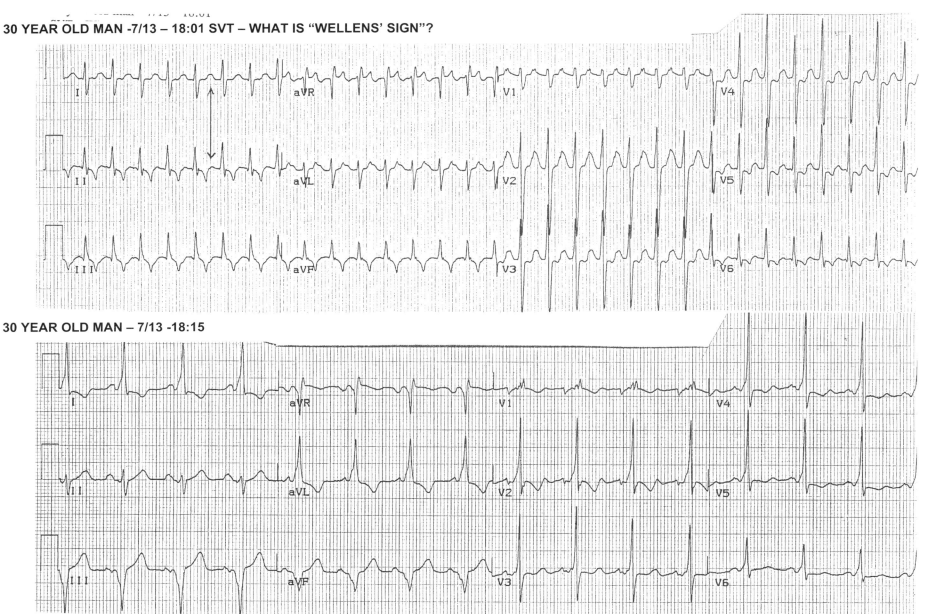

30 YEAR OLD MAN – 7/13 -18:15

An example of a supraventricular tachycardia at 200/min. due to AV reentry, utilizing an accessory pathway. There are a number of diagnostic clues. Note the timing of the T wave in lead I and compare it to lead II (arrow). The prominent trough in II is a negative P wave, located eighty msec. after the QRS complex. The tardy appearance of the P wave indicates it is not a "pseudo s wave" and is a strong point against AVNRT. Dr. Hein Wellens indicated that the presence of <u>electrical alternation</u> of the QRS (note lead V4) is often seen in A-V reentrant tachycardia and is a helpful sign. The decisive diagnosis awaits conversion of the arrhythmia. The lower tracing shows typical WPW morphology, proving the presence of an accessory pathway.

Depicted is a contrast of the anatomy of AVNRT and AVRT. Differences include:

1. The reentrant path with the larger circuit can tolerate faster heart rates. Because of its size, it has increased time for the pathways to recover before the impulse returns. Thus, it is evident that AV reentrant tachycardia usually has a more rapid rate (often 200/min. or faster) then AVNRT (usually less than 200/min.).

2. AVNRT does not <u>require</u> atrial or ventricular participation to maintain its cycling, but both are required for AV reentry to continue.

AV NODE REENTRY

ATRIOVENTRICULAR REENTRY

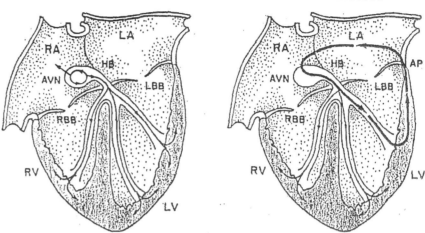

22 YEAR OLD WOMAN
SVT=222/MIN-MECHANISM??

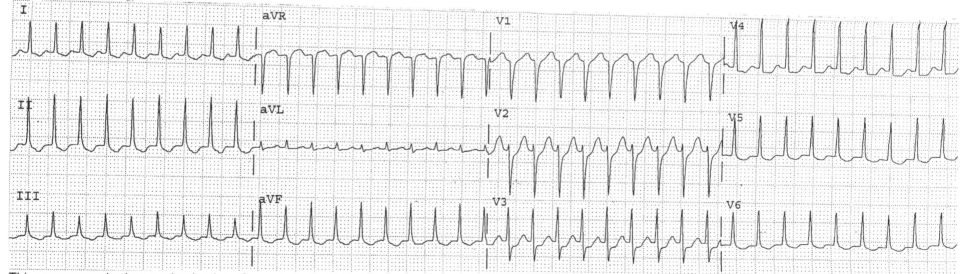

This young man had several episodes of symptomatic SVT, with a rate that always exceeded 200/min. This ECG shows a regular mechanism with slight, but definite, "QRS alternation" in leads III and aVF. There is diffuse ST segment depression, with ST elevation in lead aVR. The rate of 222/min, the alternating amplitude, and repolarization changes all point to an accessory pathway tachycardia. After conversion, typical WPW complexes were present. Ablation of the pathway was accomplished.

PR
QRSD   76
QT   196
QTc   395
--AXES--
P
QRS   59
T

+ Supraventricular tachycardia, rate = 244
- Diffuse ST-T abnormalities
-

- ABNORMAL ECG -

31 YEAR OLD WOMAN. PLEASE PROVIDE 3 OBSERVATIONS THAT HELP IDENTIFY THE MECHANISM OF THIS S.V.T.

--ALTERNATING BEATS--

UNCONFIRMED

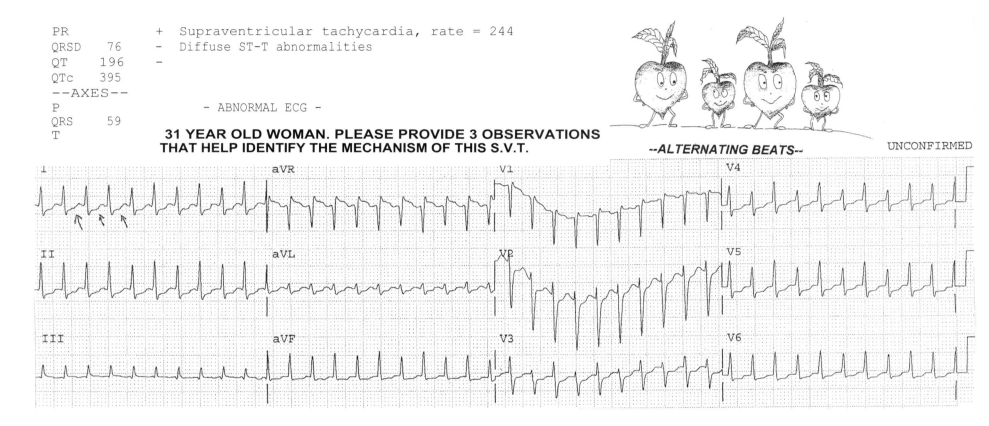

Given a rapid narrow complex rhythm, the computer rarely concludes other then "supraventricular tachycardia"--correct but not very informative! This young woman has three features that allow the conclusion that the SVT is due to <u>atrioventricular reentrant tachycardia</u> utilizing an accessory pathway.

1. The regular rhythm at the extreme rate of 244/min. would be evidence against *AVNRT* and ectopic atrial tachycardia, but it might be due to atrial flutter with 1:1 conduction.

2. The obvious QRS alternation ("Wellens' sign") is important evidence of AVRT and is supported by the probable retrograde P' waves (arrows) 80msec. after the end of the QRS complex.

3. The widespread 2 mm ST segment depression and elevation in aVR provides supportive evidence.

31 YEAR OLD MAN
S.V.T –VARIETY?? – WHAT IS A CONCEALED ACCESSORY PATH??

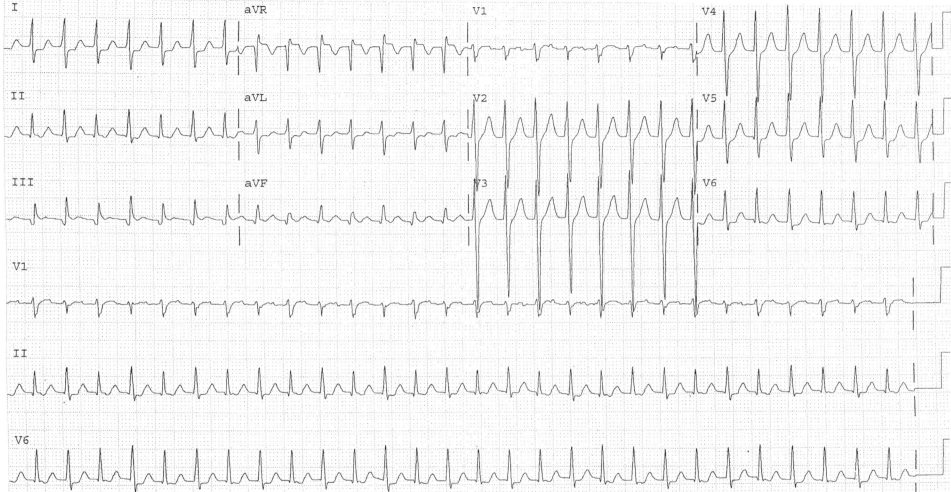

The obvious alternation of the QRS complex during this SVT identifies "Wellen's sign," providing evidence that the reentrant circuit involves an accessory pathway, ant that the arrhythmia is atrio-ventricular tachycardia. One would anticipate that upon conversion, features of "WPW morphology" would be present. However, in a significant number of patients, the accessory pathway never conducts anterogradely, and yet it remains available for retrograde participation during the tachycardia. Thus, its presence is unknown during sinus rhythm and it is termed a "concealed accessory pathway."

28 YEAR OLD WOMAN-S.V.T
ANY CLUES TO THE MECHANISM??

```
PR            +   Supraventricular tachycardia, rate = 170 [Now Present]
QRSD   72     -   RSR' in V1 or V2
QT     243    -   Consider LVH with ST-T abnormalities [Now Present]
QTc    409    -   [Now Absent] Nonspecific Anterolateral region T abnormalities
--AXES--
P                      - ABNORMAL ECG -
QRS    60
T      120
```

The small divots in the ST segment (arrows) can be construed to be retrograde P waves, occurring approximately 80 msec. after the QRS complex. This timing suggests that the reentrant circuit is utilizing an accessory pathway. QRS alternation (Wellens' sign) in lead V3 helps to support the conclusion that the tachycardia is due to *atrioventricular reentry*. Alternate diagnoses will be carefully considered before being discarded.

VENTRICULAR ARRHYTHMIAS

Perhaps the commonest abnormality noted in EKGs is the presence of one or more premature ventricular extrasystoles. These are ectopic beats arising in a ventricle and they are premature, i.e., they occur before the next expected beat of the regular rhythm that they interrupt. Since they begin in one or other ventricle, they activate the ventricle of origin first and then spread through the septum to activate the second ventricle. They therefore produce a QRS-T pattern rather similar to bundle branch block: a wide, bizarre QRS complex followed by an ST segment that slopes off in the direction opposite to the last part of the QRS complex. The terminology for these varies: "ventricular premature contractions"; and "ventricular premature beats," but perhaps the best term, since we are not dealing with a mechanical event but only an EKG waveform, is "ventricular premature <u>complex.</u>" However, the term preferred by an individual is less important than an understanding of the mechanism for their production.

In previous times, it was thought that the mechanism for ventricular ectopy was an "irritable focus" competing with a normally conducted impulse (i.e.-disturbed impulse <u>formation</u>). Evidence against this came about by the observation that the VPC was married to the previous conducted beat with a "fix-coupled interval."

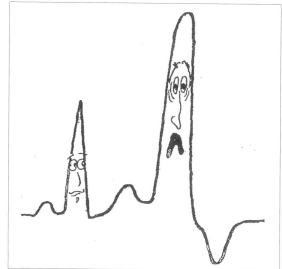

Compare the timing of the ventricular extrasystoles in these two patients. In segment (**A**) the underlying rhythm is sinus with VPCs that are "coupled" to the sinus impulses at an interval of 0.50 sec. This relationship might be coincidental, but it is more likely "cause and effect". Proving the issue is the patient recorded in (**B**). His underlying rhythm is *atrial fibrillation* and, despite the irregularity of the conducted response, the VPCs are "fixed-coupled" to them at 0.44 sec. Obviously, this consistent relationship cannot be merely a coincidence and it supports the conclusion that the majority of VPCs do not arise in an independent focus. The evidence now is that the majority of VPCs owe their origin to disturbed impulse <u>conduction</u>-- a reentrant circuit.

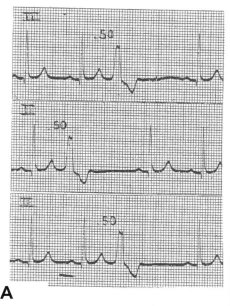

A

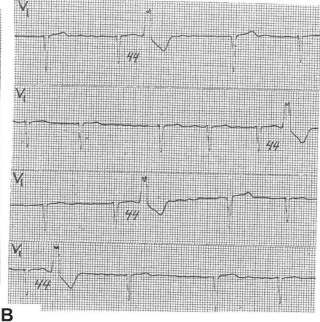

B

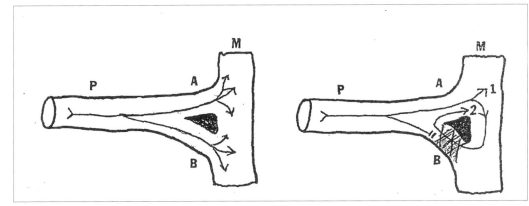

The illustration above depicts a reentrant circuit regarded as the basis for the majority of ventricular extrasystoles. A Purkinje fiber (**P**) divides into limbs A and B to reach the myocardium (**M**). If their conduction velocity and refractory period are equal, a stimulus will be conducted over both limbs, and there will be one normal ventricular activation. However, if one limb (**B**) is less responsive because of a longer refractory period, the stimulus will be blocked in it. When the impulse conducts through limb A and provides a normal activation, it can pass retrogradely up limb B. When the timing is "just right" the impulse may find limb A responsive and can "reenter" over it and activate the ventricle abnormally, resulting in an "extrasystole," appearing as a fixed-coupled VPC. Such a reentrant circuit can exist in any portion of either ventricle. If the impulse makes one revolution, an extrasystole results; but if the refractory periods of the two pathways are appropriately "synchronized," there is nothing to stop the wavefront from continuing to circulate, and a tachycardia is born.

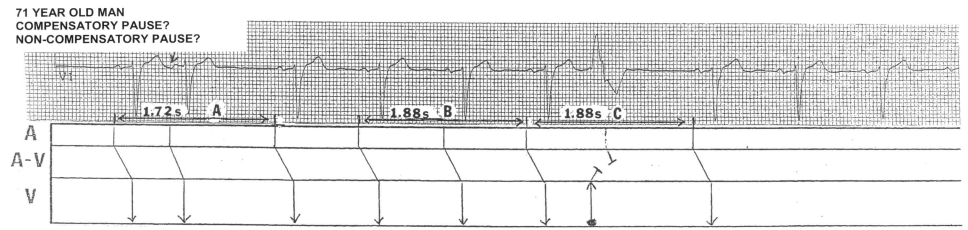

71 YEAR OLD MAN
COMPENSATORY PAUSE?
NON-COMPENSATORY PAUSE?

Although some VPCs conduct retrogradely to the atria, many do not and, therefore, do not discharge the sinus node. These ventricular extrasystoles are followed by a so-called <u>compensatory pause</u>. These cycles "compensate" for the VPC prematurity; the next sinus beat occurs exactly when it would have if there had been no intervening premature beat (segment B = C in the diagram). If the VPC does conduct retrogradely to the atria, or if there is an APC (arrow) the sinus node is depolarized ahead of its schedule. The next sinus beat appears before its scheduled return and the pause is less than compensatory (segment A).

228

69 YEAR OLD MAN
WHAT IS AN INTERPOLATED PVC?
WHAT IS RETROGRADE CONCEALED
CONDUCTION?

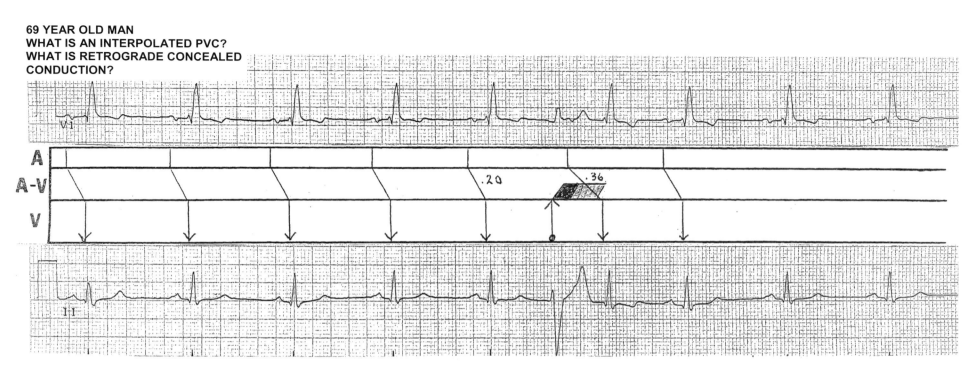

If the sinus rate is slow, a ventricular extrasystole may "sandwich" itself between two consecutive sinus beats-termed an "interpolated" VPC. Even if the ventricular stimulus does not reach the atrium, its spread depolarizes the AV junction and the next sinus impulse may encounter refractoriness and be delayed in its transmission. Although the influence of the VPC on the junction cannot be seen, its effect is shown by the prolonged PR interval of the next beat (0.36 sec). This phenomenon is called "retrograde concealed conduction."

FUSION BEATS When two separate impulses simultaneously enter the ventricles via different approaches-usually a descending sinus impulse and an ectopic impulse arising in the ventricle-they each activate only part of the ventricles and the resulting ventricular complex is called a fusion beat. Their morphology is a blend of the normal complex and the ventricular ectopic impulse. Their main importance is that they are virtually diagnostic of ventricular ectopy. More of these will be seen in the subject of wide complex tachycardias.

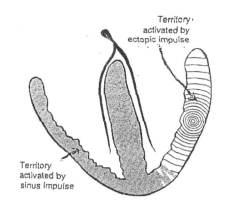

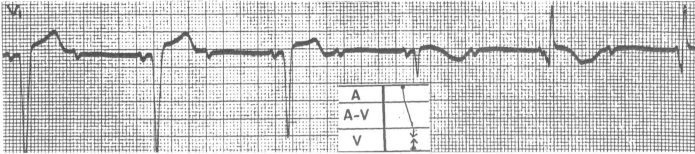

The strip begins with 2:1 A-V block and left bundle branch block and ends with two beats of a left ventricular rhythm. The intervening two beats are fusion complexes. The fourth beat represents a "normalized" complex because the ectopic left ventricular impulse activates the left ventricle, while the descending sinus impulse simultaneously activates the right.

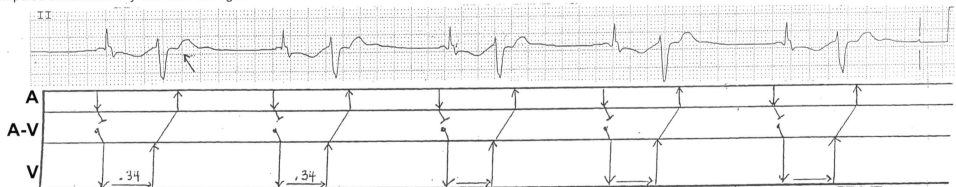

The ladder diagram depicts the rhythm-there are P waves present, but they are "too close" to the QRS complex to be conducted. The first complex in the pair is "junctional," and is married to a VPC with a constant coupling interval of 0.34 seconds. The ventricular bigemini in this woman provided a number of problems which were additive. The extrasystole was sufficiently early that ventricular filling for it was inadequate and it was mechanically ineffective. The bedside pulse rate was recorded at 30/min. When the VPC conducted retrogradely, the resultant atrial contraction occurred during ventricular systole and could not provide contribution to ventricular filling. Retrograde activation also discharged the sinus node and delayed its return, permitting the junctional focus to remain in command.

230

61 YEAR OLD WOMAN
YOUR OBSERVATIONS PLEASE

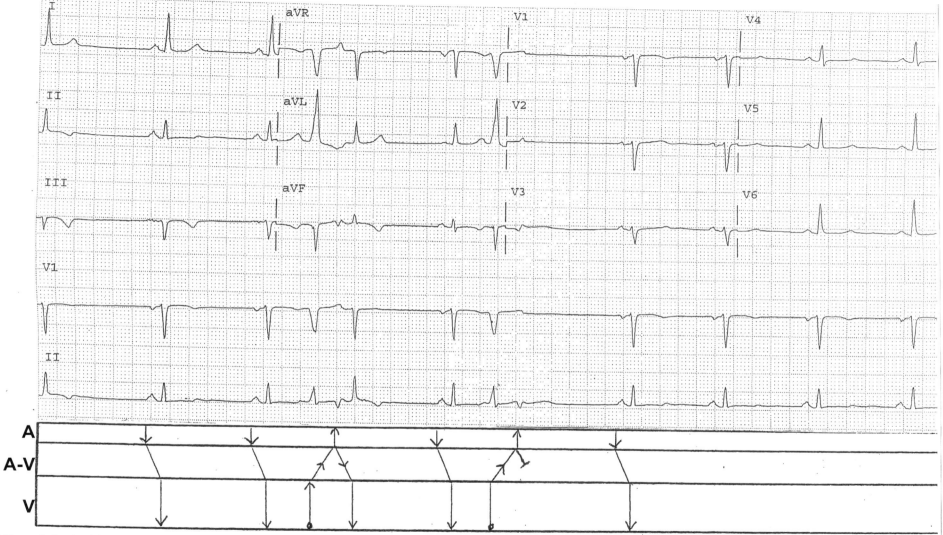

Although the incidence is uncertain, many ventricular premature stimuli are conducted retrogradely to the atria. This example shows an additional possibility. After three sinus beats, a VPC occurs. It is conducted back to the atrium and, finding a "reflection point," turns around and returns to the ventricle. After another sinus beat, another VPC occurs and again is transmitted to the atrium, this time without the returning impulse.

WHAT IS THE LOCUS OF THE FOCUS?

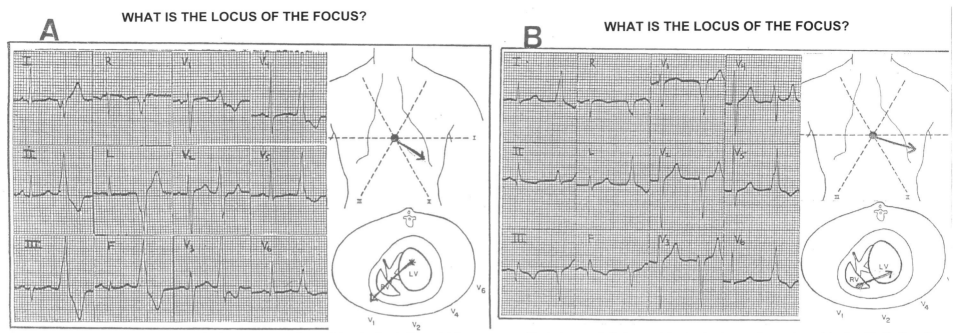

A

B

There seems little doubt that ventricular extrasystoles arising in the left ventricle are more likely to precipitate ventricular tachycardia and ventricular fibrillation than those arising in the right ventricle. It is therefore worthwhile to recognize they ventricle of origin. For this purpose 12 lead EKGs are important, but the single best lead by far is lead V1. In this lead, LV- VPCs conduct from left to right ventricle and are almost always predominantly positive and resemble <u>RBBB</u> (**example A**); whereas right ventricular beats are generally negative in V1 and resemble <u>LBBB</u> (**example B**).

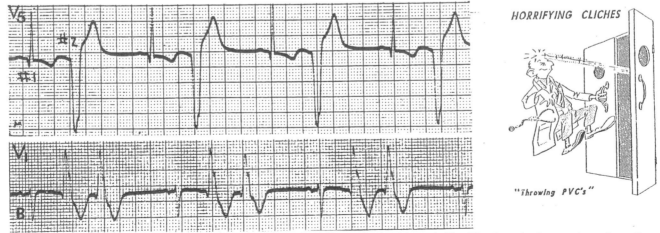

HORRIFYING CLICHES

"Throwing PVC's"

When every sinus beat is followed by a VPC, the rhythm is said to be bigeminal ("ventricular bigemini"). The terminology arises from the word "Gemini," meaning twin. In the strip of V5 twin #1 is the sinus impulse and twin #2 is the VPC. When a sinus impulse is followed by two VPCs (V1 strip) the rhythm is said to be ventricular *trigemini*.

232

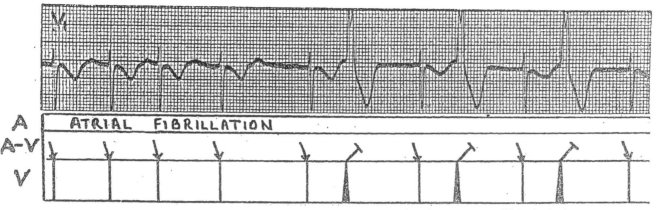

A

A-V

V

ATRIAL FIBRILLATION

When ventricular bigemini is observed, a frequent finding is that it is preceded by a pause. This led observers to postulate the "rule of bigemini." Consider: coupled bigeminal VPCs are related to <u>reentry</u> and that one limb of the involved circuit has a longer refractory period than the other. When a pause occurs, the recovery time is further prolonged, including the limb already depressed (The "Ashman effect"). A subsequent atrial stimulus then initiates a fixed coupled VPC. The retrograde concealed conduction of the VPC into the A-V junction, as diagrammed, results in another pause and another VPC occurs. Thus, the abnormal sequence may be self-perpetuating.

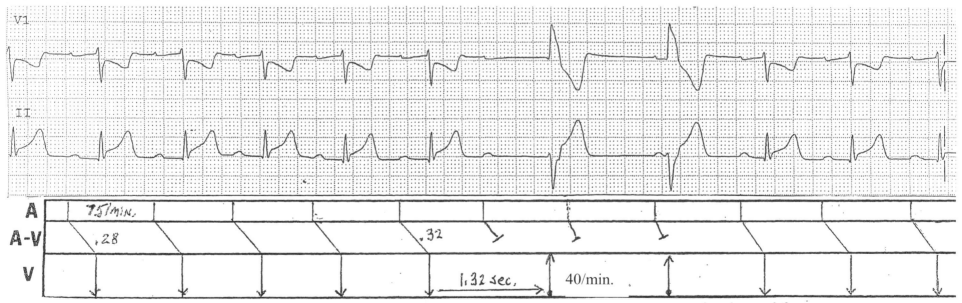

V1

II

A

A-V

V

75/min.

.28

.32

1.32 sec.   40/min.

Sometimes, ventricular ectopy serves a useful purpose. This man had sustained an inferior myocardial infarction and the accompanying vagal response resulted in A-V nodal Wenckebach block. The resulting pause of 1.32 seconds prompts an "escape" ventricular focus to surface at 40/min. The blocked P wave, hiding in the ST segment of the ventricular beat, results in another pause, permitting the ventricular focus to fire again. It's certainly better to have an escape ventricular beat than nothing!

It is generally agreed that the majority of VPCs are due to altered impulse conduction (i.e. reentry). However, a minority are due to abnormal impulse formation. Two varieties can be identified:

1. An automatic and independent ventricular focus resulting in what is termed "ventricular parasystole."

2. An ectopic pacemaker site provoked by "triggered activity." The illustration depicts this phenomenon. In A, a normal cellular action potential is shown with an appropriate resting membrane potential (RMP) and threshold level (TP). In B, there is "hyperpolarization" early in recovery (**a**) and a "rebound" that approaches, but does not reach threshold (**b**). In C, the returning signal reaches the threshold level (**b**), giving rise to an action potential, termed a "triggered" VPC. The sequence repeats with another VPC. Subsequent oscillations in the electrical activity are subthreshold and gradually recede. Triggered activity is thought to be an important mechanism in the genesis of arrhythmias due to digitalis toxicity. Triggered phenomenon can also be a function of *early* "after-depolarizations" that interrupt the descending limb of the action potential. In the example below, an early ventricular extrasystole occurs in the downslope of the T wave (arrow). When it repeats, there is a burst of irregular multiform ventricular complexes, which may be due to triggered activity.

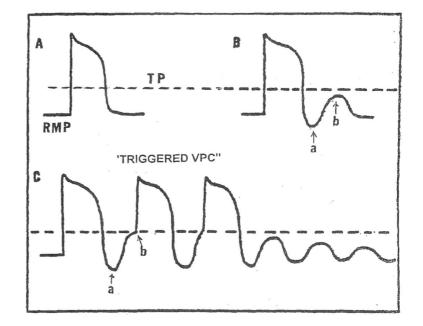

'TRIGGERED VPC"

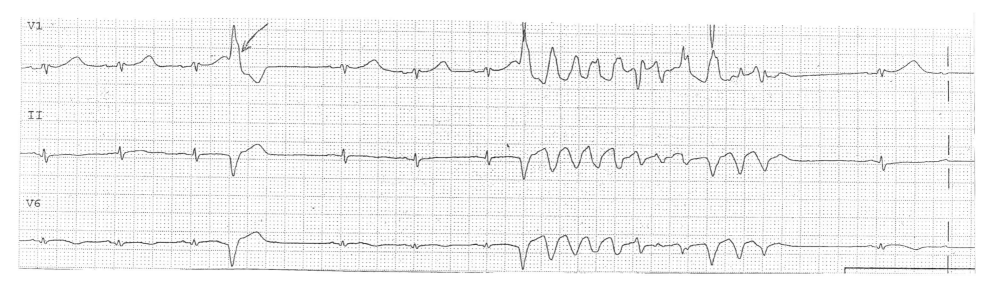

60 YEAR OLD MAN-HYPERTENSION
MECHANISM OF THE ECTOPIC
VENTRICULAR FOCUS?

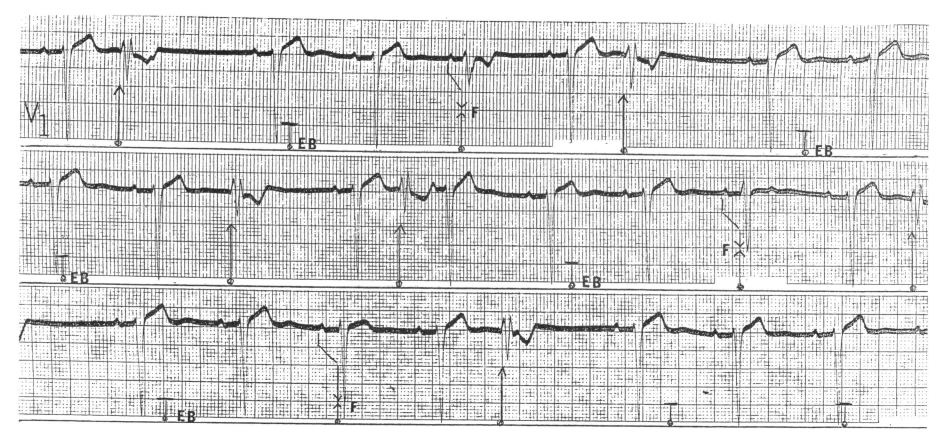

VENTRICULAR PARASYSTOLE. Criteria for the diagnosis include:
1. Lack of a "fixed coupling" of the ventricular beats to the sinus impulses, indicating the independent existence of the focus.
2. Relatively constant "interectopic intervals" reflecting the discharge rate of the focus.
3. "Entrance block"-meaning the parasystolic focus is protected from discharge by the conducted beats.
4. "Exit block"-indicating that the ectopic impulse cannot surface during the refractory period after sinus impulses.
5. Coincidental simultaneous arrival of the sinus and parasystolic impulses that can result in fusion complexes.
   In the example above, the evident ventricular ectopy is due to a parasystolic focus discharging at a reasonably constant rate of 32/min, in competition with the sinus rhythm. Fusion complexes are marked **F** and the point where exit block occurs are indicated by **EB**.

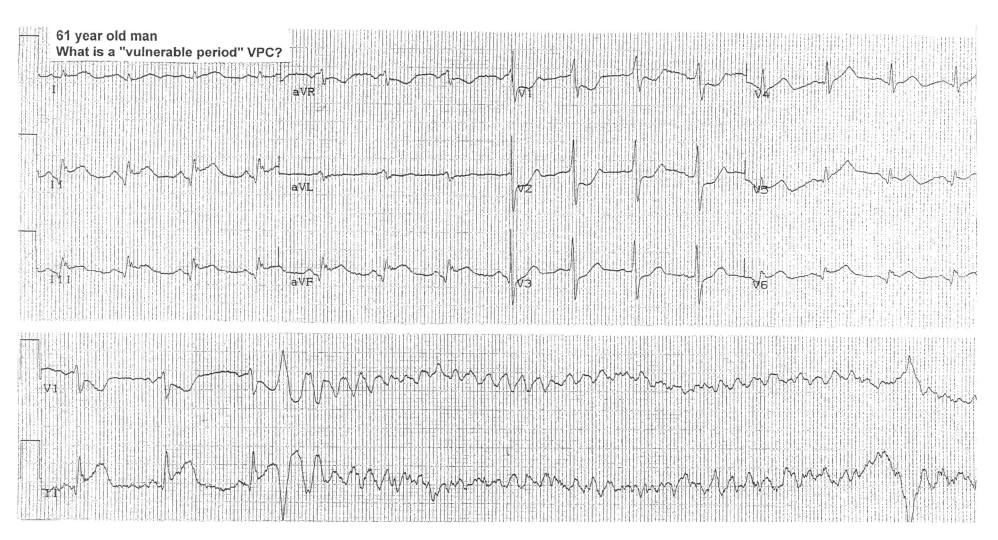

61 year old man
What is a "vulnerable period" VPC?

In the top tracing, an acute inferior-posterior-lateral myocardial infarction is evident. It has been known for decades that one can induce ventricular fibrillation with a stimulus introduced during ventricular repolarization at or near the dome of the T wave. This "vulnerability" is increased during acute myocardial infarction. The tracing above demonstrates that a single VPC, properly timed, can initiate a lethal arrhythmia.

WIDE-QRS TACHYCARDIAS

Perhaps the most startling and frightening EKG encountered in the Emergency Department or I.C.U. is a rapid wide-QRS tachycardia. The clinical setting is usually a man >45 years presenting with chest pain, or one with known heart disease. The initial (and best) reaction is that the diagnosis is ventricular tachycardia; this will be correct in the majority of cases. However, supraventricular mechanisms may be the cause. Possibilities for a SVT with a wide-QRS rhythm include:

    1. Established bundle branch block
    2. Rate related bundle branch block
    3. Aberrant ventricular conduction
    4. Antegrade use of an accessory pathway

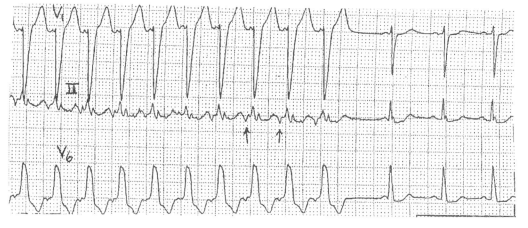

Note the polarity of the P waves in lead II (arrows) during the tachycardia, compared to those after rhythm conversion. This woman had recurrent episodes of ectopic atrial tachycardia. During the rapid rate, the ventricular conduction was always LBBB, but it was normal during sinus rhythm. This is an example of rate dependent bundle branch block.

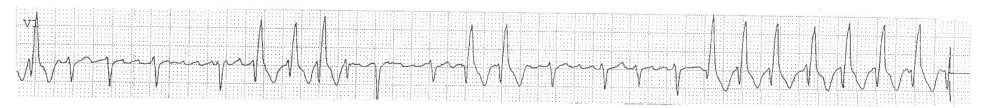

As seen in the strip above, in atrial fibrillation, variation in A-V nodal conduction promote changes in the refractory period of conducting pathways. When a pause occurs, an increased recovery time of the right bundle branch results (Ashman effect) leading to aberrant conduction, with typical RBBB morphology. This may occur once or repeat a number of times, causing bursts of wide-QRS tachycardia. The illustration provides an explanation for continuing aberrant conduction of the atrial stimuli. If the impulse blocks in the RBB, it is conducted via the left branch, activating the left ventricle and crossing the interventricular septum to depolarize the right ventricle. If this impulse also invades the RBB, the next atrial stimulus will find it refractory, and will continue to conduct aberrantly.

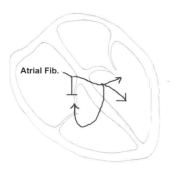

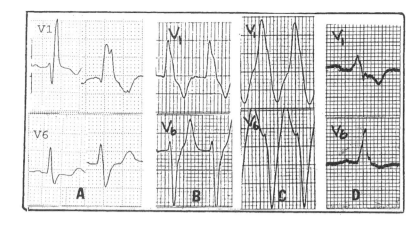

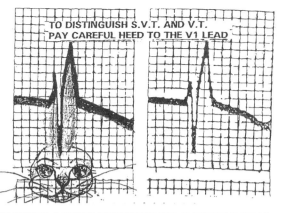

IN RBBB ABERRANCY THE RT. RABBIT EAR IS USUALLY TALLER, BUT IN V.T –PLEASE SEE THAT RABBIT EAR IS USUALLY SMALLER.

If ectopic impulses arise in the left ventricle, the sequence of activation will be from L.V to R.V. The QRS morphology will, therefore, *resemble* right bundle branch block. However, although the QRS complex will be predominantly positive in lead V1, it will not be *typical* RBBB. Variations in morphology simulating RBBB in V1 and V6 are presented. In segment A, the first QRS complex shows the morphology of typical RBBB in leads V1 (rSR') and V6 (broad, shallow s wave). Adjacent to this is a complex which is "RBBB-like". Note the initial q wave, the larger left peak ("rabbit ear") in V1 and deep broad S wave in V6.

In B, the taller R wave in V1 on the left, and the deep S wave in V6 combine to indicate that the waveform is not RBBB.

In C, the monophasic R wave steeple in V1 and huge QS trough in V1 deny RBBB.

In D, the V1 morphology is predominantly positive with a broad biphasic Rs complex and a notched R wave in V6.

Clearly, none of these waveforms is RBBB.

Similarly, right ventricular ectopy conducts right to left as though there was left bundle branch block.

In A, typical LBBB is seen. Features in V1 include minimal, if any, initial r wave; rapid descent to the nadir of the S wave; and delay in the upstroke of the S wave. In V6, a rapid rise to the top of the R wave is characteristic.

In B, the fat initial R wave in V1 and delayed upstroke in V6 indicate that the morphology is not LBBB.

In C, the broad notch in the downstroke of the QRS complex in V1 and slow R wave ascent in V6 deny LBBB.

In D, slurring in the downstroke of the S wave in V1 and marked delay in R wave rise in V6 are evidence that the wide-QRS complex is not LBBB.

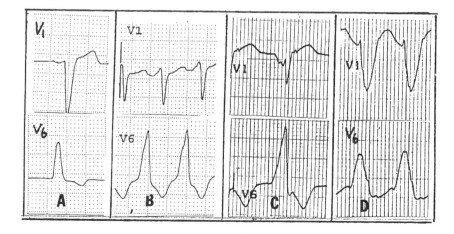

EKG Clues That Favor Ventricular Tachycardia

Most clues are obvious at a glance; some by themselves are diagnostic; others are additive to permit a reasoned diagnosis.

1. *__Regularity__*: Ventricular tachycardia is virtually always quite regular. Exceptions are encountered, and usually represent conducted atrial impulses. Examples will be shown.

2. *__Duration__*: If atrial impulses are conducted with bundle branch block, the QRS will be wide (approximately 0.12 sec.), but if they arise in the ventricle, the width will be significantly increased (> 0.14 sec). Most ventricular ectopy is *"wide-wide."*

3. *__Polarity__*: Conduction of supraventricular stimuli can occur with normal, left, or right axis. Impulses arising in the ventricle are often directed superiorly into the right upper quadrant in the frontal plane; a zone which has been termed "no man's land."
   A wide-QRS tachycardia predominantly negative in both leads I and aVF is diagnostic of VT.

4. *__Concordance__*: If all of the QRS complexes in the precordial leads are predominantly positive (positive concordance) or negative (negative concordance) there is support for a diagnosis of ventricular tachycardia.

5. *__AV dissociation__*: During a wide-complex tachycardia, the presence of dissociated atrial events is strong evidence of VT.
   These can be manifested as: a) Independent P waves
   b) Fusion complexes
   c) Early non-aberrant capture beats

   This feature has been emphasized in the diagnosis of VT and it is a valuable observation. Its drawback is that it frequently requires valuable time to determine-- time spent at the expense of the patient who is often unstable. In addition, atrial fibrillation may be present or the ventricular impulse may conduct retrogradely to the atria. Therefore, to rely upon Independent atrial activity to make a diagnosis of ventricular tachycardia, as many recommend, is like waiting for the rattle to recognize a rattle snake!

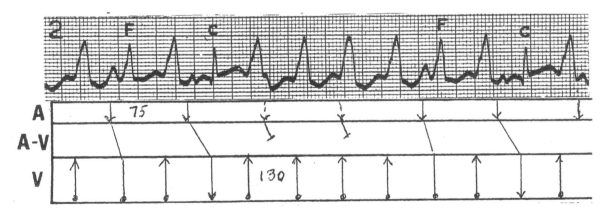

The ventricular rate is 130/min; the independent P waves are easily identified at 75/min. At the slow ventricular rate there is ample opportunity for ventricular fusion (**F**) and capture beats (**C**) to appear.

6. *__Ventriculo-atrial association__*: If the wide-QRS rhythm can be established to conduct retrogradely to the atrium, it virtually always is ventricular in origin.
7. *__Morphology__*:
   Global. If the stimuli are conducted from the atria with a wide-QRS morphology, the QRS must appear as <u>typical</u> bundle branch block. Atypical examples will help provide a diagnosis during a wide-QRS tachycardia and are potent evidence that the mechanism is ventricular tachycardia.

The latest addition to diagnostic criteria for ventricular tachycardia was provided by the Brugada brothers. These are based on the QRS morphology in the precordial leads. In the first criterion (Brugada #1 —**example A**), if <u>none</u> of the chest leads have an R/S configuration, VT is supported. In the second (Brugada #2—**example B**), if there are R/S complexes, and the separation from the beginning of the R wave to the nadir of the S wave exceeds <u>100 milliseconds</u>, strong evidence of VT is present.

Brugada, Pedro et. al. Circulation 1991, 83 1649-59

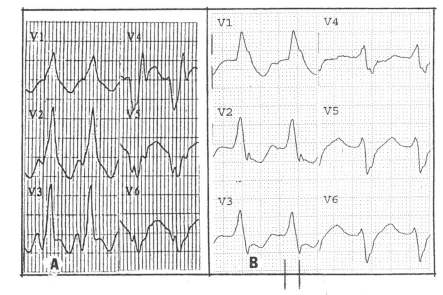

130msec

Common Problems That Impair Diagnosis

1. Attempting diagnosis from single rhythm strips. Unless the patient is unstable, a 12 lead tracing should always be obtained.
2. Failure to compare prior tracings for QRS morphology.
3. Accepting that irregularity in the tachycardia supports VT. The ventricular complexes are usually quite regular, despite the widespread doctrine that irregularity helps to identify ventricular tachycardia.
4. Believing that ventricular tachycardia cannot be well tolerated. *The patient's hemodynamic status on presentation does not provide a reliable separation of VT and SVT. Many patients with VT are stable when initially seen.*

Ventricular tachycardia (VT) may be either ectopic (a rapidly firing focus) or reentrant. If it is reentrant, it may involve a microscopic Purkinje circuit (microentry), or it may enjoy a wider sweep (for example, traveling down one division of the left bundle branch and up the other). It is impossible to distinguish these from the clinical tracing.

Evidence of A-V dissociation during the tachycardia can sometimes be determined by "bedside" observations. When atrial activation is divorced from ventricular events, its contraction frequently occurs during ventricular systole. Since the A-V valves are closed, the energy of the atrial contraction propels a wave ("cannon A wave") into the superior vena cava and it is visible as thrusts in the jugular veins. Similarly, atrial contraction may coincide with passive ventricular filling and the forceful contribution can result in intermittent third heart sounds. Thus, although the pulse is regular, the sounds seem irregular. These observations require only a few moments and can be helpful in diagnosis.

A number and variety of wide-QRS tachycardias follow. It is suggested that the problem EKG be analyzed before reading the interpretation at the bottom of the tracing. A scheme of diagnostic elements is provided with the majority of tracings.

MCL1

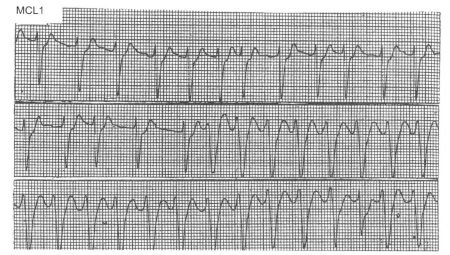

In the top strip and the first part of the second, there is *atrial fibrillation* with *LBBB*. The abrupt development of a fat initial r wave in the sixth beat in the second strip with regularization of the ventricular rhythm signals the development of *right ventricular tachycardia.*

62 YEAR OLD MAN – CHEST PAIN AND PALPITATIONS
"WIDE QRS TACHYCARDIA" – DIAGNOSIS? –Rx?

-REGULAR R-R CYCLE?
-WIDE-WIDE DURATION?
-QRS AXIS?
-RBBB-LBBB LIKE?

- (+) or (-) CONCORDANCE?
- BRUGADA 1 OR 2?
- AV DISSOCIATION?
- CAPTURE FUSION COMPLEXES?

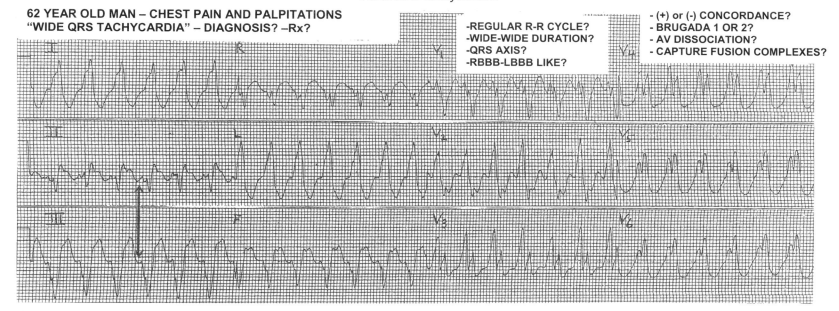

This example deserves several check marks in the diagnostic outline. The tachycardia is regular and "wide-wide." The axis is not helpful. The QRS morphology in V1 is pretending to be left bundle branch block, but clearly is atypical. The broad initial r wave, delay in the downstroke, and the tardy rise to the summit of the R wave in V6 combine to deny LBBB. The delay in the R/S of 120 msec. in lead V2 satisfies Brugada criterion #2. The apparent P waves in lead II (arrow) are really the beginning of the QRS complex. No P waves are evident, but are unnecessary. The diagnosis is clearly ventricular tachycardia at 150/min.

241

51 YEAR OLD MAN IN THE E.D.
AWARE OF "FAST HEART BEAT"
BP=120/90 DX? RX?

-REGULAR R-R CYCLE?
-WIDE-WIDE DURATION?
-QRS AXIS?
-RBBB-LBBB LIKE?

- (+) or (-) CONCORDANCE?
- BRUGADA 1 OR 2?
- A-V DISSOCIATION?
- CAPTURE OR FUSION COMPLEXES?

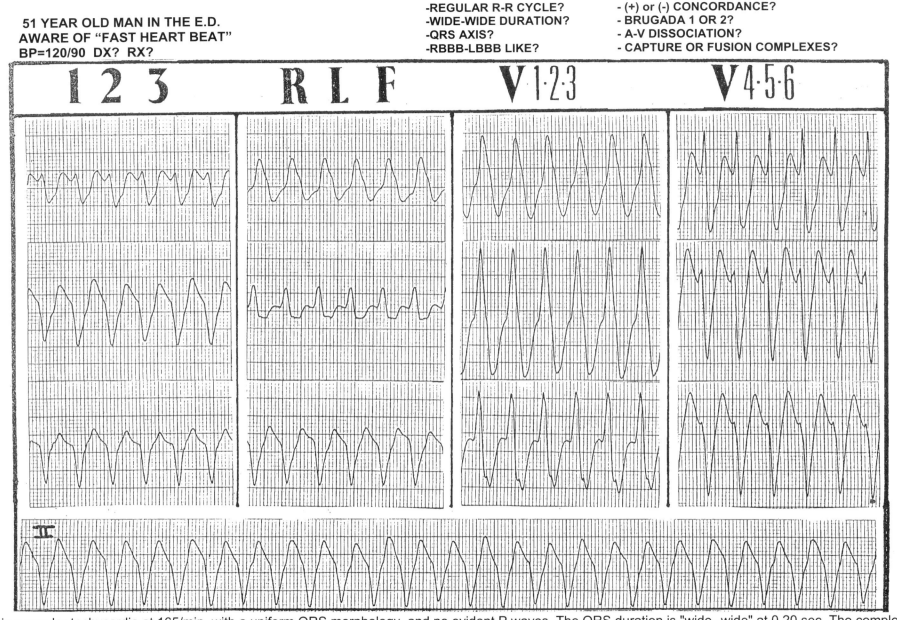

This is a regular tachycardia at 165/min. with a uniform QRS morphology, and no evident P waves. The QRS duration is "wide--wide" at 0.20 sec. The complexes are dominantly negative in leads I and aVF, and, thus, the QRS's axis is in "no man's land." The QRS complex in V1 is a monomorphic positive deflection and in V6 deeply negative. The overall configuration is certainly not that of the "typical RBBB." The evident diagnosis is that this patient has ventricular tachycardia, and one should not be reassured by a blood pressure of 120/90. The attending physician at another hospital interpreted the tracing as "SVT with aberration" and gave IV verapamil. The patient's blood pressure "bottomed out" and he required precordial shock and CPR. He did not survive to give everyone a second chance.

242

PR   + Serial comparison not performed -previous ECG within 30 minutes
QRSD   147 - Tachycardia, ? origin, rate 145 - Absent P waves, rate >= 130
QT   351 - Rightward axis - QRS axis 91 to 110
QTc   545 - Nonspecific intraventricular conduction delay - QRS 120 mS or wider
--AXES--   - Consider LVH with ST-T abnormalities - LVH voltage, ST-T neg. age < 35
P   - Q's in I, aVL, V5-V6; probably normal for age -Male under 31 or female under 40
QRS   93
T   -84

28 YEAR OLD WOMAN
HISTORY OF COCAINE USE COMPUTER INTERPRETATION HELP?

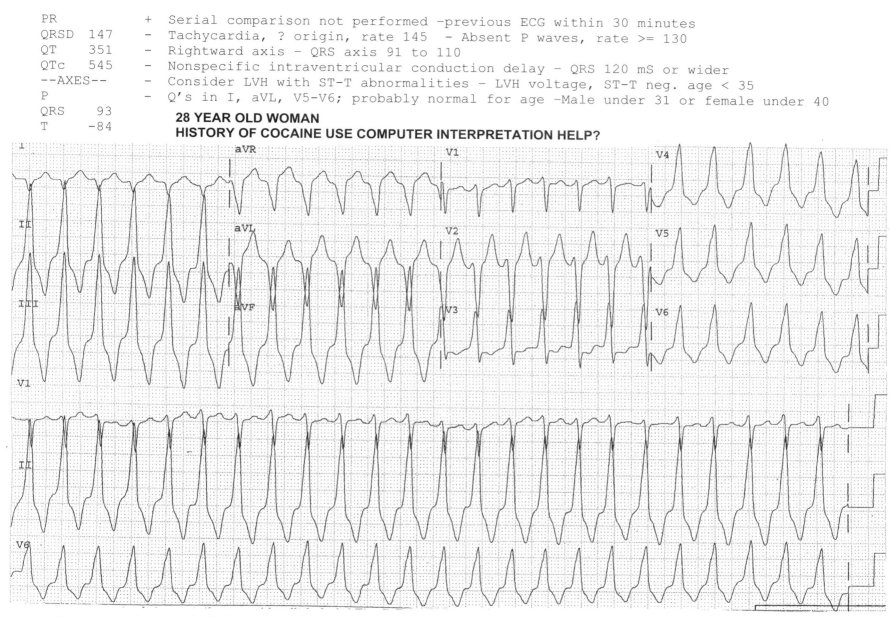

The computer interpretation provides little help! The R-R cycle is regular at 145/min, with "wide-wide" QRS complexes. The right axis supports, but does not prove ventricular tachycardia. The QRS morphology in lead V1 is predominantly negative (LBBB "like") but the fat initial r wave indicates a ventricular origin. The R/S duration in leads V1--2--3 exceeds 100 millisec. (Brugada criterion #2). Although no convincing dissociated P waves are seen, the combination of the observations above supports a diagnosis of ventricular tachycardia, arising in the right ventricle. Daily cocaine use can be arrhythmogenic!

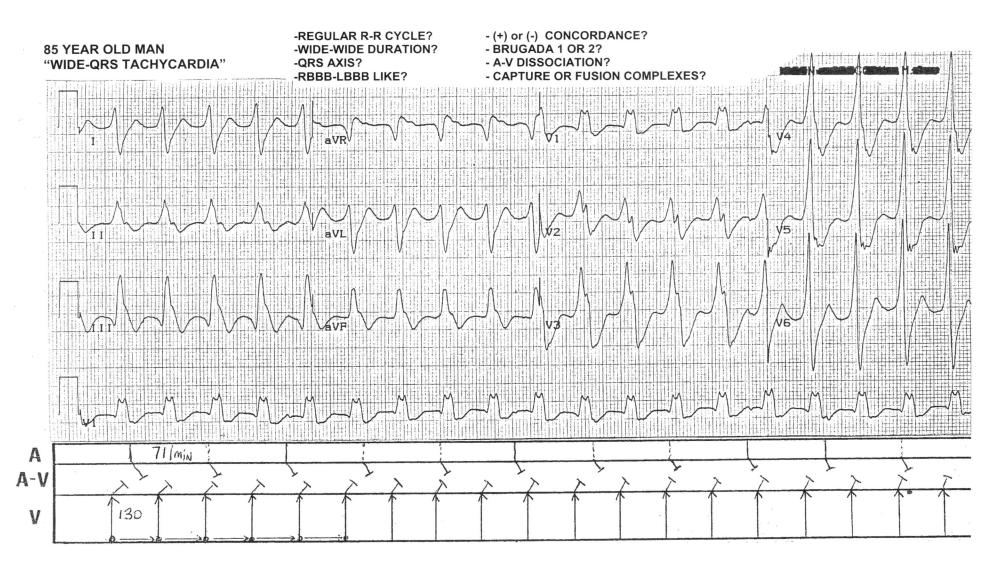

85 YEAR OLD MAN
"WIDE-QRS TACHYCARDIA"

- REGULAR R-R CYCLE?
- WIDE-WIDE DURATION?
- QRS AXIS?
- RBBB-LBBB LIKE?

- (+) or (-) CONCORDANCE?
- BRUGADA 1 OR 2?
- A-V DISSOCIATION?
- CAPTURE OR FUSION COMPLEXES?

This "wide-wide" complex tachycardia is regular at 130/min. with an axis of (+) 120°. So far not very decisive! However, the ladder diagram depicts the dissociated P waves marching along at 71/min. The morphology of the complex in V1 is "right bundle like" but clearly not the typical RBBB pattern. The predominant QRS configuration in all precordial leads shows positive concordance. In addition, note the Brugada criterion in lead V3--the onset of the R wave to the nadir of the S wave greatly exceeds 100 milliseconds. Clearly this man has ventricular tachycardia of left ventricular origin.

244

70 YEAR OLD MAN
KNOWN ISCHEMIC HEART DISEASE

-REGULAR R-R CYCLE?
-WIDE-WIDE DURATION?
-QRS AXIS?
-RBBB-LBBB LIKE?

- (+) or (-) CONCORDANCE?
- BRUGADA 1 OR 2?
- A-V DISSOCIATION?
- CAPTURE OR FUSION COMPLEXES?

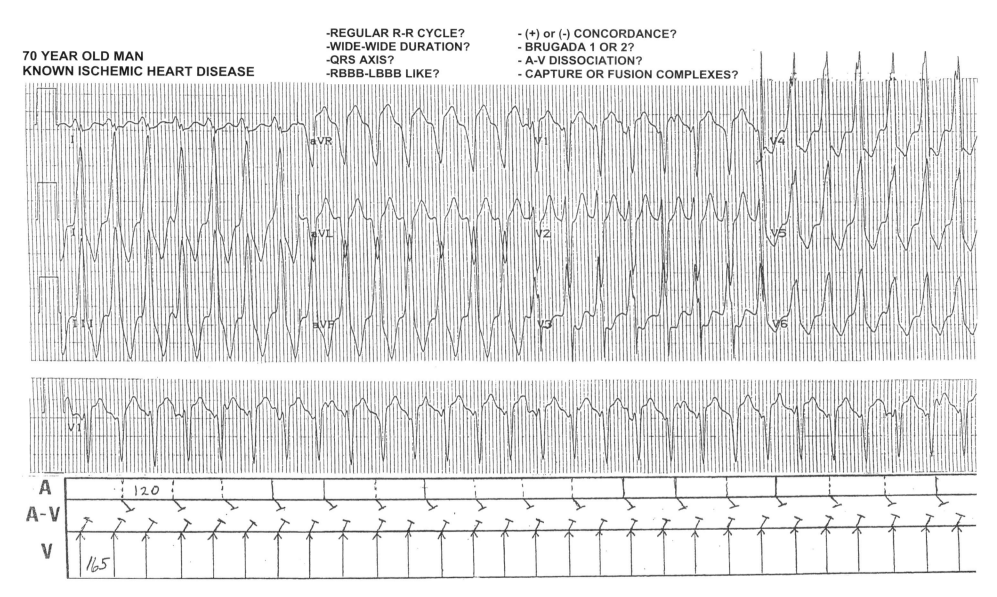

The wide QRS rhythm is regular at 120/min. with an axis of (+) 80°. So far nothing conclusive. The QRS morphology in V1 is predominantly negative, but atypical for LBBB because of the "notching and slurring" of the downstroke. Although there is no precordial concordance, the R/S duration in V3-4 exceeds 100 milliseconds (Brugada criterion #2). The ladder diagram demonstrates P waves at 120/min. which are dissociated from the ventricular mechanism of 165/min., proving that the arrhythmia is ventricular tachycardia originating in the right ventricle.

PR
QRSD 152
QT   305
QTc 496
--AXES--
P
QRS   9
T   164

+ Ventricular Tachycardia, rate = 159
- No further analysis will be attempted
              -ABNORMAL ECG-

71 YEAR OLD MAN
DO YOU AGREE WITH THE COMPUTER
INTERPRETATION?

-REGULAR R-R CYCLE?   - (+) or (-) CONCORDANCE?
-WIDE-WIDE DURATION?   - BRUGADA 1 OR 2?
-QRS AXIS?   - A-V DISSOCIATION?
-RBBB-LBBB LIKE?   - CAPTURE OR FUSION COMPLEXES?

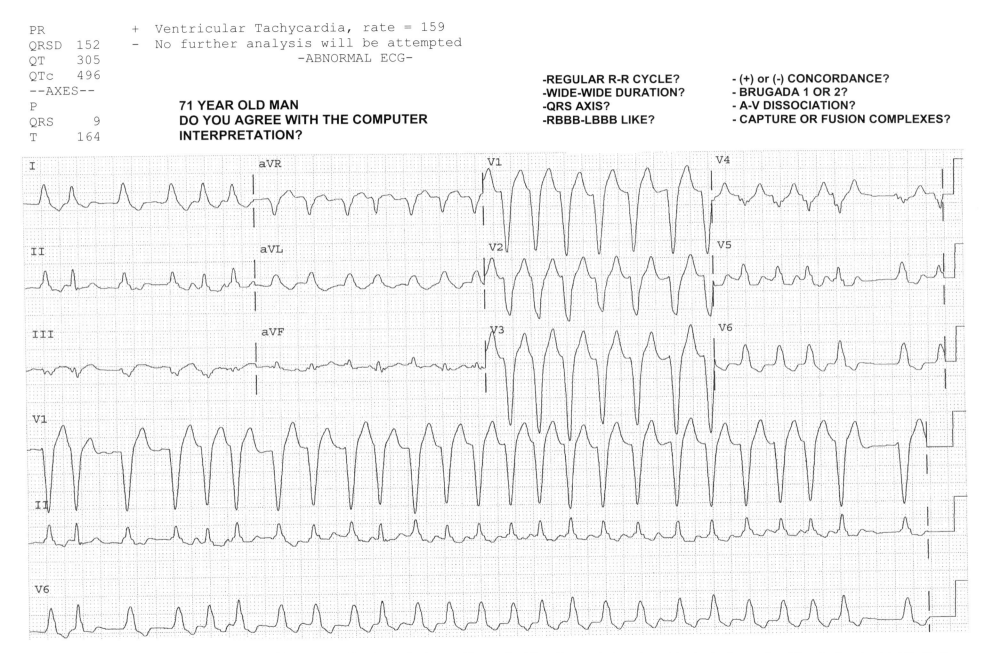

The obvious irregularity of the rhythm provides strong, if not conclusive, evidence that the diagnosis is not ventricular tachycardia. The rhythm is atrial fibrillation conducted with typical LBBB.

```
RATE   142    +  Tachycardia with unusual P axis, rate 142
PR     150    -  Bifascicular block: RBBB & LAFB
QRSD   164    -  Right atrial enlargement
QT     372    -  Borderline low voltage in frontal leads
QTc    572    -  Anterolateral injury (ACUTE INFARCT)
--AXIS--
P      -41
QRS    -80
T       64
```

80 YEAR OLD MAN
DO YOU AGREE WITH THE COMPUTER??

-REGULAR R-R CYCLE?   - (+) or (-) CONCORDANCE?
-WIDE-WIDE DURATION?   - BRUGADA 1 OR 2?
-QRS AXIS?   - A-V DISSOCIATION?
-RBBB-LBBB LIKE?   - CAPTURE OR FUSION COMPLEXES?

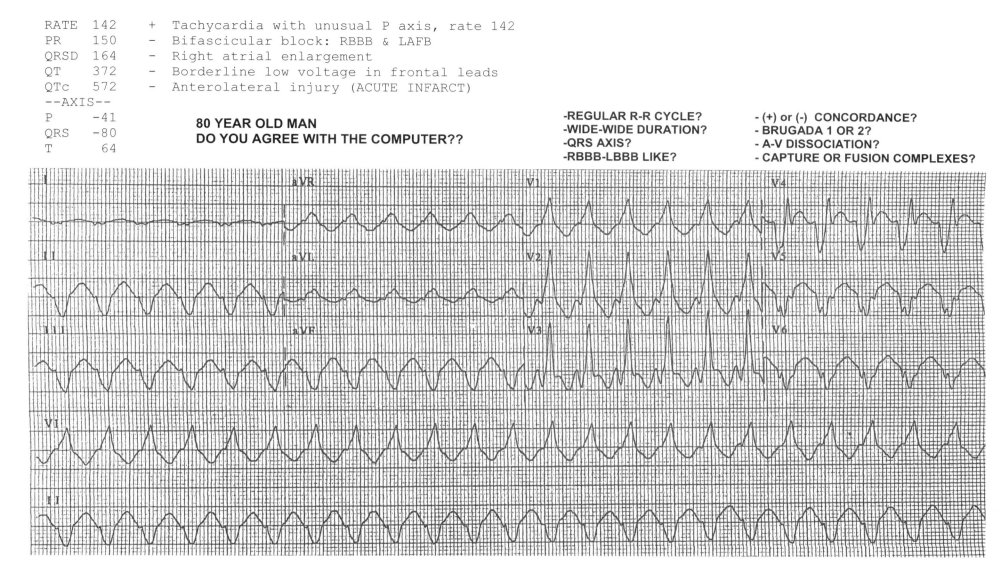

The computer made a gallant effort with five conclusions--all of which are wrong! The rhythm is regular with a marked QRS duration of 0.20 sec.; an axis in "no man's land"; a V1 morphology which is a poor facsimile of RBBB; and no precordial complexes of R/S pattern (Brugada criterion #1). There are no P waves to be found. The evident diagnosis is ventricular tachycardia originating in the left ventricle.

```
PR          +  Extreme tachycardia, rate = 170
QRSD  138   -  Bifascicular block: RBBB & LAFB
QT    317   -  Poor R-wave progression
QTc   372
--AXIS--
P
QRS   -88
T      87
```

70 YEAR OLD WOMAN-4/3 -14:05

-REGULAR R-R CYCLE?   - (+) or (-) CONCORDANCE?
-WIDE-WIDE DURATION?   - BRUGADA 1 OR 2?
-QRS AXIS?   - A-V DISSOCIATION?
-RBBB-LBBB LIKE?   - CAPTURE OR FUSION COMPLEXES?

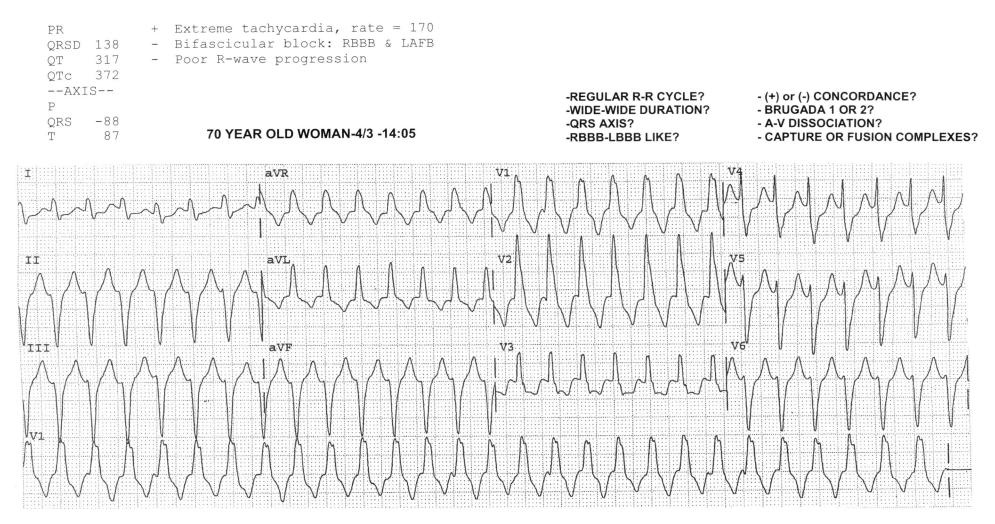

The computer interpretation is uninformative, to say the least! Features indicating ventricular tachycardia include: regular cycle at 170/min; wide-wide duration; marked left axis deviation (almost "no man's land"); and morphology in V1 simulating, but not right bundle branch block. The lack of precordial concordance and Brugada's sign is quickly offset by the evident dissociated P waves in the rhythm strip. Conclusion: the "extreme tachycardia" represents V.T. of left ventricular origin.

87 YEAR OLD MAN
A NIFTY EXAMPLE OF V.T.!!
WHAT FEATURES INDICATE THIS??
WHAT OTHER Dxs??

-REGULAR R-R CYCLE?
-WIDE-WIDE DURATION?
-QRS AXIS?
-RBBB-LBBB LIKE?

- (+) or (-) CONCORDANCE?
- BRUGADA 1 OR 2?
- A-V DISSOCIATION?
- CAPTURE OR FUSION COMPLEXES?

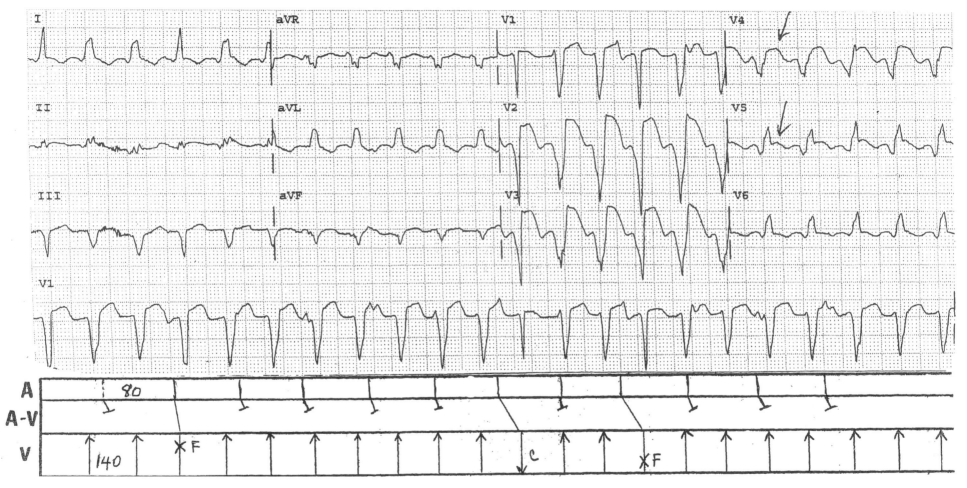

The duration is "wide-wide" and the axis is normal at (-) 30°. In lead V1, the QRS morphology is "LBBB-like" but the "slur" on the downstroke suggests that it represents ventricular ectopy originating in the *right ventricle*. The major diagnostic features of ventricular tachycardia are AV dissociation with discrete P waves, fusion complexes (**F**) and capture beats (**C**). Absence of R/S complexes in the precordial leads (Brugada's #1 sign) is supportive. Note the ST segment elevation and Q waves of the capture beat in V1-2-3, indicating that the arrhythmia is occurring in the throes of acute anterior infarction.

249

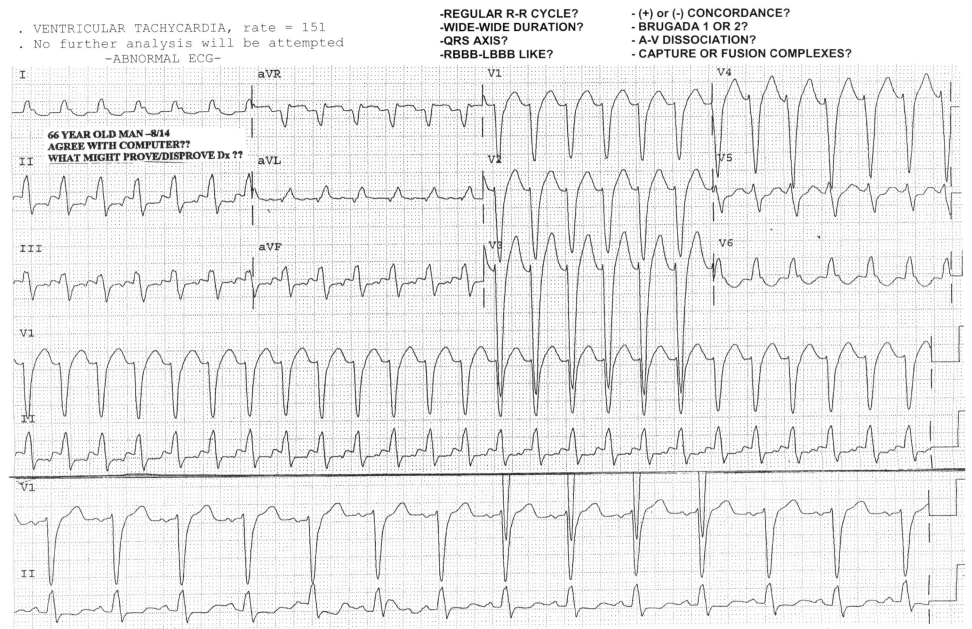

. VENTRICULAR TACHYCARDIA, rate = 151
. No further analysis will be attempted
           -ABNORMAL ECG-

-REGULAR R-R CYCLE?   - (+) or (-) CONCORDANCE?
-WIDE-WIDE DURATION?   - BRUGADA 1 OR 2?
-QRS AXIS?   - A-V DISSOCIATION?
-RBBB-LBBB LIKE?   - CAPTURE OR FUSION COMPLEXES?

66 YEAR OLD MAN –8/14
AGREE WITH COMPUTER??
WHAT MIGHT PROVE/DISPROVE Dx ??

Although the QRS duration is "wide-wide" (0.16 sec.) none of the other diagnostic features of V. T. and apply. The axis is 0° and the QRS morphology in V1 is typical left bundle branch block. There is no precordial concordance, Brugada sign, or evidence of AV dissociation. The conclusion should be that this is a variety of <u>supraventricular tachycardia</u>. The value of a previous EKG in sinus rhythm (below) is obvious. The morphology of the QRS is identical, proving the diagnosis. The supraventricular tachycardia turned that to be atrial flutter with 2:1 conduction.

250

80 YEAR OLD MAN
"WIDE QRS TACHYCARDIA"
S.V.T.? V.T.? WHY?

-REGULAR R-R CYCLE?
-WIDE-WIDE DURATION?
-QRS AXIS?
-RBBB-LBBB LIKE?

- (+) or (-) CONCORDANCE?
- BRUGADA 1 OR 2?
- A-V DISSOCIATION?
- CAPTURE OR FUSION COMPLEXES?

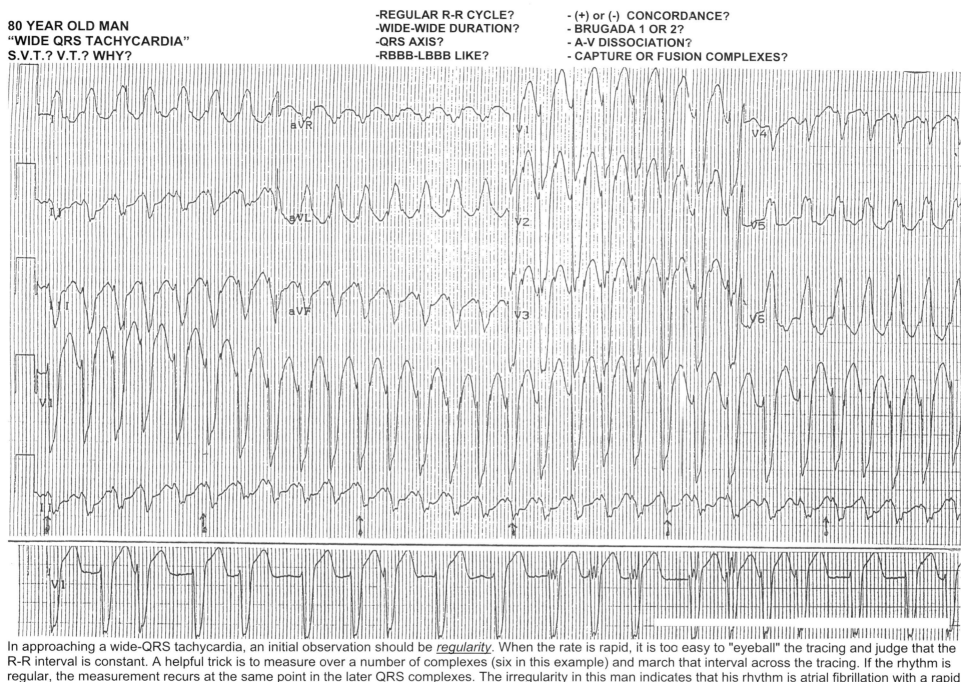

In approaching a wide-QRS tachycardia, an initial observation should be _regularity_. When the rate is rapid, it is too easy to "eyeball" the tracing and judge that the R-R interval is constant. A helpful trick is to measure over a number of complexes (six in this example) and march that interval across the tracing. If the rhythm is regular, the measurement recurs at the same point in the later QRS complexes. The irregularity in this man indicates that his rhythm is atrial fibrillation with a rapid ventricular response, conducted with typical LBBB. His rhythm one hour later, with better rate control, shows an identical V1 morphology.

251

```
TACHYCARDIA, ? JUNCTIONAL ORIGIN, RATE 114
BIFASCICULAR BLOCK (RBBB & LAFB)
WITH REPOLARIZATION CHANGES                -REGULAR R-R CYCLE?        - (+) or (-) CONCORDANCE?
ACUTE EXTENSIVE ANTERIOR INFARCT           -WIDE-WIDE DURATION?       - BRUGADA 1 OR 2?
WITH RECIPROCAL ST DEPRESSION              -QRS AXIS?                 - A-V DISSOCIATION?
NONDIAGNOSTI INFERIOR ST ELEVATION         -RBBB-LBBB LIKE?           - CAPTURE OR FUSION COMPLEXES?
BASELINE WANDER IN LEAD(S): V3, X, Y, Z
```

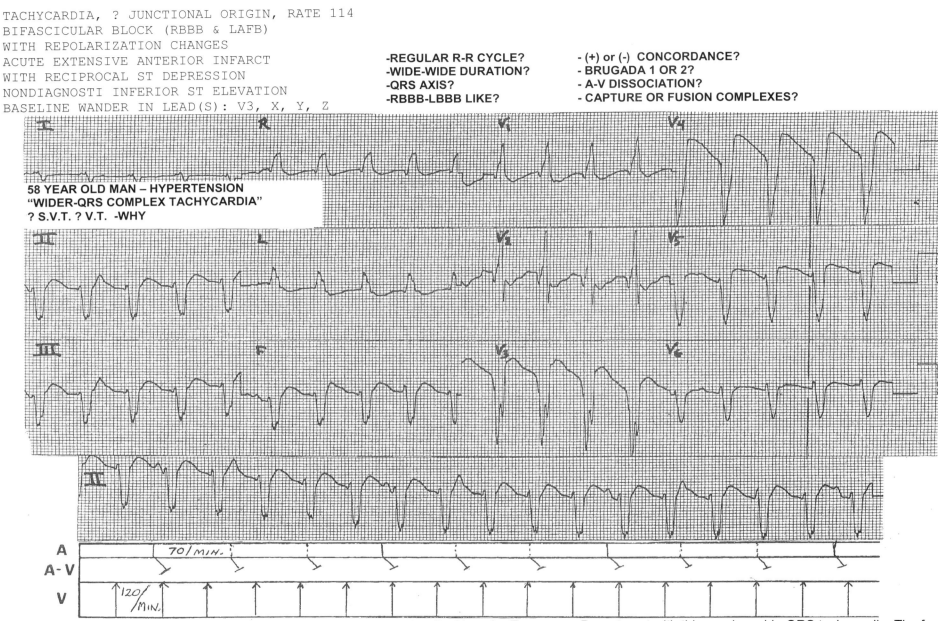

58 YEAR OLD MAN – HYPERTENSION
"WIDER-QRS COMPLEX TACHYCARDIA"
? S.V.T. ? V.T. -WHY

This man sustained a myocardial infarction in the preceding year, and walked into the Emergency Department with this regular, wide-QRS tachycardia. The frontal plane axis is negative in leads I and aVF ("no man's land")--already evidence that the rhythm is ventricular tachycardia. Additional support is the atypical "RBBB-like" morphology in V1, indicating that the tachycardia originates in the *left ventricle*. There is no precordial QRS concordance, but none of the leads have an R/S pattern (Brugada criterion #1). In the rhythm strip, the dissociated P waves are evident at a rate of 70 per minute.

39 YEAR OLD MAN – "HEART RACING"

-REGULAR R-R CYCLE?
-WIDE-WIDE DURATION?
-QRS AXIS?
-RBBB-LBBB LIKE?

- (+) or (-) CONCORDANCE?
- BRUGADA 1 OR 2?
- A-V DISSOCIATION?
- CAPTURE OR FUSION COMPLEXES?

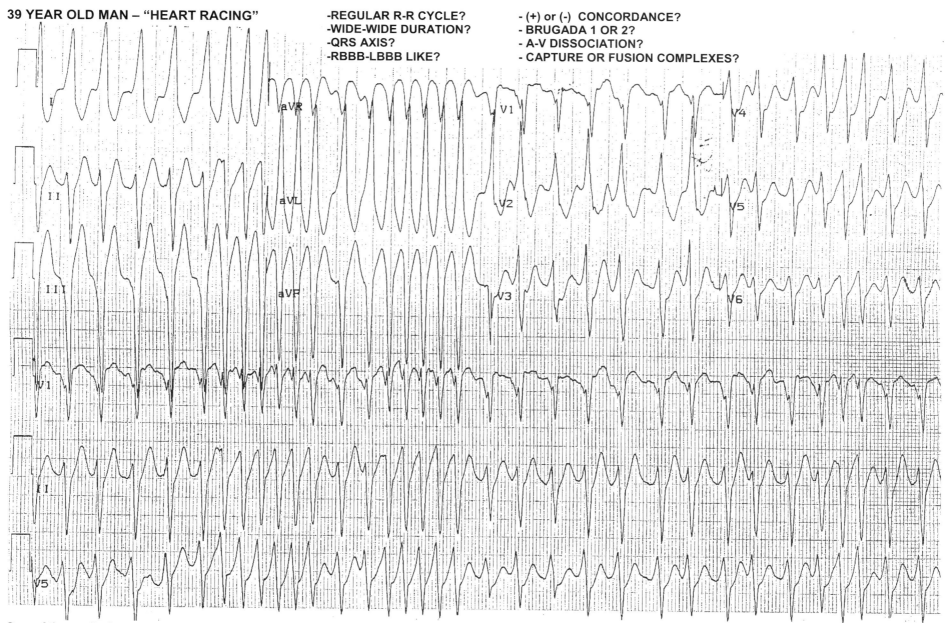

One of the perils for someone with an accessory pathway is the development of atrial fibrillation. With this arrhythmia, a myriad of atrial impulses may be rapidly transmitted over the abnormal communication, rather than the normal A-V bridge. The QRS complexes will be broad and bizarre, and the morphology confused with ventricular tachycardia. The obvious clue is the gross irregularity of the QRS rhythms. Early reports of this arrhythmia were misinterpreted, and led to an incorrect conclusion that V.T. could be irregular.

35 YEAR OLD MAN
POSSIBILITIES FOR THIS TACHYCARDIA INCLUDE

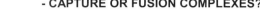

-REGULAR R-R CYCLE?   - (+) or (-) CONCORDANCE?
-WIDE-WIDE DURATION?   - BRUGADA 1 OR 2?
-QRS AXIS?   - A-V DISSOCIATION?
-RBBB-LBBB LIKE?   - CAPTURE OR FUSION COMPLEXES?

VENTRICULAR TACHYCARDIA, RATE = 201. No further analysis will be attempted

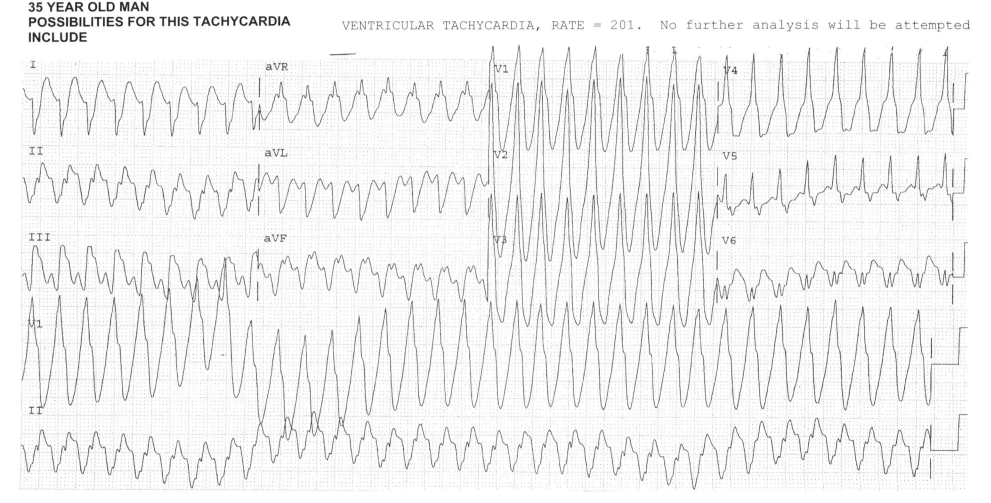

This wide-QRS tachycardia is regular at 200/min. Leads I and aVF are both negative and, therefore, the QRS axis is in "no man's land." Lead V1 shows a mountainous monomorphic R wave, clearly not typical RBBB. Although there is no precordial concordance, there is an R/S ratio > 100 msec. (Brugada criterion #2). Every day in the week this should be regarded as an example of ventricular tachycardia—but beware! This young man has an accessory pathway which is being used as the <u>anterograde</u> limb to the ventricle, resulting in this bizarre QRS morphology. The impulse completes the circuit by returning to the atrium over the A-V bridge. This variety of A-V reentrant tachycardia has been termed "antidromic tachycardia," and it can perfectly simulate V.T. Post-conversion, sinus rhythm was restored and typical WPW complexes were present. His accessory pathway was successfully ablated.

254

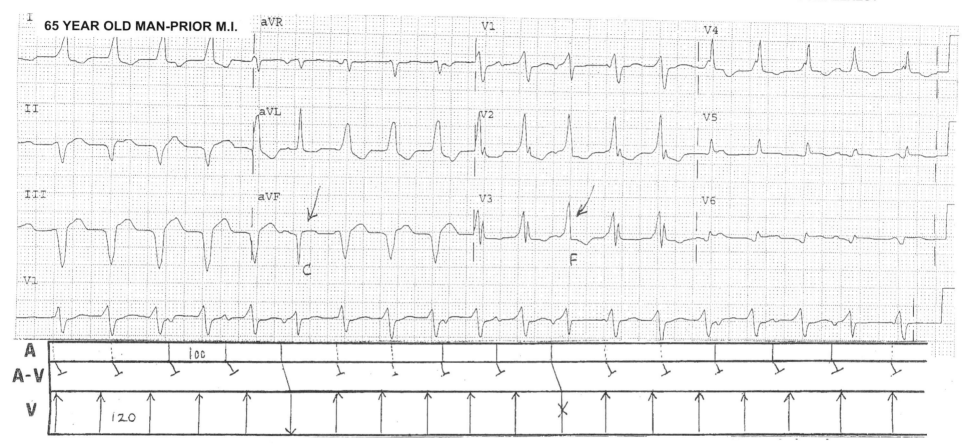

-REGULAR R-R CYCLE?
-WIDE-WIDE DURATION?
-QRS AXIS?
-RBBB-LBBB LIKE?

- (+) or (-) CONCORDANCE?
- BRUGADA 1 OR 2?
- A-V DISSOCIATION?
- CAPTURE OR FUSION COMPLEXES?

65 YEAR OLD MAN-PRIOR M.I.

The rhythm is a regular wide-QRS tachycardia at 120/minute, with an inconclusive left axis of (-) 55°. The V1 morphology is neither typical RBBB nor LBBB, but the broad R/S in that lead provides Brugada criterion #1. The precordial complexes are "almost concordant." The most compelling evidence is provided by the dissociated P waves resulting in a capture beat (**C**) and fusion complex (**F**), proving that the mechanism is ventricular tachycardia.

37 YEAR OLD MAN-THIS WIDE QRS COMPLEX TACHYCARDIA REPRESENTS V.T. OR S.V.T WITH ABERRATION?

-REGULAR R-R CYCLE? - (+) or (-) CONCORDANCE?
-WIDE-WIDE DURATION? - BRUGADA 1 OR 2?
-QRS AXIS? - A-V DISSOCIATION?
-RBBB-LBBB LIKE? - CAPTURE OR FUSION COMPLEXES?

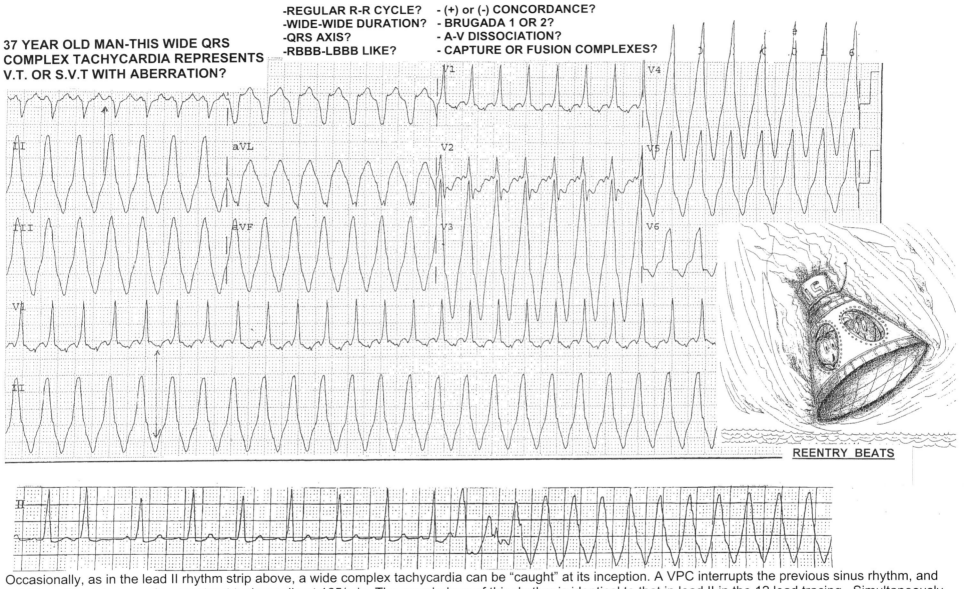

REENTRY BEATS

Occasionally, as in the lead II rhythm strip above, a wide complex tachycardia can be "caught" at its inception. A VPC interrupts the previous sinus rhythm, and quickly settles into a regular, reentrant tachycardia at 165/min. The morphology of this rhythm is identical to that in lead II in the 12 lead tracing. Simultaneously recorded leads are essential for the timing of the QRS onset/offset, and for the occurrence of the P wave, otherwise the little "blips" in leads I + V1 (arrows) could be mistaken for P waves. Even without the lucky catch, the atypical QRS morphology, Brugada criterion, and (+) concordance identify ventricular tachycardia.

57 YEAR OLD MAN
"WIDE TACHYCARDIA"
S.V.T.?? –V.T.??

-REGULAR R-R CYCLE?   - (+) or (-) CONCORDANCE?
-WIDE-WIDE DURATION?   - BRUGADA 1 OR 2?
-QRS AXIS?   - A-V DISSOCIATION?
-RBBB-LBBB LIKE?   - CAPTURE OR FUSION COMPLEXES?

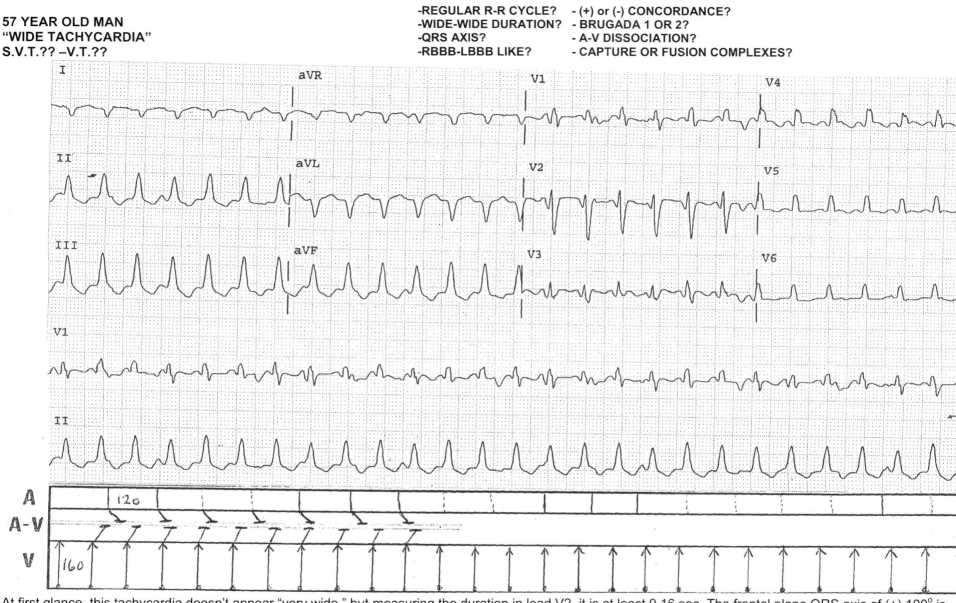

At first glance, this tachycardia doesn't appear "very wide," but measuring the duration in lead V2, it is at least 0.16 sec. The frontal plane QRS axis of (+) 100° is suggestive of V.T., but not diagnostic. The precordial lead morphology is neither typical RBBB nor LBBB, which is also suggestive. None of the precordial complexes have an R/S morphology (Brugada criterion #1). The ultimate proof lies in the rhythm strip. There are P waves at 120/min. dissociated from the QRS complexes, establishing the diagnosis as ventricular tachycardia.

257

```
PR          +   Junctional tachycardia, rate 109 [Remains]
QRSD  189   -   Right axis deviation [Now Present]
QT    421   -   Right bundle branch block [Remains]
QTc   567   -   Inferior infarct, age indeterminate [Remains]
--AXIS--    -   [Now Absent] Superior axis
P           -   [Now Absent] Borderline low voltage in frontal leads
QRS   151   -   [Now Absent] Anterolateral region infarct, age indeterminate
T     -35           -ABNORMAL ECG-
```

-REGULAR R-R CYCLE?   **- (+) or (-) CONCORDANCE?**
-WIDE-WIDE DURATION? **- BRUGADA 1 OR 2?**
-QRS AXIS?   **- A-V DISSOCIATION?**
-RBBB-LBBB LIKE?   **- CAPTURE OR FUSION COMPLEXES?**

71 YEAR OLD MAN
DO YOU AGREE WITH COMPUTER?

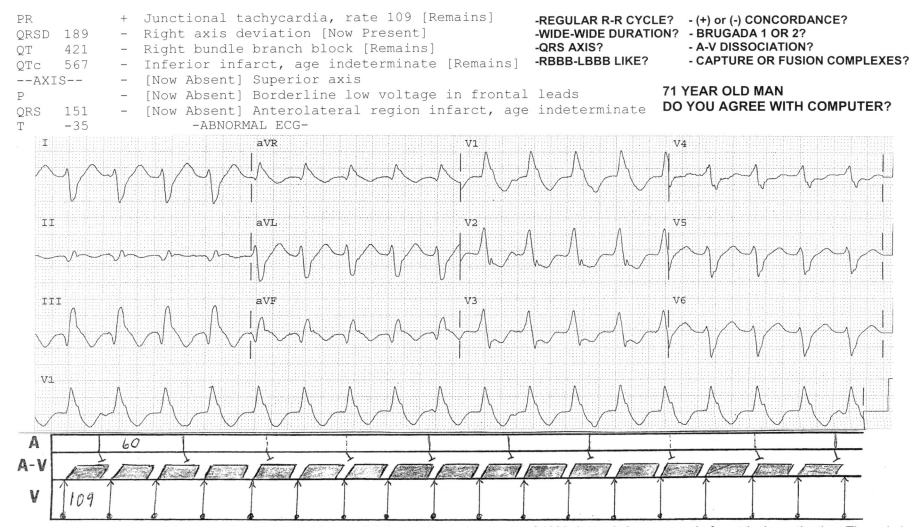

Let's disagree with the computer. A regular ventricular focus, slightly accelerated to a rate of 109/minute, is in command of ventricular activation. The axis is abnormal at (+) 180°. The QRS morphology is "RBBB-like," but clearly atypical. The taller initial R wave in V1, and deep broad S wave in V6 indicate this is not right bundle branch block. The R/S measurement is 160 msec. in V3 (Brugada criterion #2). The ladder-diagram is "icing on the diagnostic cake," showing that the P waves are dissociated and marching through the QRS complexes at 60/min. The ventricular discharge repetitively enters and depolarizes the junctional bridge. The resulting lengthy zone of refractoriness prevents all atrial impulses from crossing to the ventricle.

69 YEAR OLD MAN
Dx? Rx?

-REGULAR R-R CYCLE?   - (+) or (-) CONCORDANCE?
-WIDE-WIDE DURATION?   - BRUGADA 1 OR 2?
-QRS AXIS?   - A-V DISSOCIATION?
-RBBB-LBBB LIKE?   - CAPTURE OR FUSION COMPLEXES?

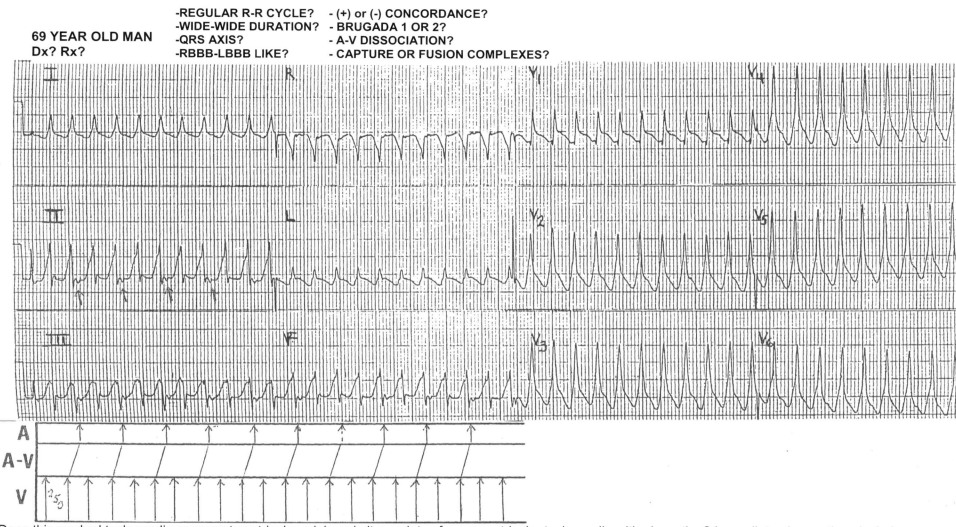

Does this marked tachycardia represent ventricular origin or is it a variety of supraventricular tachycardia with aberration? Immediate observations include:

#1: The QRS axis is normal at (+) 45°--this could be VT or SVT.

#2: The QRS duration although appearing to be narrow in a number of leads, in reality is at least 0.14 sec in leads II, III, and aVF. This could support VT.

#3: The QRS complexes are upright across the entire precordial leads--a "positive concordant pattern"--an observation in favor of VT.

#4: The morphology in lead V1 is positive, but in no way resembles typical RBBB. #5 Absence of R/S pattern in all precordial leads (Brugada's criterion #1) strongly favors VT. #6.The most compelling point is provided in the ladder-diagram. There are retrograde P waves following *every other QRS complex*. This represents ventriculo-atrial conduction--"VA Association"--and makes VT a virtual certainty.

259

53 YEAR OLD MAN –VALVULAR HEART DISEASE
WIDE QRS TACHYCARDIA – SVT? VT?
ANY A-V RELATIONSHIP?

-REGULAR R-R CYCLE?   - (+) or (-) CONCORDANCE?
-WIDE-WIDE DURATION?   - BRUGADA 1 OR 2?
-QRS AXIS?   - A-V DISSOCIATION?
-RBBB-LBBB LIKE?   - CAPTURE OR FUSION COMPLEXES?

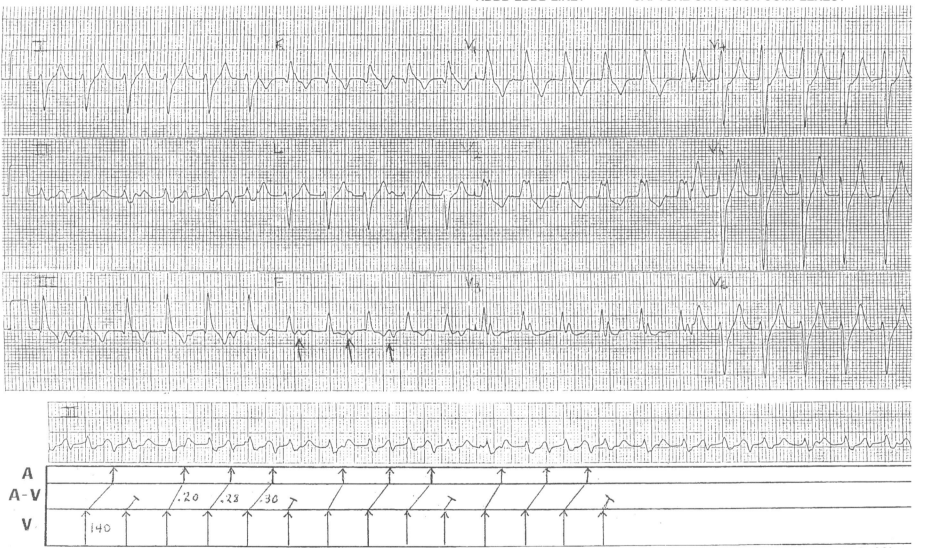

An example of "guilt by association"--The rhythm is regular at 140/min. with an axis of (+) 130°. The QRS morphology in V1 is "RBBB-like," with a taller left "rabbit ear," and in V6 there is a deep S wave. The combination indicates that this is <u>not</u> RBBB. There is no precordial concordance and no Brugada sign. Once again, the problem is solved by the rhythm strip. There are P waves intermittently present, but they are negative in leads II, III, and aVF (arrows). The wide-QRS tachycardia of 140/min. is transmitted retrogradely to the atrium--(V-A) conduction. Note the changing R-P intervals, consistent with Wenckebach prolongation, until a "dropped P wave" occurs. Thus, the conclusion is: the rhythm is ventricular tachycardia of L.V. origin with 4:3 Wenckebach V-A conduction. The ventriculo-atrial <u>*association*</u> proves that the ventricle is in command.

260

52 YEAR OLD MAN
WHO IS IN CHARGE HERE??

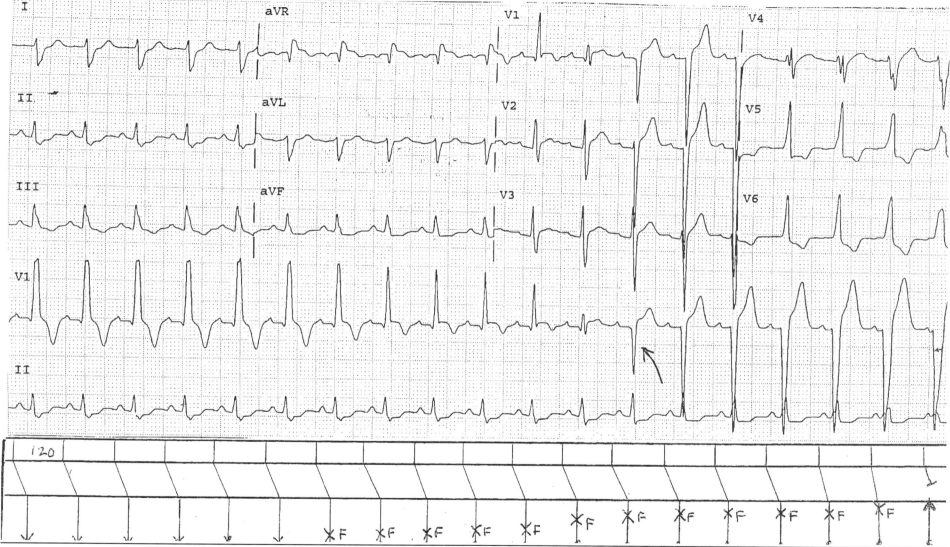

A FASCINOMA! The tracing *begins* with a sinus tachycardia of 120/min. and a wide QRS. The morphology and frontal plane axis indicate that this is due to bifascicular--RBBB + left posterior fascicular block. It *ends* with an accelerated ventricular focus with LBBB morphology, at a very similar rate. The configuration during this rhythm suggests that the ectopic site is probably in the right ventricle. When its discharge is coincident with the arrival of sinus impulses, ventricular fusion beats result. In the middle portion of the tracing, a number (12) of these are present. Their changing configuration demonstrates the variable participation of the conducted and ectopic stimuli. Of particular interest, when the RV focus discharges at "just the right time," it cancels the RBBB and a normal QRS complex results (arrow). The next day the accelerated ventricular focus was gone and only the bifascicular block remained.

261

```
PR              +  Accelerated junctional rhythm, rate 69 [Now Present]
QRSD    189     -  Right axis deviation [Now Present]
QT      411     -  Right bundle branch block [Now Present]
QTc     440     -  Inferior T wave abnormalities [Now Present]
--AXIS--        -  Consistent with ischemia
P               -  [Now Absent] Consider left atrial enlargement
QRS      99
T       -63             -ABNORMAL ECG-
```

-REGULAR R-R CYCLE?   - (+) or (-) CONCORDANCE?
-WIDE-WIDE DURATION?   - BRUGADA 1 OR 2?
-QRS AXIS?   - A-V DISSOCIATION?
-RBBB-LBBB LIKE?   - CAPTURE OR FUSION COMPLEXES?

82 YEAR OLD MAN
AGREE WITH THE COMPUTER?
WHAT IS POSITIVE CONCORDANCE?

UNCONFIRME

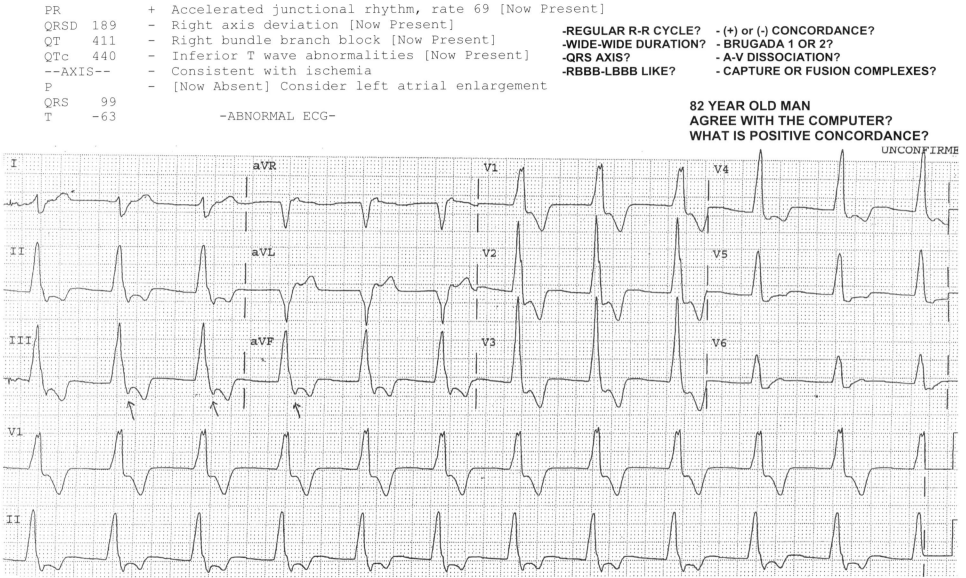

Although the QRS duration is "wide-wide," the rate is only 69/min. Nonetheless, most of the other diagnostic features of ventricular origin apply. The morphology is not typical RBBB; there is (+) concordance; and absence of R/S in the precordial leads (Brugada criterion #1). These features combine to indicate an ectopic impulse arising in the left ventricle. In the limb leads, the sharp negative deflection at the end of the QRS complex strongly suggests a retrograde P wave (arrows). The diagnosis is: _accelerated ventricular rhythm_ with a 1:1 V-A conduction.

REPOLARIZATION ABNORMALITIES
"The pure and simple truth is rarely pure and never simple."
-Oscar Wilde-

Repolarization abnormalities are extremely common in the clinical EKG. Possible causes are numerous; some are well-defined; others are less certain; some are of serious import; others less so. Very often, and unfortunately, minimal information is provided the interpreter. Lacking the indication for the study, the patient's symptoms, and drugs being taken, the proper analysis is jeopardized. The interpreter may retreat to a diagnosis of "nonspecific repolarization changes," or "probable ischemia."
When appropriate information is available, a more thoughtful and conclusive diagnosis is possible.

The components of repolarization are well known. The ST segment begins at the end of the QRS complex, and correlates with phase 2 of the action potential. The point at which it "takes off" from the QRS is called the J (junction) point. Two features of the ST segment should be observed: its level relative to the baseline, i.e., whether it is elevated or depressed; and its shape. Normally it is on the same level as the T-P segment, i.e., it is isoelectric or only slightly above or below it. In shape, the ST segment normally curves gently and imperceptibly into the proximal limb of the T wave. It should not form a sharp angle with this limb, nor pursue a frankly horizontal course. "Horizontality" of the ST segment is highly suspicious of myocardial ischemia.

The T wave represents phase 3 of the action potential; i.e., the recovery period of the ventricles, when they recruit their spent electrical forces (repolarization). Three of its features should be noted: its direction, its shape, and its height.
The T wave *direction* in the frontal plane tends to parallel that of the QRS vector and, generally, is upright in leads in which the QRS is positive. It is more variable in the precordial leads, but should be upright in leads V 4-6. In adults, the normal T wave is commonly negative in V1 and sometimes in V2.
In *shape*, the T wave is normally slightly rounded and asymmetrical, with a shallow upslope and a steeper downslope. When the T waves are sharply pointed or grossly notched, they should be regarded with suspicion, though either of the characteristics may sometimes occur in the precordial leads as a normal variant. A sharply pointed symmetrical T wave (upright or inverted) is suspicious of acute myocardial infarction.
The *height* of the T wave is also important. They are normally not above 5 mm in any standard lead; and not above 10 mm in any precordial lead (an exception is seen in youth when the T wave in the precordial leads may equal 15 mm or more). Unusually tall T waves suggest myocardial infarction or potassium excess. Tall T waves are also seen in myocardial ischemia without infarction.

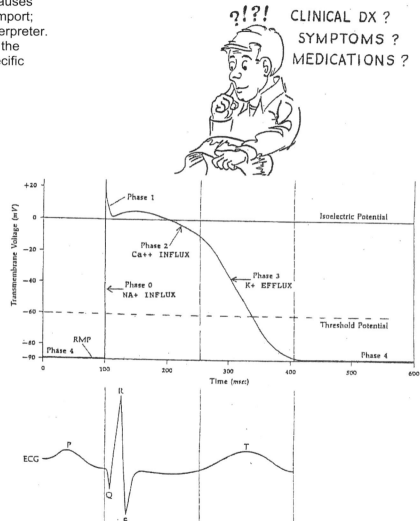

263

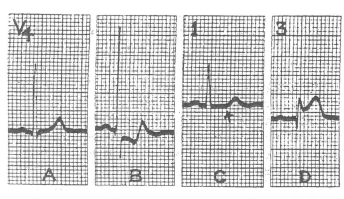

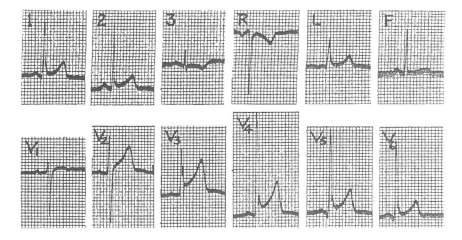

ST segments, (**A**) normal. (**B**) same lead, same patient as in A; two minutes after exercise, showing ST segment depression reflecting induced myocardial ischemia. (**C**) ST segment is minimally depressed but is horizontal and forms a rather sharp angled junction with the proximal limb of the T wave (compare with A). (**D**) ST segment elevation from myocardial injury (an acute infarction).

From a normal 29-year-old black man. Note the marked ST segment elevation in the precordial leads, without reciprocal ST depression or PR segment depression. The tracing is characteristic of "early repolarization."

```
PR      209   = Normal sinus rhythm, rate 67 [Remains]
QRSD    72                    -NORMAL ECG-
QT      433
QTc     457
```

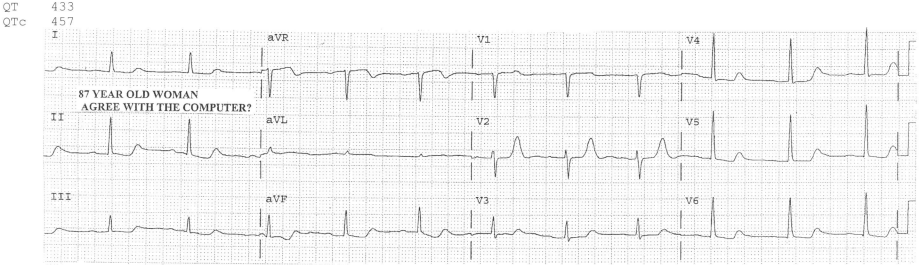

87 YEAR OLD WOMAN
AGREE WITH THE COMPUTER?

The computer is too easily satisfied and is badly mistaken! The downsloping and depressed ST segments, in the majority of leads, are evidence of ongoing myocardial ischemia; recorded in this woman during an episode of angina.

264

70 YEAR OLD WOMAN -12/25 -12:47
E.R. – CHEST PAIN
ANYTHING ABNORMAL??

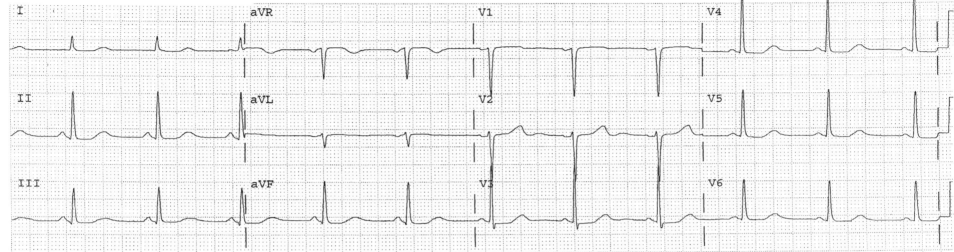

12/25 -22:23 NOW WHAT??

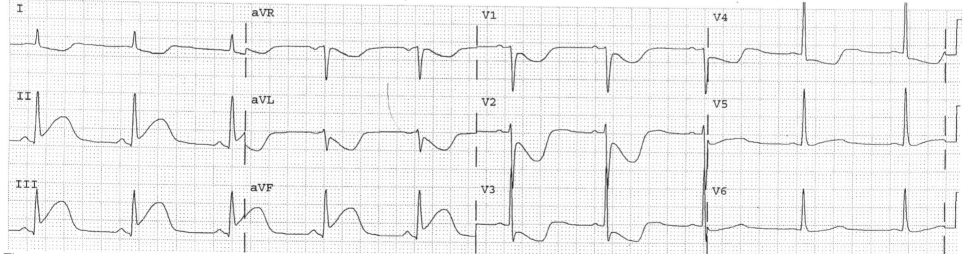

The woman presented to the Emergency Department with symptoms initially thought to be "reflux." Her EKG showed only linear and slightly downsloping ST segments. Cardiac enzymes were normal, but she was admitted for "observation." 10 hours later, her chest discomfort returned, and repeat EKG showed an acute inferior-posterior infarct. Emphasis: many patients with an acute "coronary syndrome" present with tracings that may be normal or non-diagnostic. The physician's clinical judgment should outweigh any EKG result.

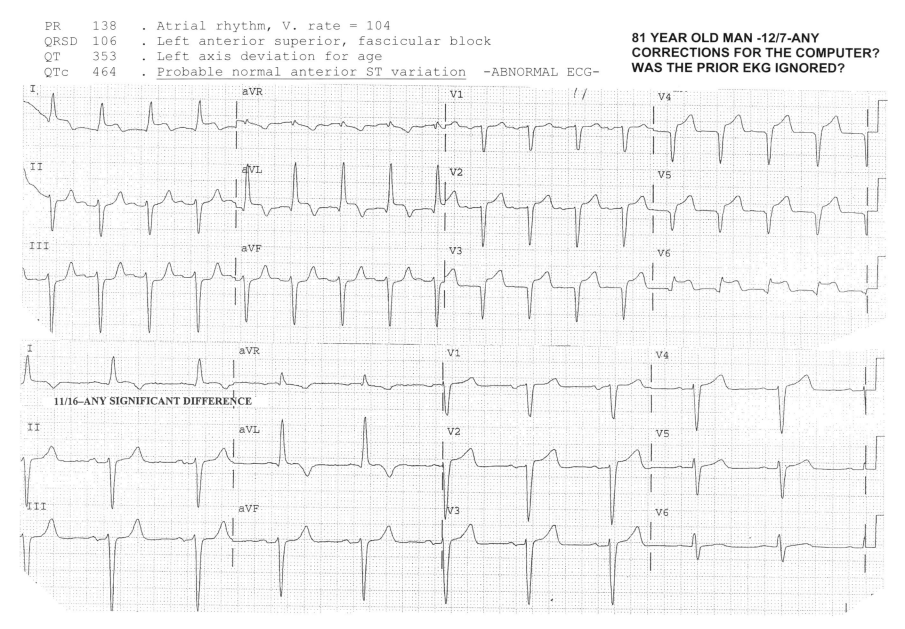

```
PR    138   . Atrial rhythm, V. rate = 104
QRSD  106   . Left anterior superior, fascicular block
QT    353   . Left axis deviation for age
QTc   464   . Probable normal anterior ST variation  -ABNORMAL ECG-
```

81 YEAR OLD MAN -12/7-ANY CORRECTIONS FOR THE COMPUTER? WAS THE PRIOR EKG IGNORED?

11/16–ANY SIGNIFICANT DIFFERENCE

The computer has made a grievous error, which if not recognized, could be life-threatening. In the frontal plane in the top tracing, the ST segment elevation in leads I and aVL is accompanied by reciprocal depression in leads III and aVF, indicating an acute lateral wall myocardial infarction. The "probably normal anterior ST variations" are really the ST elevations of acute anterolateral infarction, not present in the earlier EKG at the bottom. The computer is, allegedly, programmed to compare the *current and prior* EKGs, but it ignores the marked difference between the two tracings.

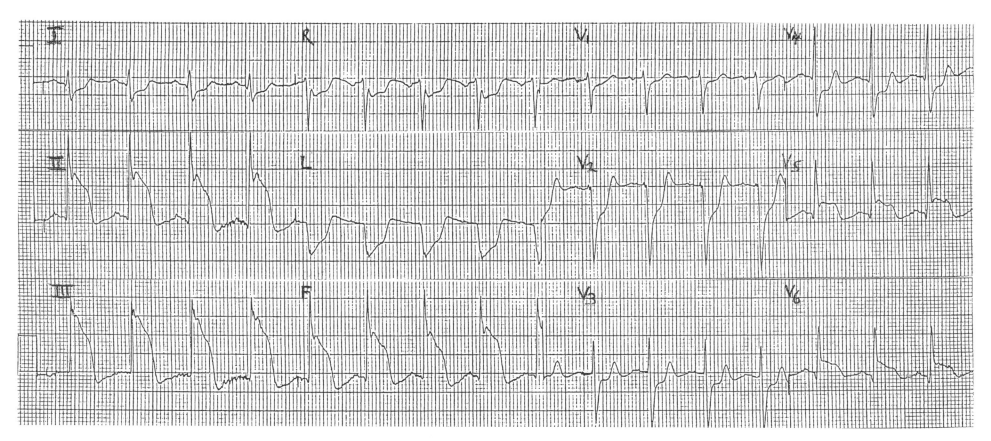

This 50-year-old man had recurrent exercise-induced chest pain for the preceding three months. His resting EKG was normal. Treadmill exercise test was performed and, at five minutes, he developed his chest sensation and the tracing shown above. The striking ST segment elevation is directed inferiorly in the frontal plane, and posterolaterally in the horizontal plane, consistent with significant disease in a dominant right coronary artery. Despite explanation and counseling, he refused cardiac catheterization and was lost to followup.

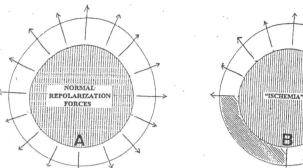

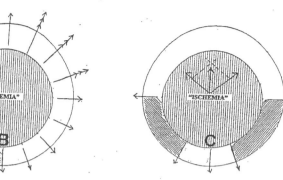

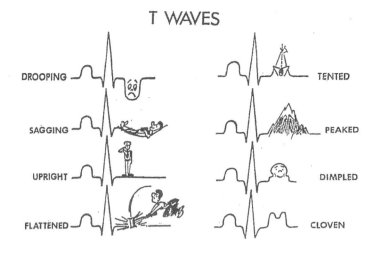

T WAVES

DROOPING

SAGGING

UPRIGHT

FLATTENED

TENTED

PEAKED

DIMPLED

CLOVEN

Since all portions of the ventricular myocardium must repolarize, opposing areas, as depicted by vector arrows (**A**), result in a significant cancellation of some forces by those in other zones. The resulting surface T wave is the summation of these "counterbalance" vectors. If a given area does not produce normal repolarization ("ischemia"), the resulting T wave vector is oriented away from the abnormal zone (**B**). This has led to the axiom: "*the T wave vector points away from the abnormal area.*" Although this is a useful rule, there is often a problem, as depicted in (**C**). If two, or more areas are abnormal, the T wave orientation represents a composite of these vectors and will not localize the involved zones.

In the bygone years, when "pattern" electrocardiography was the rule, some interesting and picturesque labels were assigned to the morphology of the T waves. Unfortunately, the correlation of the T wave pattern and clinical conditions was poor, if any.

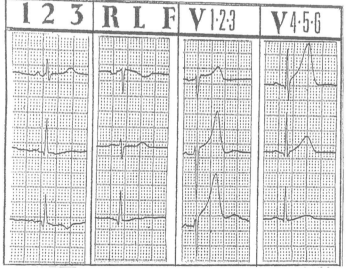

An interesting term applied to the repolarization abnormality in this tracing is "Hyperacute T waves," indicating that the tall T waves are reflecting an acute infarction is in progress.

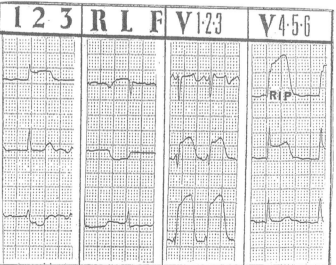

An evident anteroseptal-lateral M.I. Is present and accompanied by atrial fibrillation. Early interpreters were reminded of familiar objects and labeled the striking repolarization changes as "tombstone T waves," reflecting the *grave* prognosis at the time.

268

T WAVES

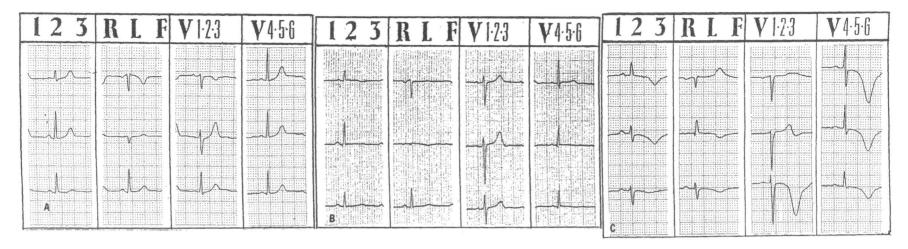

T wave abnormalities can be indicated by changes in direction, amplitude, or breadth. In the normal young individual (**A**), the T wave *direction* in the frontal plane parallels that of the QRS complex. The axis of the QRS is (+) 70° and the T wave (+) 50° - resulting in a narrow "QRS-T angle" of 20° (less than the normal limit of 60°). In the horizontal plane, the T wave is normally inverted in leads V1 and sometimes in V2, and upright in the other precordial leads.

In patient (**B**) the frontal plane T wave amplitude and direction are abnormal. The QRS axis is normal at (+) 60° and that of the T wave (+) 150°-a wide QRS-T angle indicating a <u>primary</u> T wave abnormality. The precordial leads show that the T wave has an anterior direction and is prominently positive in lead V1 and flat in lead V6. An old axiom states: when the T wave amplitude in V1 exceeds that in V6, a repolarization abnormality is present. This woman was in shock secondary to hemorrhage. In patient (**C**) the T wave is broad and diffusely inverted in both frontal and horizontal planes. Although there are other possible causes, the most common is ongoing serious myocardial ischemia. This man presented with chest pain and elevated troponin indicating an acute myocardial infarction.

Abnormalities of depolarization are always accompanied by abnormalities of repolarization. These are expected and are referred to as "secondary" repolarization events. They occur with myocardial ischemia/infarction, ventricular enlargement (LVH or RVH), and accessory pathway activation of the ventricle (WPW). When ventricular conduction delay occurs-RBBB or LBBB-and increases the ST-T changes become more marked. The vectoral direction of the ST-T becomes oriented opposite to that of the last part of the QRS complex. The "degree" of block determines the accompanying repolarization abnormality. Note that in examples A, B, and C, depicting degrees of RBBB, the amount of ST sagging and T wave inversion in lead V1 parallels the terminal delay (the R') in the QRS complex.

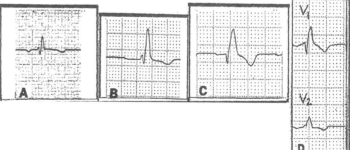

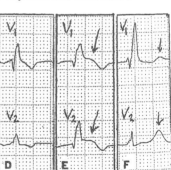

In (**A**) it is minimal; it increases in (**B**) and is maximal in (**C**). In segment (**D**), the QRS and ST-T morphology is typical for complete RBBB. Contrast the repolarization in V1 and V2 with that in E and F. The ST segment elevation (arrows) in (**E**) should not be present with RBBB and is indicative of acute anterior infarction. In segment (**F**), the T wave is upright in V1 and V2, (arrows) indicating that the <u>expected</u> T wave abnormality has been negated--an example of an anticipated *secondary* T wave abnormality altered by a superimposed *primary* abnormality. The reason for this demands clinical correlation.

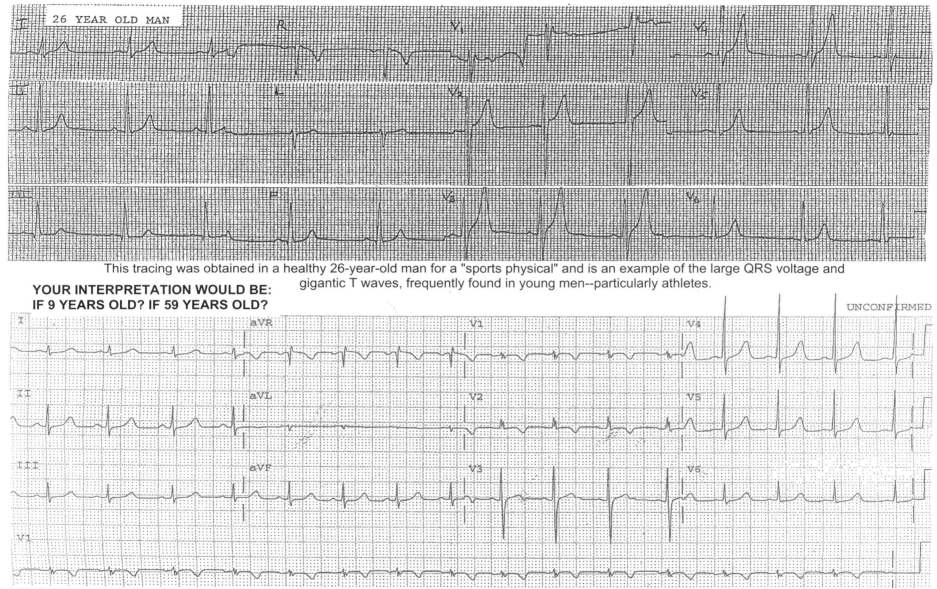

26 YEAR OLD MAN

This tracing was obtained in a healthy 26-year-old man for a "sports physical" and is an example of the large QRS voltage and gigantic T waves, frequently found in young men--particularly athletes.

**YOUR INTERPRETATION WOULD BE:
IF 9 YEARS OLD? IF 59 YEARS OLD?**

UNCONFIRMED

The EKG during childhood differs from that of the adult. Persistence of RV dominance in children results in repolarization changes reflected by T wave inversions in V1-V2, and often in V3. The transition form a negative to a positive T wave frequently results in a diphasic morphology, such as seen in lead V3. This is a tracing obtained on a normal nine-year-old child. If it was recorded in a 59-year-old man, the same T waves would be abnormal and regarded as "anterior ischemia."

The expected <u>secondary</u> repolarization abnormalities that accompany LBBB (**A**) include ST-T direction opposite that of the QRS complex. Leads that are predominantly positive, such as lead I and V6, have STT changes that are negative. Those that are negative, such as V1, have a repolarization direction that is positive. When the direction of the ST-T vector is reversed (**B**), a <u>primary</u> repolarization abnormality has appeared to replace the expected St-T change, indicating that an additional problem is present, and requiring further evaluation.

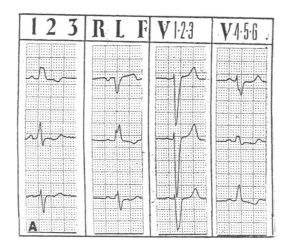

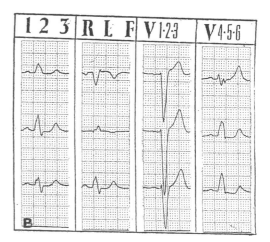

CONCORDANT ST SEGMANT ELEVATION

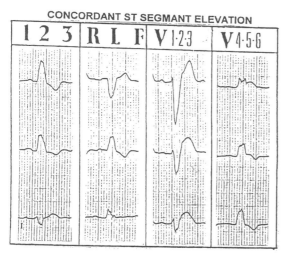

ST SEGMENT DEPRESSION IN V1 or V2 or V3

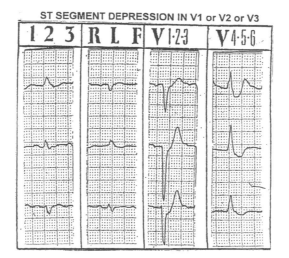

DISCORDANT ST SEGMENT ELEVATION

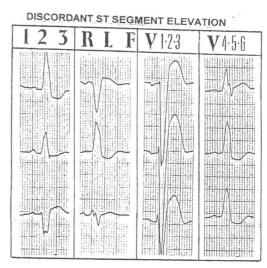

EKG Dx of M.I. with LBBB

IS THERE ST SEGMENT ELEVATION 1MM IN ANY LEAD THAT IS CONCORDANT WITHT THE QRS COMPLEX?

IS THERE ST SEGMENTDEPRESSION IN LEAD V1 OR V2 OR V3?

IS THERE ST SEGMENT ELEVATION 5MM THAT IS DISCORDANT WITH THE QRS COMPLEX?

Sgarbossa et. Al. N. Eng. J. Med. 334: 481, 1996.

The diagnosis of acute MI in the presence of LBBB can be provided by the "GUSTO criteria" (reference cited). They reflect *inappropriate* repolarization, indicating the presence of an "injury current." In the upper left example, note the ST segment elevation in leads V4-5 <u>concordant</u> with the QRS complexes. In the middle tracing, the ST segment is depressed in V1-2-3, leads in which the QRS is negative and the ST-T segment should be elevated. The right upper example shows exaggerated ST segment elevation in leads V1-3 > 5 mm, as well as concordant ST elevation in lead V4. Any of these patterns is consistent with acute myocardial infarction.

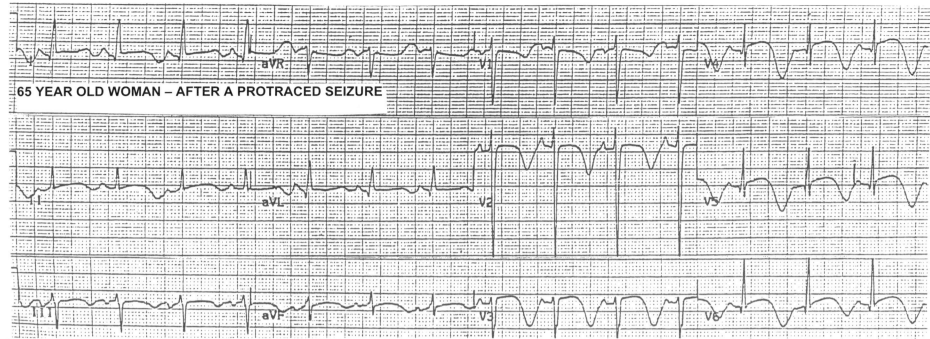

65 YEAR OLD WOMAN – AFTER A PROTRACED SEIZURE

This tragic woman was found by family members in the throes of a grand-mal seizure. It persisted during EMS transport to a distant hospital, and was controlled only with large doses of anticonvulsant medication. Her EKG in the Emergency Department is shown. The abnormality, at a glance, is that there is striking QT prolongation with diffuse and deep T wave inversion. She was subsequently found to have a malignant brain tumor, which was the cause of her seizure. This bizarre EKG pattern can be seen in any condition causing an increase in intracranial pressure, and has been called the "pattern of CNS disease." The reason why this *extracardiac* stimulus results in such striking EKG change is unclear.

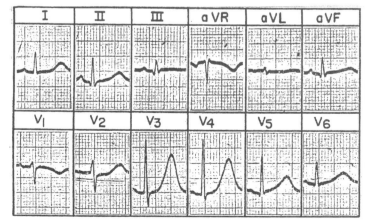

Occasionally, the EKG abnormality due to "CNS disease" presents as broad <u>upright</u> T waves. This 23 year old woman had a subarachnoid hemorrhage from a ruptured AV malformation. When the blood was removed, her tracing returned to normal.

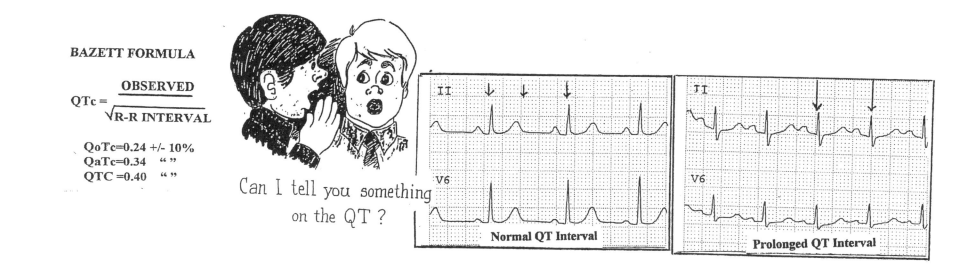

BAZETT FORMULA

$$QTc = \frac{OBSERVED}{\sqrt{R\text{-}R\ INTERVAL}}$$

QoTc=0.24 +/- 10%
QaTc=0.34 " "
QTC =0.40 " "

Can I tell you something on the QT ?

Normal QT Interval

Prolonged QT Interval

The QT interval, measured from the beginning of the QRS to the end of the T-wave, represents the time required from the onset of myocardial depolarization to the completion of repolarization. It is known as the "action potential duration." The QRS complex requires a minor portion of the total interval, and the ST and T waves are the major contributors. The QT is not a stable measurement, but varies with the heart rate, i.e., as the rate slows and the R-R cycle lengthens, the QT lengthens; as the rate accelerates, the QT shortness. A useful and easy rule is that the interval should be _less than half the R-R interval_. A formula for correction of the QT (Bazett formula) may be applied in questionable cases, but is infrequently required. The diagnostic value of the QT duration is seriously limited by the technical difficulties of measuring it exactly. The end of the T wave is not always a crisp landmark, and it is prudent to compare measurements of the QT in several leads. The EKG computer often seriously errors in its measurement. A prolonged QT means that there is delayed repolarization of the ventricular myocardium. This is associated with an increased predisposition to reentry, favoring the development of serious ventricular tachyarrhythmias, syncope, and sudden death. Numerous conditions, including drugs, have been incriminated as causing QT prolongation.
A number of examples will be shown.

CAUSES OF Q-T PROLONGATION

A. Primary-"Idiopathic"
B. Secondary
    a. Drugs: Antiarrhythic Drugs
        i. Antidepressants
        ii. Phenothiazines
        iii. Antihistamines
        iv. Antibiotics
    b. Electrolyte Derangements
        (Hypo K^+ Hypo Ca^{++} Hypo Mg^{++})
    c. Myocardial Ischemia
    d. Autonomic Effects
    e. CNS Lesions
    f. Hereditary/Genetic Disorders

88 YEAR OLD WOMAN-DID THE COMPUTER ACCURATLEY DETERMINE THE QT INTERVAL?

```
PR    178    +  Sinus bradycardia, rate 49 [Now Present]
QRSD   88    -  Nonspecific ST-T abnormalities [Now Present]
QT    495    -  [Now Absent] QT interval long for rate
QTc   447    -  [Now Absent] Diffuse ST-T abnormalities
--AXIS--
P      64
QRS    -2
T                     -OTHERWISE NORMAL ECG-
```

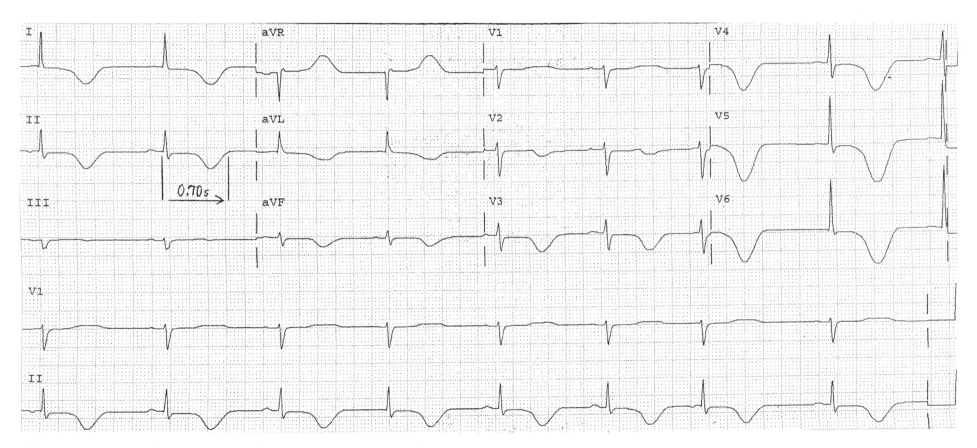

This woman presented with chest pain of three hours duration and elevated cardiac enzymes. The broad and deep T waves are accompanied by marked QT prolongation. For some reason, and despite the clear onset of the QRS and end of the T waves, the computer measures the QT interval at 0.495 sec.; and regards the repolarization abnormality as "nonspecific." In reality the QT is 0.70 sec. and the marked T wave troughs indicate serious and ongoing myocardial ischemia. Although there are a number of other potential causes, ischemic heart disease remains the most common explanation for the striking ST-T changes.

274

An important aspect of the repolarization is the interlude in recovery when the limb of phase 3 passes through the threshold potential to reach the resting membrane potential (approximating the apex of the surface T wave). This brief time has been termed the "vulnerable period" (lower arrow). A stimulus at this point will find the ventricular myocardium with marked repolarization "inhomogeneity." There will be cells that have completely recovered, some that are just beginning to recover, and still others that have not begun the process. Thus, this point will have the myocardium divided into a myriad of islands that are out of phase with each other--a perfect set up for a reentrant arrhythmia. Reports of tragic sudden death in athletes struck in the mid chest with a soccer ball, helmet, etc. are frequent, and carry the interesting description of death due to "commotio cordis." If this phase of cellular recovery is prolonged (dashed lines) by drugs or electrolyte imbalance, the vulnerable period is significantly increased (upper arrow) and the likelihood of a lethal arrhythmia is increased.

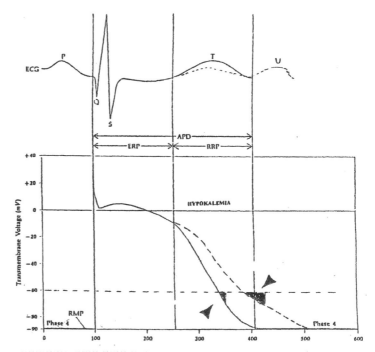

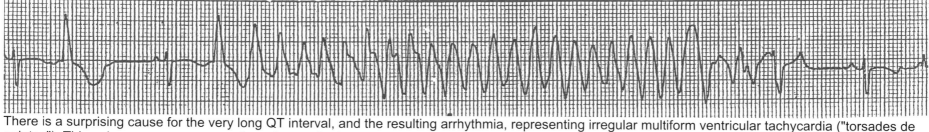

37 year old man - ER tracing

There is a surprising cause for the very long QT interval, and the resulting arrhythmia, representing irregular multiform ventricular tachycardia ("torsades de pointes"). This unhappy young man swallowed an entire bottle of an antihistamine (terfenadine) in a suicide attempt. This drug joins an increasingly long list of other drugs that prolong repolarization and can lead to this lethal arrhythmia. It is now "off the market."

49 YEAR OLD WOMAN-SYNCOPE OBSERVATIONS?? NEXT TRACING MAY REVEAL THE CAUSE??

RATE	96	+	Normal sinus rhythm, rate 96
PR	160	-	Diffuse ST-T abnormalities
QRSD	74		
QT	322		
QTc	407		

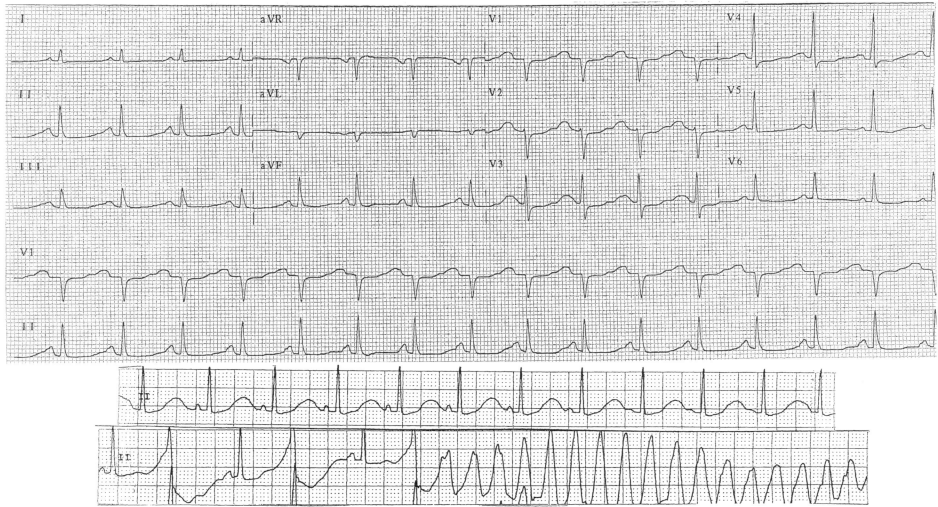

There is marked prolongation of the QT interval in the 12 lead tracing, and the top rhythm strip of lead II. This set the stage for the arrhythmia in the second segment. In this strip, sinus beats are following by VPCs that interrupt the delayed T wave. The third ectopic beat initiates an irregular, multiform ventricular tachycardia. This rhythm carries the term "torsades de pointes"--"twisting of the points." The number of causes which can result in QT prolongation, and this arrhythmia continues to increase. (and will be further discussed in another chapter). This woman was taking a polypharmacy" of medications, including large doses of methadone. She required 18 emergency cardioversions in the first 24 hours, and it was day after the drugs were stopped that the QT normalized.

47 YEAR OLD WOMAN-"BELLY PAIN"

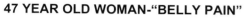

```
PR     191     +   Regular rhythm, undetermined origin, rate 98
QRSD    81     -   Diffuse ST-T abnormalities
QT     354         Possible ischemia
QTc    452         -ABNORMAL ECG-
```

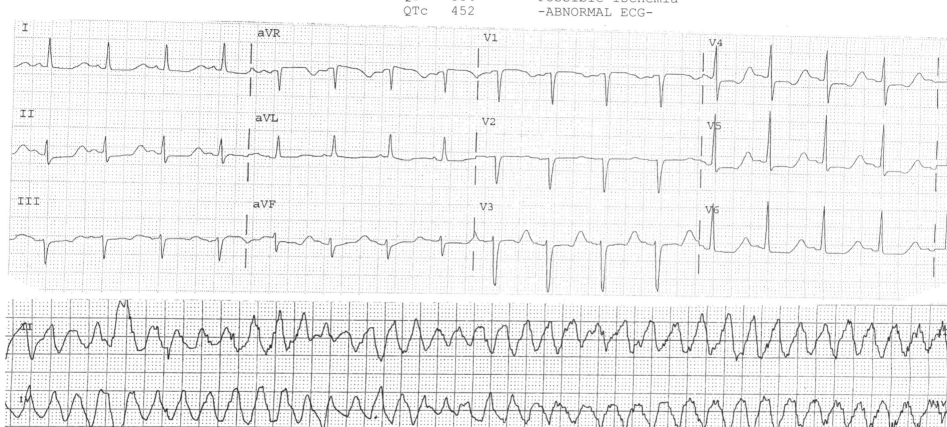

This woman presented with acute pancreatitis and an EKG showing a markedly long QT interval. The time between the onset of the QRS and the beginning of the T wave (QoT interval) is prolonged, and the T wave may be a combination of T + U waves. The electrolyte derangements of hypokalemia (2.7) and hypocalcemia (7) caused a long QT interval, and resulted in a lengthy run of irregular polymorphic ventricular tachycardia ("torsades de pointes").

277

52 YEAR OLD MAN
AFTER A VISIT TO THE DOCTOR!

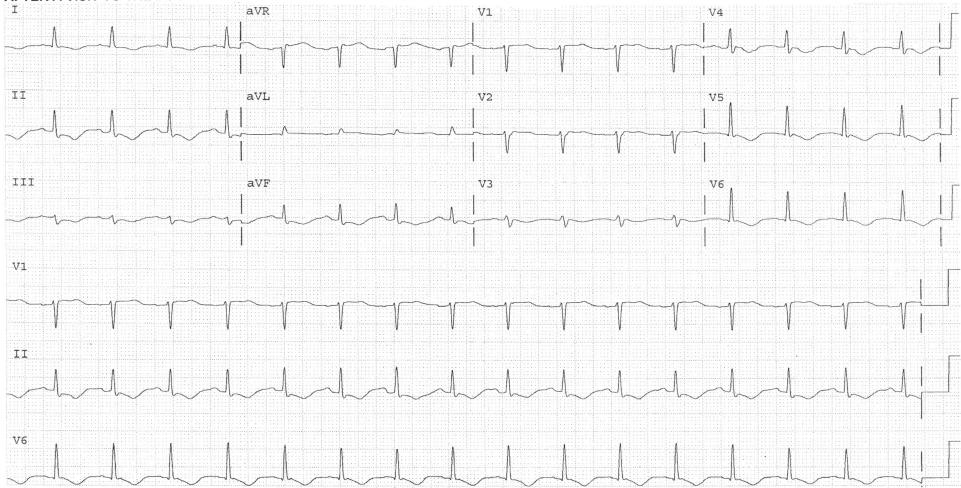

The EKG shows QT prolongation and diffuse T wave inversion-consistent with many things, but in this man it was due to "CNS disease." The doctor's "visit" involved chiropractic manipulation of the neck. It resulted in "syncope" due to cerebral artery thrombosis, and ultimately a "vegetative state." He became an organ donor. Axiom: the neck is an anatomic structure designed for neckties, necklaces, scarves, and the guillotine, and should only rarely be submitted to chiropractic manipulation!

PR   138   Normal sinus rhythm
QRSD   80   Probable LVH wit ST-abnormalities
QT   346   Poor R-wave progression, possibly due to LVH
QTc   444   ABNORMAL ECG
--AXES—
P   23
QRS   -22   **57 YEAR OLD WOMAN**
T   82   **ONCOLOGY SERVICE**
                     OBSERVATIONS?

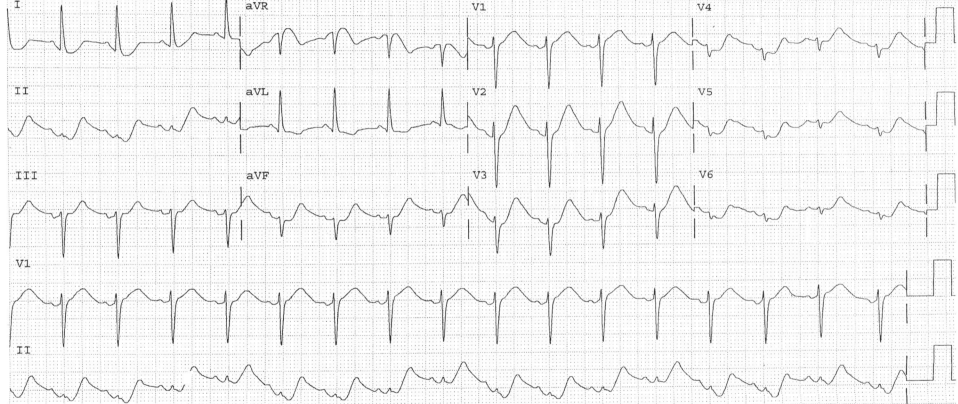

The computer diagnoses are partially correct, but the QT interval is longer than the computer measurement. "Poor R wave progression" is not due to LVH, but to the "insulating" effect of a large left pleural effusion. There is an additional problem! Cardiotoxic agents, including many of those used for cancer chemotherapy, can result in diffuse myocardial "damage." The resulting cellular abnormality may be expressed as diffuse repolarization changes, seen in most leads in this example as broad-based T waves and prolonged QT interval.

U WAVES

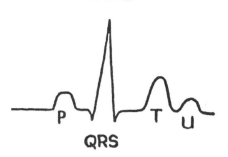

QRS

Normal U Waves
1. Same polarity as the T waves (But 5-50% of T amplitude)
2. Highest in Leads V2-V3 (Averages 0.33 mm. but may be 2 mm.)
3. U waves voltage varies directly with T wave voltage
4. Largest at slow rates (Almost imperceptible at rates greater than 90)

The U wave is a component of repolarization and is present in the normal EKG, probably representing the recovery of the Purkinje network. As indicated in the table, the normal U wave is small compared to the T wave and is upright in leads in which the T wave is recorded positive. The U wave becomes abnormal either because of its *amplitude* or *polarity*. Perhaps the most commonly recognized cause of increased U wave size is hypokalemia. Negative U waves are always abnormal, usually representing ongoing serious myocardial ischemia, less frequently hypokalemia. When the U wave is abnormal, current evidence is that it occurs because of inappropriate delay in repolarization of the middle layers of the left ventricular wall. Frequently, the U wave may blend with the late part of the T wave and be difficult to identify.

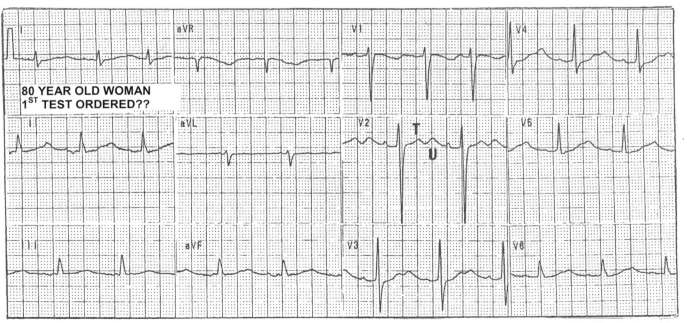

80 YEAR OLD WOMAN 1ST TEST ORDERED??

Diuretic use has resulted in this woman's hypokalemia of 2.3 mEq/L. The U wave in the precordial leads towers over the T wave and is an evident alert to the patient's electrolyte disturbance.

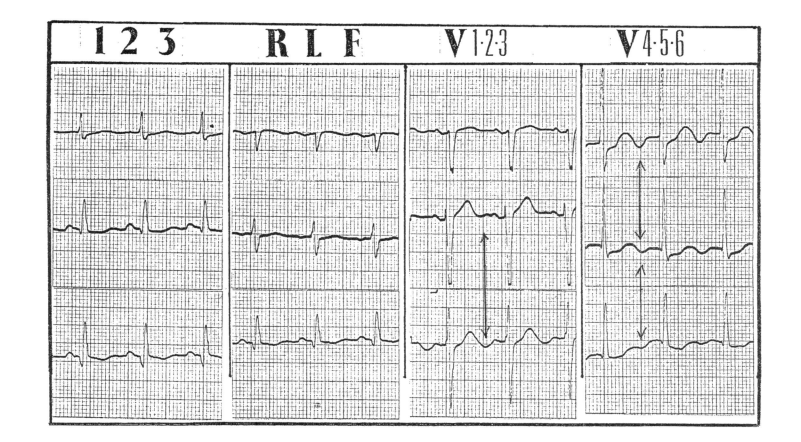

The tracing shows sinus rhythm with a frontal plane axis of (+) 70°. Q waves are present in leads II, III, and aVF reflecting a previous inferior M.I. QRS complexes in precordial leads V 1-2 and V4 exceed the limit of stylus excursion and their true amplitude is unknown, but there is probably LVH voltage. A noteworthy abnormality is prolongation of the QT-U interval with _negative U waves_ well seen in leads V3-6 (arrows). This 70-year-old man sustained an inferior infarction five years ago, and presented to the Emergency Department with increasing chest pain and the new inverted U waves. Coronary arteriography showed extensive, but operable, three vessel coronary artery disease and bypass surgery was performed.

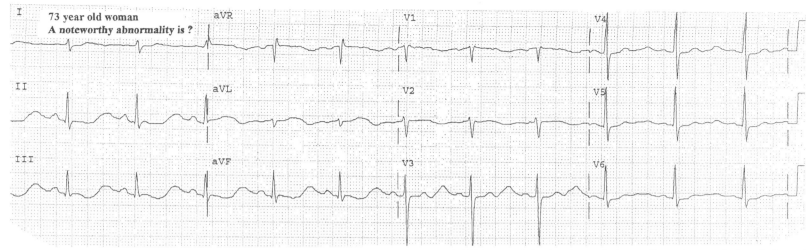

I   73 year old woman
    A noteworthy abnormality is ?   aVR   V1   V4

II   aVL   V2   V5

III   aVF   V3   V6

This EKG provides an explanation why hypokalemia is said to cause a prolonged QT interval. In the frontal plane, there is an obviously long interlude between the beginning of the QRS and the end of T wave. However, in the precordial leads V 3-5, it is apparent that the frontal plane "T wave" is an amalgam of a small T and a large U wave. The result is really a prolonged Q-T-U interval. Potassium level in this woman was 2.2, the result of diuretic therapy.

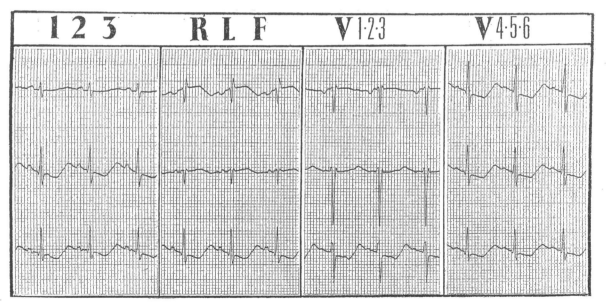

The rhythm is sinus at 95/minute, with a normal PR interval and QRS duration, and a frontal plane axis of + 90°. The ST segments are "sagging" and depressed in most leads and the QT interval is markedly prolonged, however, the apparent measurement is probably a combination of a negative T wave and a dominant positive U wave. Hypokalemia is a frequent cause of this EKG abnormality. This 24-year-old woman had the self-image that she was "too fat" and began a protracted fast, supplemented with the use of cathartics and emetics. When hospitalized she weighed 78 pounds and her serum potassium was 1.9. mEq/L.

282

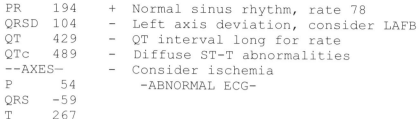

```
PR      194    +   Normal sinus rhythm, rate 78
QRSD    104    -   Left axis deviation, consider LAFB
QT      429    -   QT interval long for rate
QTc     489    -   Diffuse ST-T abnormalities
--AXES—        -   Consider ischemia
P        54         -ABNORMAL ECG-
QRS     -59
T       267
```

80 YEAR OLD WOMAN
AGREE WITH THE COMPUTER?

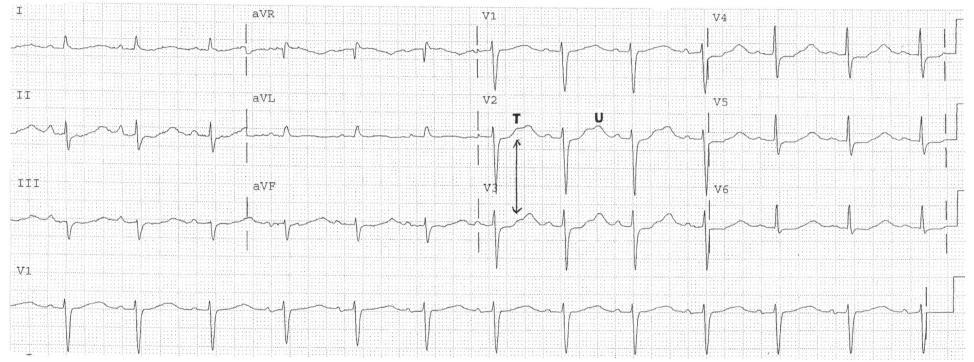

Sometimes, we join the computer in the inability to accurately measure the QT interval, and such is the case in this example. In leads V2-3, it is evident that the T wave is closely followed by a dominant U wave, and the actual end of the T wave is not seen, and, therefore, the QT interval is not evident. The tracing should raise concern that a drug effect or electrolyte imbalance is present. Her serum (K^+) was found to be 2.2, due to diuretic therapy. Her EKG normalized with potassium repletion.

The tracings to follow represent "patterns" of repolarization that, although not specific, are suggestive of an underlying problem or disease. You are invited to review them and suggest a diagnosis before reading the analysis provided. Obviously, clinical information is essential before the most thoughtful interpretation is possible.

Digitalis provides repolarization features that are reasonably characteristic. Unlike most cardioactive drugs, digitalis *shortens* the recovery time of the ventricular myocardium, and, thus, shortens the QT interval. The ST segment slopes downward and ends in a negative T wave. The P-R interval lengthens; mild prolongation is likely due to the vagal effect of the drug. These are not indications of digitalis *toxicity* but rather simple digitalis *effect*.

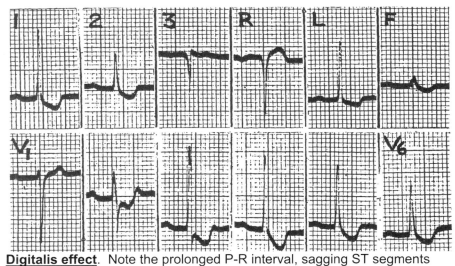

Digitalis effect. Note the prolonged P-R interval, sagging ST segments in most leads, with short Q-T interval.

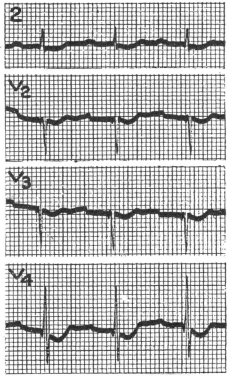

Digitalis effect. Note the sagging ST segments, even in leads that have negative QRS complexes; also the short Q-T interval and first-degree A-V block (P-R = 0.26 sec).

284

32 YEAR OLD MAN
DIFFERENTIAL DIAGNOSIS?

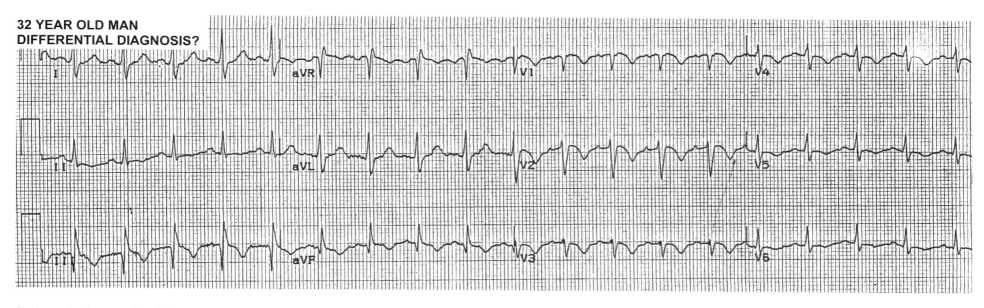

An important example of abnormal depolarization and repolarization. In the frontal plane, the Q waves in leads II, III, and aVF are accompanied by inverted T waves, consistent with an inferior wall infarction. In the horizontal plane, the inverted T waves in V1-6 are associated with abnormal R wave development, consistent with anterior MI. In reality, the EKG is that of serious pulmonary embolization--the so-called "McGinn-White pattern" of S1-Q3-T3, with anterior T wave inversion. An important axiom is: "when the frontal plane leads suggest inferior infarction and the precordial leads anterior infarction-think acute cor pulmonale." Pulmonary arteriogram in this young man showed major occlusive thrombi.

```
Sinus tachycardia, rate 111 [Remains]
Probable early repolarization pattern [Remains]
          -OTHERWISE NORMAL ECG-
```

32 YEAR OLD WOMAN-5/27
DO YOU AGREE?

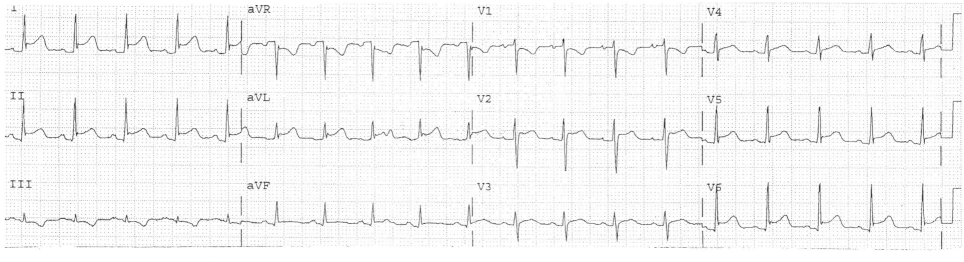

12/20-BASED ON YOUR DX ABOVE-
WHAT ARE SPODICK'S PHASES??

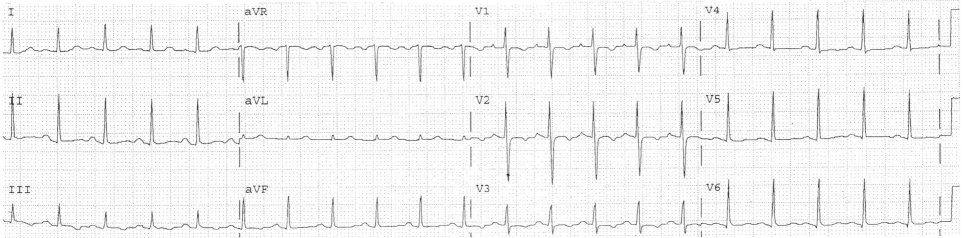

The tracing is a textbook EKG showing "pericarditis," with diffuse ST segment elevation and PR segment depression. Dr. David Spodick has been a student of pericardial disease for many years. He catalogued the diagnostic features in the top tracing as stage 1. In stage 2, the elevated ST segment returns to the baseline. In stage 3, the T waves invert, and the inversion may persist for many months after the acute episode (It lasted for seven months in this woman). In stage 4, the EKG returns to normal.

Spodick, D.H. Electrocardiogram in Acute Pericarditis   Am J. Cardiol. 1974: 33,470

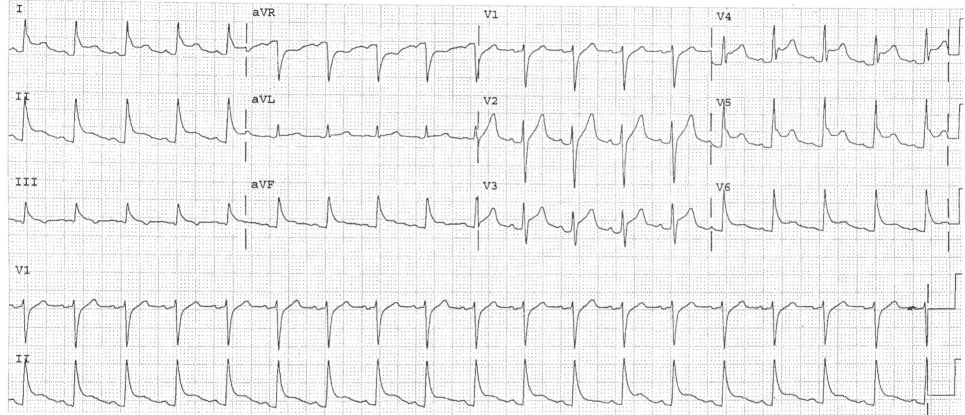

Note the diffuse ST segment elevation and PR segment depression, typical of pericarditis. The most impressive EKG examples in this condition tend to be in patients with uremic and purulent pericarditis. This man had a bloodstream infection, and the process involved the pericardium; 300 ml of frank pus was removed by pericardiocentesis.

67 YEAR OLD MAN – 7/12

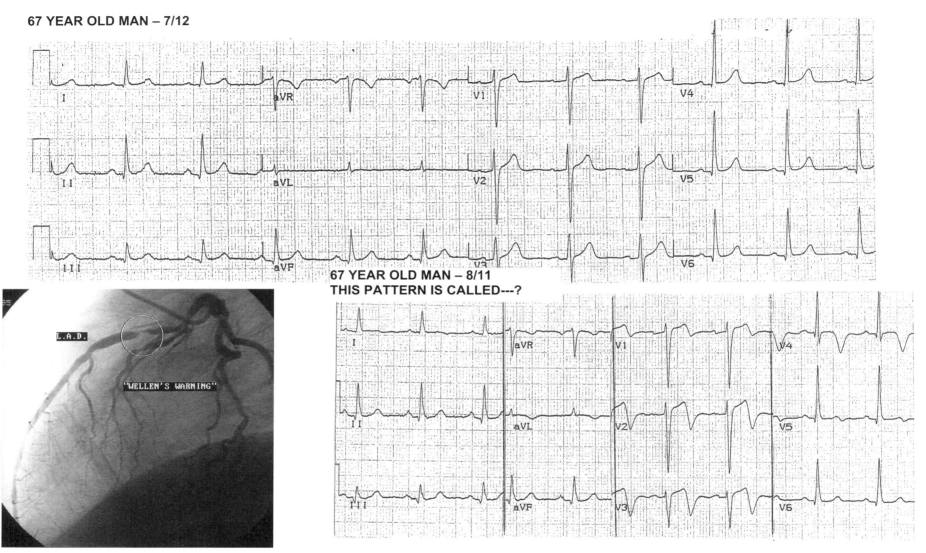

67 YEAR OLD MAN – 8/11
THIS PATTERN IS CALLED---?

Dr. Hein Wellens and his colleagues in 1987 described an EKG pattern with an important correlation. This man had sustained an inferior wall infarction four years earlier, with minimal EKG residuals. He presented to the Emergency Department on 7/12 complaining that he had had chest pain the preceding day. Since he was asymptomatic, his tracing unchanged from prior, and enzymes "negative," he was reassured and advised to return if the symptoms recurred. He returned on 8/11 with chest discomfort and the tracing shown. The noteworthy and evident abnormality is a slight ST segment elevation, and the initial positive portion of the T wave, followed by a sharp and precipitous descent to the bottom. This pattern was described by Wellens as correlating with a high grade and proximal obstruction of the left anterior descending coronary artery. The suggested term for this EKG pattern is "Wellens' warning." Note the angiographic lesion in this man; a threatening 90% occlusion of his LAD.   Am. Heart J. 1989; 117: 657.

61 YEAR OLD WOMAN
WHAT TYPE OF "ALTERNATION"?

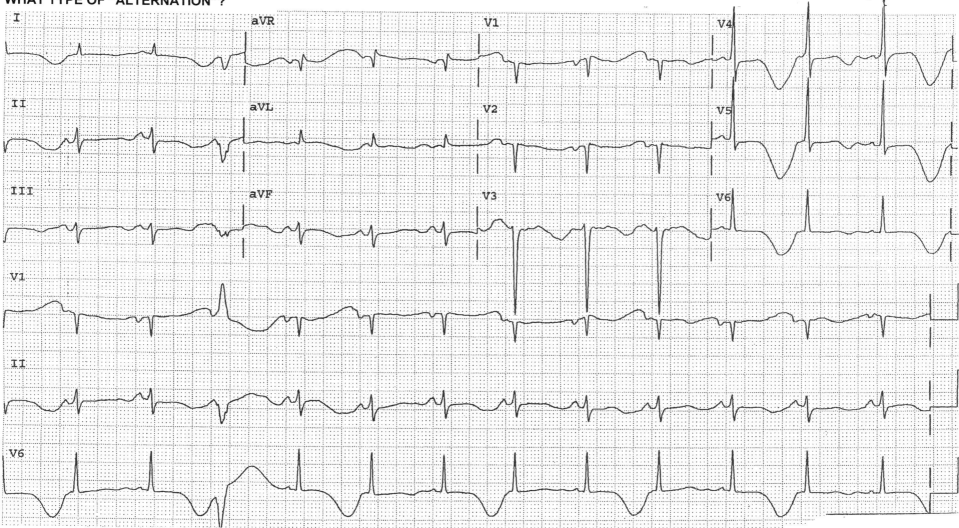

The markedly long QT interval is accompanied by evident alternation of the T-wave depth. Repolarization "alternans" is most often reported as due to serious myocardial ischemia, and less often to drugs or electrolyte derangements. This woman was admitted to the CCU and subsequently evolved an acute anterior wall infarction.

23 YEAR OLD WOMAN
WHAT IS THE "JERVELLE-
LANGE-NIELSEN SYNDROME?"

```
PR    283    +  Atrial pacer rate 90
QRSD   64    -  Diffuse Nonspecific T abnormalities
QT    188       -ABNORMAL ECG-
QTc   230
```

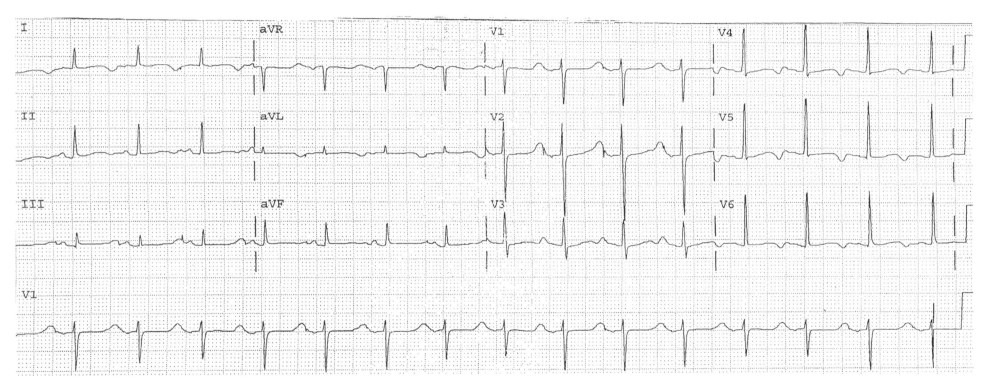

The syndrome is congenital deafness accompanying a long QT interval and, sadly, is associated with sudden arrhythmic death. This young woman has had several episodes of aborted sudden death. Note the incorrect computer measurements of the QT and rate-related QTc. The real numbers should be QT = 0.48 and the QTc = 0.60 (normal= 0.40). The atrium is being paced, but the QRS represents A-V conduction of the atrial stimulus.

290

84 YEAR OLD MAN -8/31-WHAT IS REPORTED TO BE EVIDENCE OF LEFT MAIN COR. ART. DISEASE??

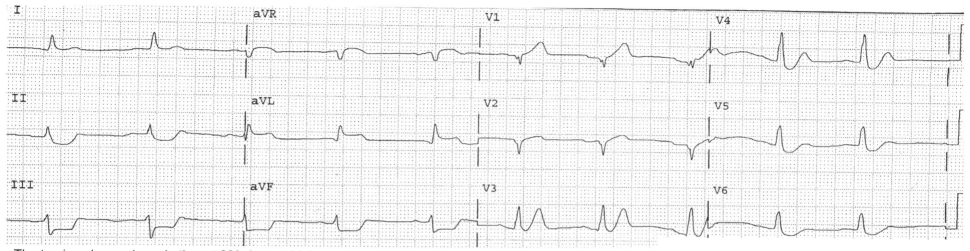

The tracing shows sinus rhythm at 60/minute with low-voltage QRS complexes and diffuse repolarization abnormality. The frontal plane leads show evidence of acute lateral wall infarction and the precordial leads probable septal M.I. Anything else? There have been several articles indicating ST segment elevation in <u>lead aVR</u>, more than that in lead V1, provides evidence that there is left main coronary artery occlusive disease. Consider this: if there is left main obstruction, both the left anterior descending and circumflex arteries are compromised. The ST segment "injury" vector becomes the resultant of <u>two wave fronts</u>--as depicted in the diagram. This vector is oriented to the *right and superior*, and would be recorded positive in lead aVR. Cardiac catheterization in this man revealed almost complete left main obstruction with minimal downstream flow. He died on the cath. table.

Yamaji, H et. al. Prediction of Acute Left Main Coronary Artery Obstruction by 12 Lead Electrocardiography
        J Am Coll Cardiol 2001; 5: 1348.

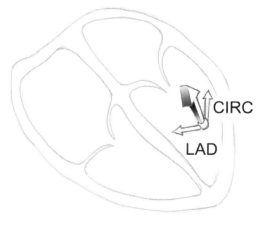

CIRC

LAD

79 YEAR OLD MAN-WHAT IS "APICAL HYPERTROPHIC CARDIOMYOPATHY"??

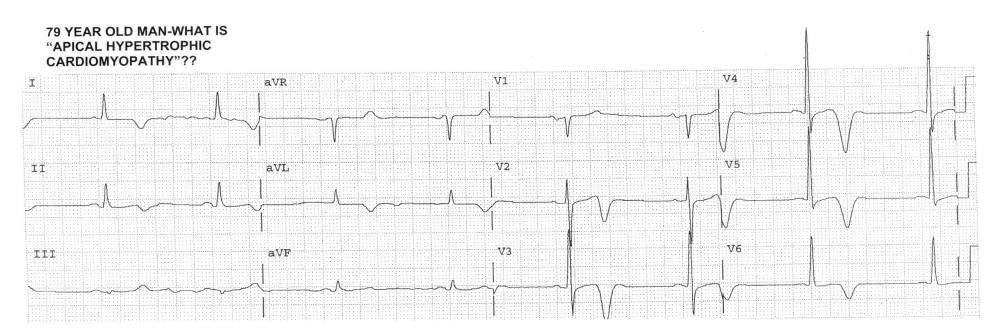

Sinus bradycardia of 50/min. is accompanied by precordial QRS voltage of LVH and diffuse marked T wave inversion. This pattern is seen with an unusual variety of "nonobstructive cardiomyopathy," with predominant apical hypertrophy. It was first described by Japanese authors in 1979, and since that time there have been many reports of cases throughout the world. As depicted in the illustration, angiograms show marked systolic obliteration of the LV apex. These EKG findings are regarded as characteristic of the problem. This patient has carried the same EKG for at least 10 years.

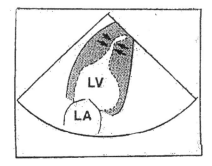

61 YEAR OLD MAN-"FOUND DOWN" HIS
SEASONAL PROBLEM IS??

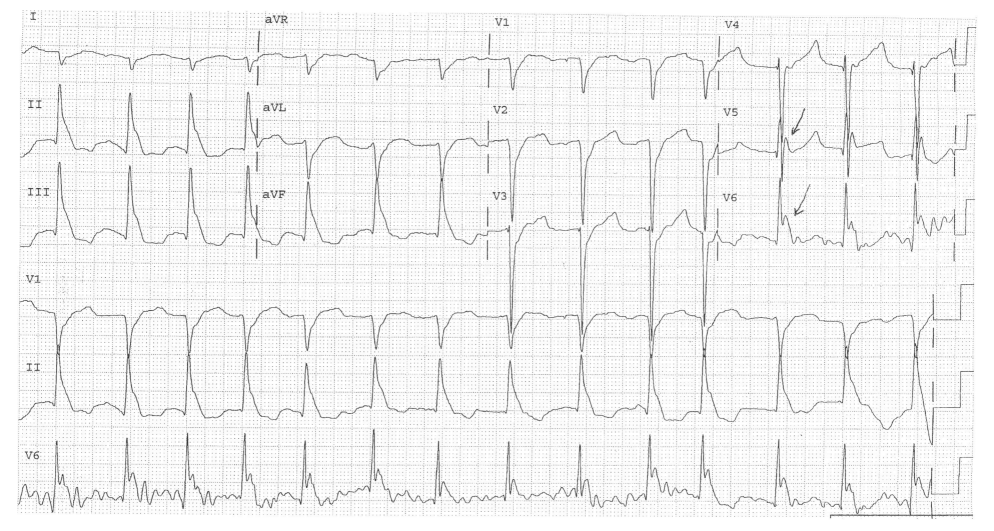

The "seasonal problem" was winter time cold. Although the tracing is technically poor, there are characteristic "Osborn waves" present and best seen in lead V6. Dr. J. J. Osborn, a cardiac surgeon, in 1953 presented the result of his experimental studies of induced hypothermia. He described the peculiar changes in the EKG and correlated them with the decrease in body temperature. Another picturesque term for this waveform is the "hypothermic hump." Other observations in this man include atrial fibrillation, LVH, and markedly increased Q-T interval. This man was found unconscious in an unheated room and, on presentation to the E.D. his rectal temperature was 84°. He arrested shortly after this tracing and could not be resuscitated.

71 YEAR OLD WOMAN
WHAT IS "TAKA-TSUBO SYNDORME"?

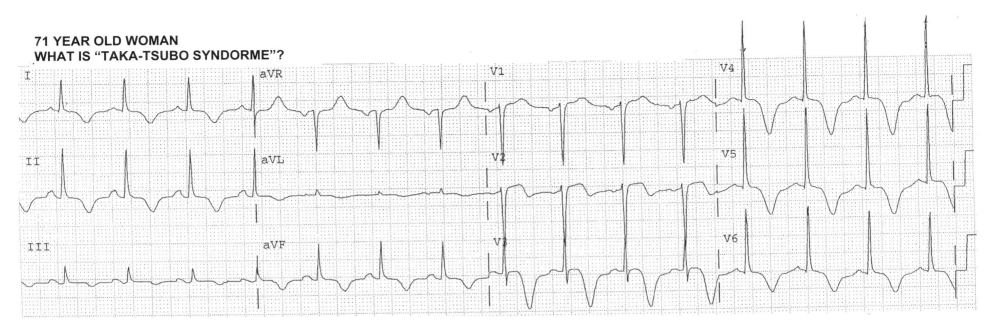

This interesting cardiac entity was described in Japan in 1970, but has been encountered worldwide. The syndrome consists of chest pain, ST segment elevation, positive cardiac enzymes, but <u>normal</u> (or mildly abnormal) coronary arteries. The left ventricle is abnormal in morphology showing apical "ballooning," resembling an octopus trap (hence the Japanese name). The cause is not yet clear, but the usual history is that the provocation is extreme emotional upset. It is postulated that there is a catecholamine surge leading to myocardial microvascular spasm. The prognosis is good, usually with normalization of LV anatomy and function in several weeks. This woman presented with substernal chest pain that began after a stressful domestic dispute. Troponin was elevated to 12.1 and her EKG is shown above. She was taken for urgent coronary arteriography, which showed only mild non-obstructive plaque in her arteries. The left ventricular ejection fraction was 30% and extensive anterior and inferior LV wall akinesis was present and thought to represent apical "ballooning." Follow-up echocardiogram one month later showed resolution of the abnormal LV morphology and an ejection fraction of 50-55%.

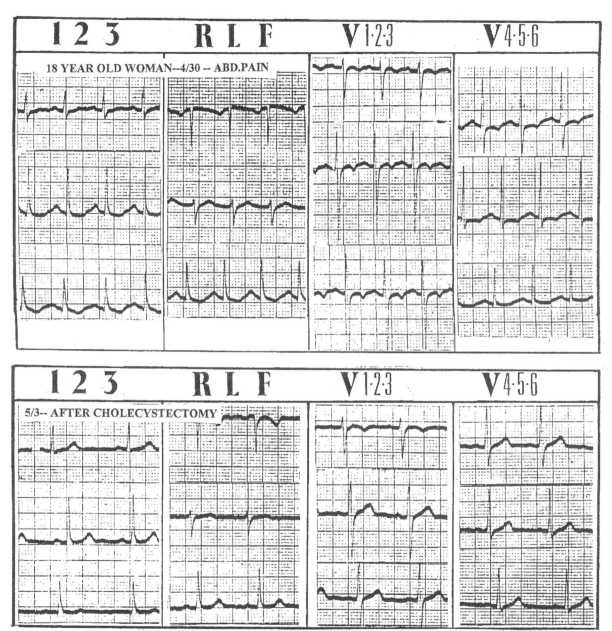

1 2 3	R L F	V 1·2·3	V 4·5·6

18 YEAR OLD WOMAN--4/30 -- ABD.PAIN

1 2 3	R L F	V 1·2·3	V 4·5·6

5/3-- AFTER CHOLECYSTECTOMY

An interesting and disturbing fact is that non-cardiac stimuli can result in EKG changes. Signals arising in the abdomen and central nervous system can significantly alter the electrocardiogram. The relationship is unclear, but is thought to represent abnormal autonomic input into the heart. The EKG above was obtained on 4/30 in a young woman with abdominal pain, due to acute cholecystitis. The ST depression and T wave inversion are evident. After cholecystectomy, the tracing on 5/3 returned to normal.

PRE-EXCITATION SYNDROMES

In 1930, Drs. Louis Wolff, John Parkinson, and Paul Dudley White collaborated on a publication which they entitled "Bundle Branch Block with Short PR interval in Healthy Young People Prone to Paroxysmal Tachycardia" (Amer. Heart J. 5: 685, 1930). Today, the abbreviation "WPW" is familiar to all. They deserve credit, but the title of the paper proves they were mistaken in the cause of the wide QRS complexes. We now know that the wide QRS complexes in WPW tracings are *not* due to bundle branch block, but to abnormal activation of the ventricles over an accessory pathway (A.P.) for impulse transmission. An unknown percentage of our population has this abnormality, but it is relatively common.

SINUS RHYTHM

As early as 1893, Kent described muscular connections between the atria and ventricles and later these became known as "bundles of Kent." The term remains a synonym for the "accessory pathway."
The illustration (**A**) depicts the anatomy that is involved. If one is born with an accessory pathway, there are two entries into the ventricle. With sinus rhythm, the atrial impulse has an option. It may cross the normal bridge and activate the ventricles normally (the dotted lines in figure (**B**). However, as an alternative, the stimulus can be transmitted over the accessory pathway and result in abnormal ventricular depolarization and repolarization. When the accessory pathway is used the familiar WPW complex is recorded.

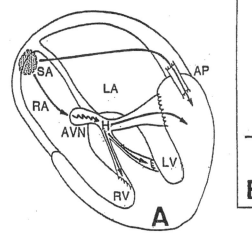
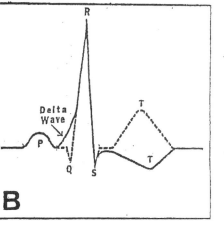

Features of WPW include:
1. A short PR interval (<0.12 sec) because the accessory pathway does not "slow" the atrial impulse as does the A-V node.
   Occasionally, the PR interval may be longer than 0.12 seconds if the accessory pathway is quite a distance from the impulse origin in the sinus node.
2. Since the accessory pathway delivers the stimulus before the normal bridge can transmit it, the ventricular is said to be "preexcited."
3. The earlier arrival of the signal via the A.P. results in premature depolarization of a variable area of the ventricular myocardium. Since the abnormal route lacks the availability of the rapidly conducting Purkinje fibers, the depolarization is slow intramyocardial conduction resulting in a delay in the initial upstroke of the QRS--the "delta wave." Depending on the degree of "preexcitation," the delta wave will increase in breadth, resulting in a variable increase in QRS duration.
4. Often, the same atrial impulse arrives via the normal A-V bridge and participates in total ventricular activation, representing "fusion" of the normal and abnormal activation impulses.
5. The abnormal sequence of ventricular activation will result in an abnormality of repolarization, with, at times, remarkable S-T changes.

It was many years before it was appreciated that the QRS might be widened either because part of the ventricular myocardium was activated _late_ (bundle branch block), or because part was activated _early_ (preexcitation). The QRS morphology in the figure contrasts typical right and left bundle branch block, and the WPW simulation of these conduction abnormalities. The arrows indicate the delay in ventricular activation-late in bundle branch block, and early in accessory pathway activation.

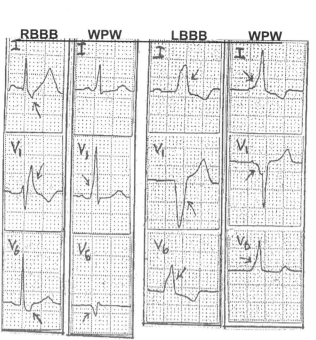

```
PR    143   .  Normal sinus rhythm, rate 60
QRSD  135   .  Left bundle branch block
QT    488   .  No previous tracing
                -ABNORMAL ECG-
```

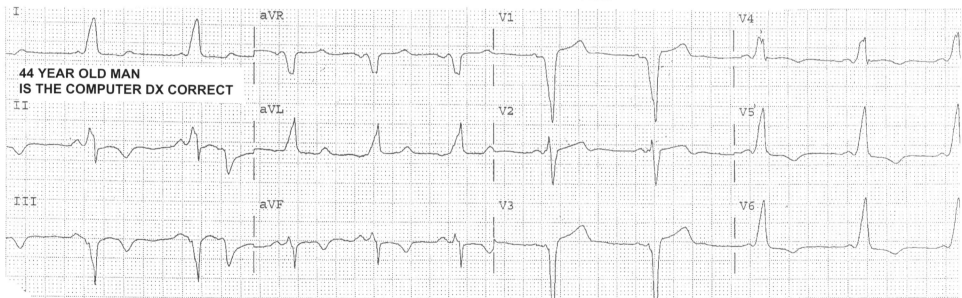

44 YEAR OLD MAN
IS THE COMPUTER DX CORRECT

An asymptomatic man applied for life insurance, and because of the size of the policy, a "routine" EKG was obtained. His application was refused because of the computer diagnosis. The simulation of "left bundle branch block" is good, but note that the major delay is in the _early portion_ of the QRS complex. The short P-R segment, and prominent delta wave in many leads, proves that the correct diagnosis should be preexcitation over an A.P. The negative deflection in V1 indicates that the pathway is situated in the right ventricle.

The "Kent bundle" was a pathway between the lateral left atrial wall, across the fibrous annulus to the left ventricle. For years it was thought that this was the only location of an accessory pathway. The advance of electrophysiologic studies demonstrated that this was not correct and that numerous pathways could be identified.

Dr. Melvin Scheinman and his colleagues have provided clarification of the zones where an A.P could be located. They identified eight areas where an AP was present (five on the right and three on the left). These are depicted in the illustration.

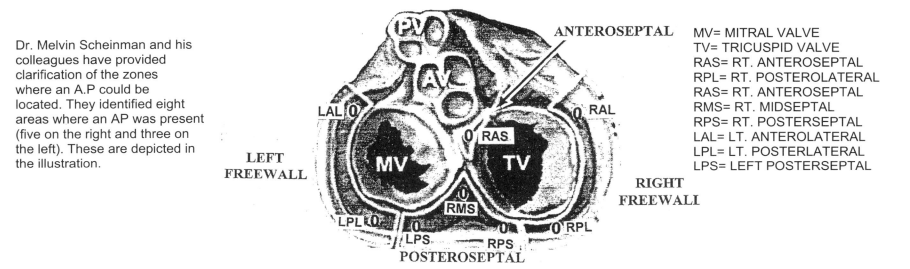

MV= MITRAL VALVE
TV= TRICUSPID VALVE
RAS= RT. ANTEROSEPTAL
RPL= RT. POSTEROLATERAL
RAS= RT. ANTEROSEPTAL
RMS= RT. MIDSEPTAL
RPS= RT. POSTERSEPTAL
LAL= LT. ANTEROLATERAL
LPL= LT. POSTERLATERAL
LPS= LEFT POSTERSEPTAL

It should be evident that the sequence of abnormal ventricular activation will depend on the delivery of the early stimulus-the location of the accessory pathway. The general location of the pathways can be surmised by simple observations.
1. If the preexcited QRS complex is predominantly positive in lead V1, resembling *RBBB*, the stimulus has arrived via a
   left sided pathway.
2. If the QRS is predominantly negative in V1, simulating *LBBB*, the "bypass tract" is right-sided in location.
3. If the delta waves are oriented to the right and, thus, negative in leads I and aVL, the accessory pathway is located in the
   left lateral atrial wall.
4. The direction of initial deflections in leads II, III, and aVF indicate, with reasonable accuracy, the location of the septal
   pathways. When they are positive, the pathway is anteroseptal; when negative it is posteroseptal.

The preexcitation of the ventricles can lead to a number of problems. Some are due to the abnormal anatomy itself and, unfortunately, others are due to incorrect diagnosis by the computer or by the interpreter.
1. The dual pathways-the AV bridge and the accessory pathway-are a perfect circuit for reentrant supraventricular tachycardias.
2. The availability of the "bypass tract" in the presence of atrial fibrillation can allow the ventricle to be bombarded by impulses passing over the abnormal pathway,
   leading to life-threatening arrhythmia.
3. The altered sequence of depolarization can *simulate*: Bundle Branch Block; Myocardial Infarction; or Ventricular Hypertrophy.
4. The repolarization abnormality due to the abnormal ventricular activation can lead to an incorrect diagnosis of "ischemia."

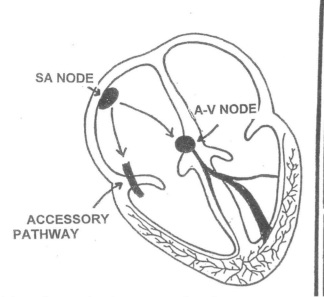

SA NODE

A-V NODE

ACCESSORY
PATHWAY

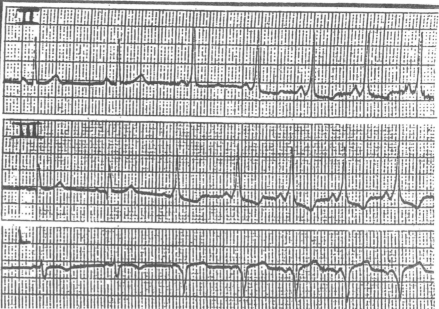

An interesting contrast occurs as sinus impulses, which are an initially normally conducted, began to cross the accessory pathway. Note that as the P-R interval shortens, the delta wave increases and the repolarization abnormality becomes more marked. In the two normal beats in lead aVL, the initial r wave is replaced by a "Q wave," which is actually a *negative* delta wave.

Sometimes the evidence of an accessory pathway is inconclusive. A simple expedient is to provide a vagatonic stimulus (e.g. carotid massage, Valsalva maneuver, etc.) to decrease AV nodal conduction. This will diminish the sinus node stimulus over the AP and increase the degree of "preexcitation." In the example to the right, carotid sinus massage was briefly applied in each lead (the dark lines). The sinus rate promptly slows, the PR interval shortens, and obvious delta waves appear with an increase in the QRS duration. Prominent repolarization abnormality accompanies the induced depolarization changes. A similar result would be expected with the AV nodal blocking drug adenosine.

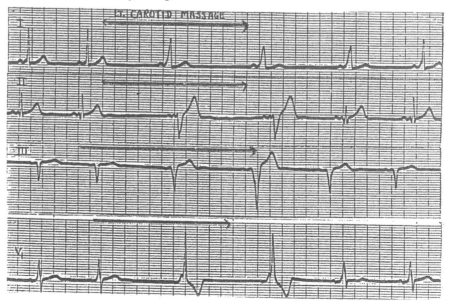

48 YEAR OLD MAN
 YOUR DIFFERENTIAL DIAGNOSIS?

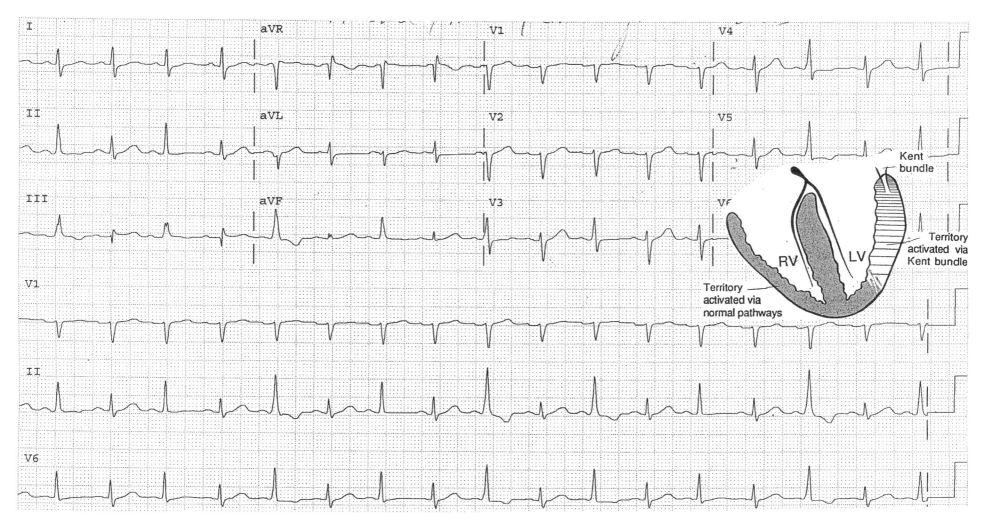

Note that alternate QRS complexes vary in morphology--Why? The availability of two pathways into the ventricle can permit an interesting array of "fusion complexes." When the sinus node impulse travels simultaneously over both limbs, the contribution over the accessory pathway may vary. This will lead to WPW complexes with a variable degree of PR interval shortening, preexcitation, and QRS duration.

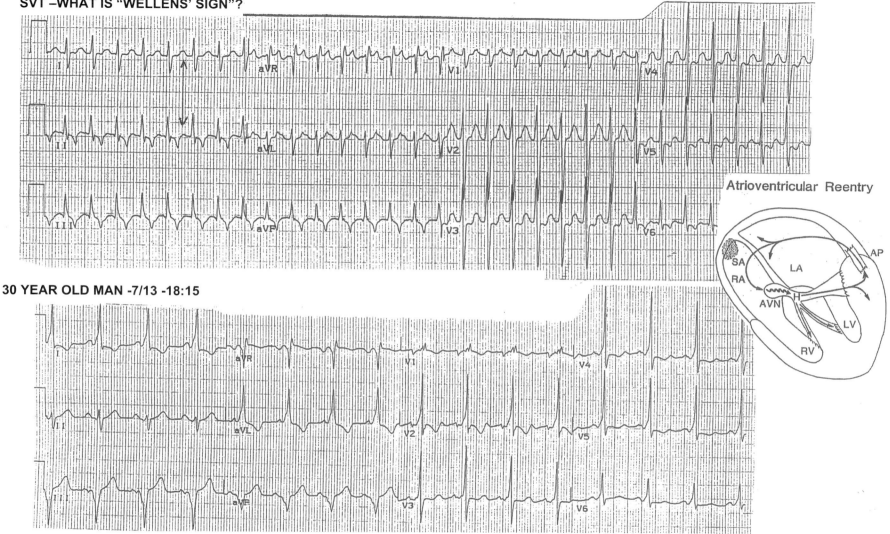

30 YEAR OLD MAN – 7/13 -18:01
SVT –WHAT IS "WELLENS' SIGN"?

Atrioventricular Reentry

30 YEAR OLD MAN -7/13 -18:15

The availability of both the normal A-V bridge and the "Kent bundle" provides a perfect reentrant circuit. The illustration shows the "anatomy" of this tachycardia. A premature atrial stimulus conducts over the normal AV connection, activates the ventricle, and crosses the accessory pathway (AP) retrogradely to return to the atrium and to continue the chase. A term for this variety of SVT is "*orthodromic* AV reentrant tachycardia." Since the reentrant impulse enters the ventricle normally, the QRS morphology is normal, unless there is pre-existing bundle branch block. A very solid clue to the diagnosis was provided by Dr. Hein Wellens. He observed that, in many examples of the A-V reentrant tachycardia, there was alternation of QRS amplitude. (Note leads V4-5). In the top tracing, there is a SVT at 200 per min. Note the timing of the T wave in lead I and compare to lead II (arrow). The prominent trough in lead II is not a T wave, but a negative P wave located 80 msec after the QRS complex. This delay is due to the time required for ventricular depolarization and passage of the retrograde stimulus over the accessory pathway to the atrium. After conversion of the tachycardia, the QRS shows typical WPW morphology, proving the presence of an accessory pathway.

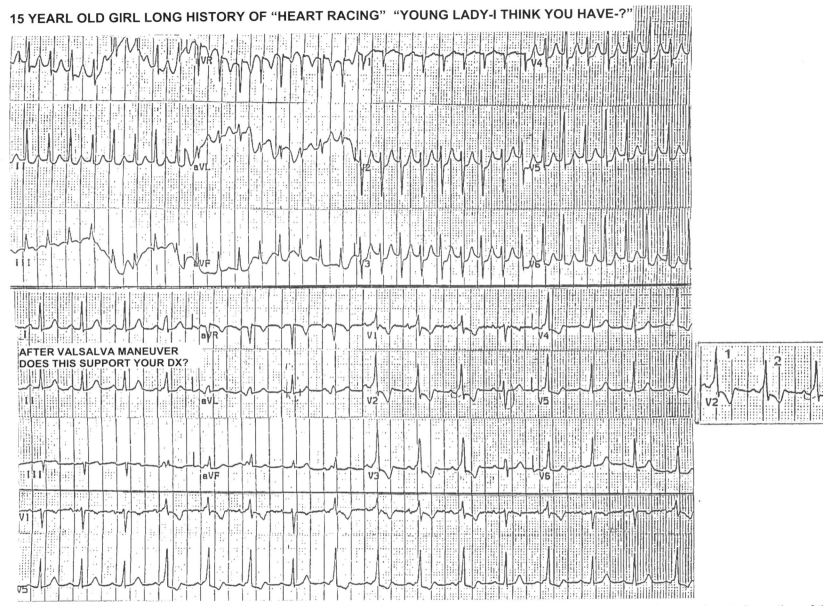

15 YEARL OLD GIRL LONG HISTORY OF "HEART RACING" "YOUNG LADY-I THINK YOU HAVE-?"

AFTER VALSALVA MANEUVER
DOES THIS SUPPORT YOUR DX?

This is an interesting example of A-V reentrant tachycardia utilizing an accessory pathway. In the top tracing, note the prominent alternation of the QRS complexes in many leads-"Wellens' sign"-evidence that this is an orthodromic tachycardia. After conversion, the sinus impulses have an option: transmission may occur over the normal A-V bridge, over the accessory pathway, or over both. The enlarged lead V2 (box) is an instructive example. QRS #1 represents maximal use of the accessory path, #4 uses the normal path, and #2 and 3 are fusion complexes representing simultaneous use of both pathways.

66 YEAR OLD MAN -8/19
MECHANISM OF THE S.V.T??

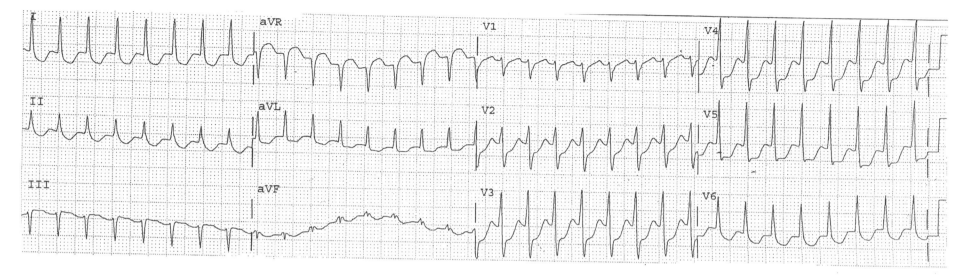

PRIOR TRACING-DOES THIS PROVIDE ANY CLUE??

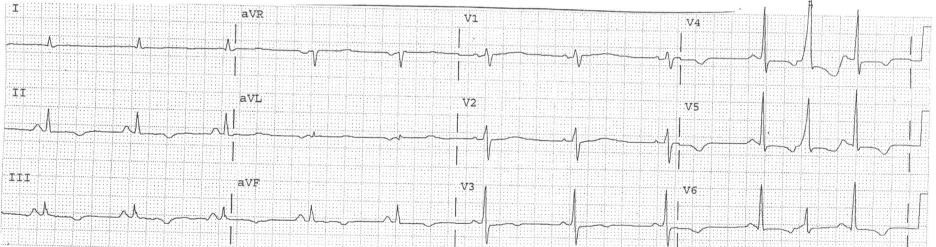

The regularity would remove atrial fibrillation and multifocal atrial tachycardia as contenders. The rate of 200/min would make atrial flutter and AV nodal reentrant tachycardia unlikely. The best bet is that the mechanism is AV reentrant tachycardia utilizing an accessory pathway. The lower tracing is a gift. Note that the APC in leads V4-6 is conducted with a short PR interval and a prominent delta wave, indicating the presence of an accessory pathway characteristic of WPW conduction. This provides proof that the tachycardia is AV reentrant.

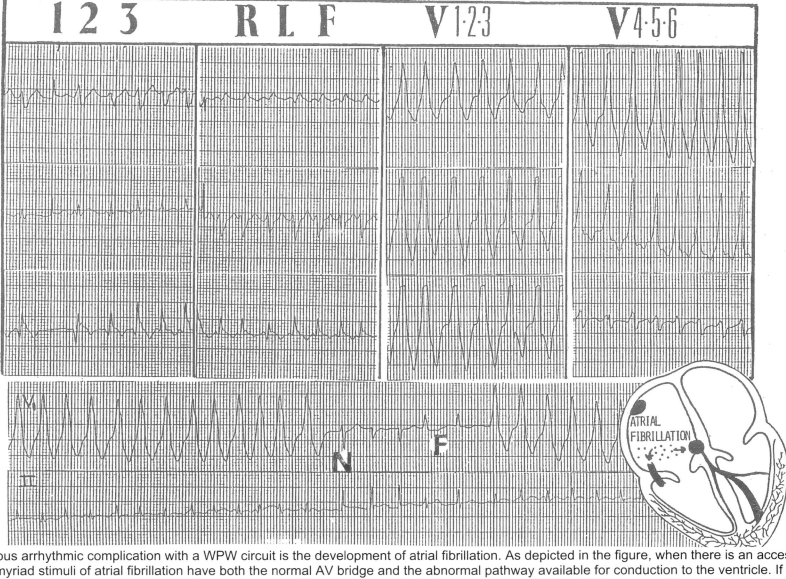

The most serious arrhythmic complication with a WPW circuit is the development of atrial fibrillation. As depicted in the figure, when there is an accessory pathway, the myriad stimuli of atrial fibrillation have both the normal AV bridge and the abnormal pathway available for conduction to the ventricle. If the refractory period of the accessory path is less than that of the AV node, or if its conduction velocity is greater, most of the atrial impulses will cross the accessory pathway. The result will be a rapid, irregular, wide complex tachycardia. If some of atrial impulses are normally conducted, the resulting QRS will be a normal (**N**). If the stimuli pass over both channels, fusion complexes (**F**) will be recorded.

29 YEAR OL MAN
YOUR DX AT A GLANCE?

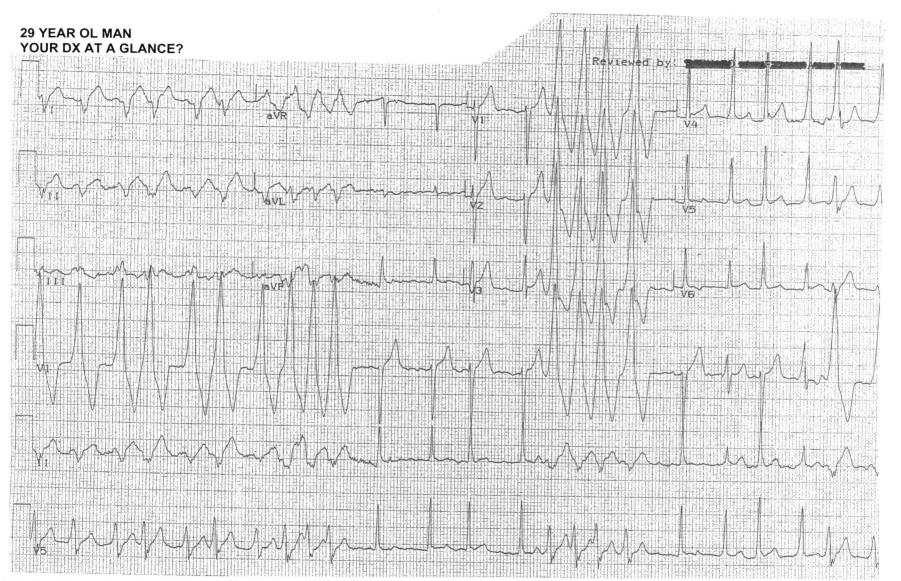

Note the bizarre, irregular, wide QRS complexes interspersed with irregular narrow ones. This is the result of atrial fibrillation in the presence of an accessory pathway. Some of the atrial impulses conduct normally, some via the A.P., and some pass over both pathway simultaneously resulting in ventricular fusion complexes. This is a very distinctive and important EKG pattern. Early observers misinterpreted the wide complexes as due to "ventricular tachycardia" leading to the incorrect conclusion that ventricular tachycardia was often irregular.

29 YEAR OLD MAN -3/25-15:17
WHAT RX HAS BEEN GIVEN??

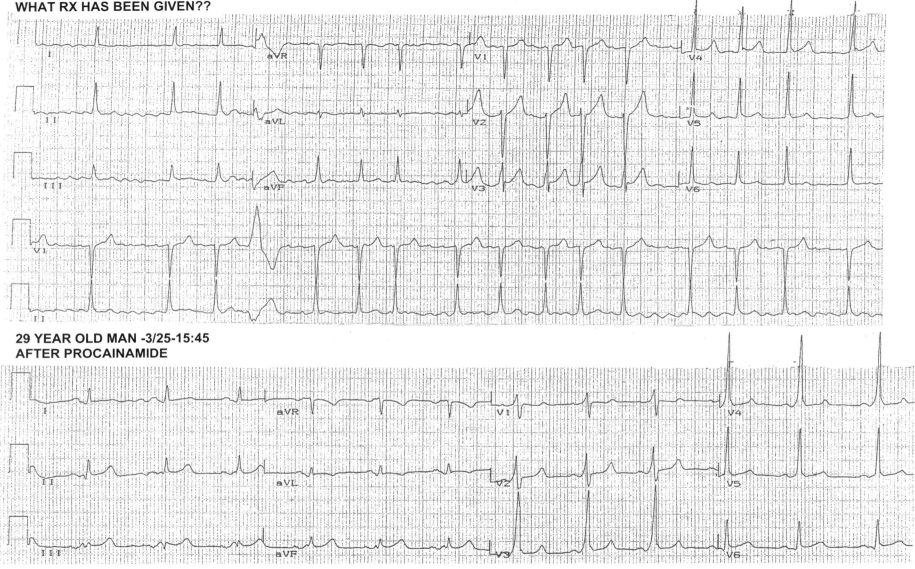

29 YEAR OLD MAN -3/25-15:45
AFTER PROCAINAMIDE

The tracing is a follow-up in the patient on the preceding page. The options for treatment are defined by the clinical condition. If the patient is unstable, <u>prompt</u> cardioversion should be accomplished. If the situation is less critical, IV procainamide can be administered. This drug will inhibit transmission over the accessory pathway and slow the ventricular rate. In the top tracing, some 20 minutes after the drug was given, the rate has decreased and the conduction is mostly over the normal A-V bridge. A single wide complex remains and has the same QRS morphology as seen in the prior EKG. In the bottom tracing, this young man has converted to sinus rhythm, with QRS morphology typical for accessory pathway activation. The negative delta waves in leads I and aVL indicate that the pathway is located in the lateral aspect of the left atrium.

26 YEAR OLD MAN
AGREE WITH THE COMPUTER?

PR		VENTRICULAR TACHYCARDIA, RATE = 164
QRSD	157	No further analysis will be attempted
QT	318	-ABNORMAL ECG-
QTc	525	

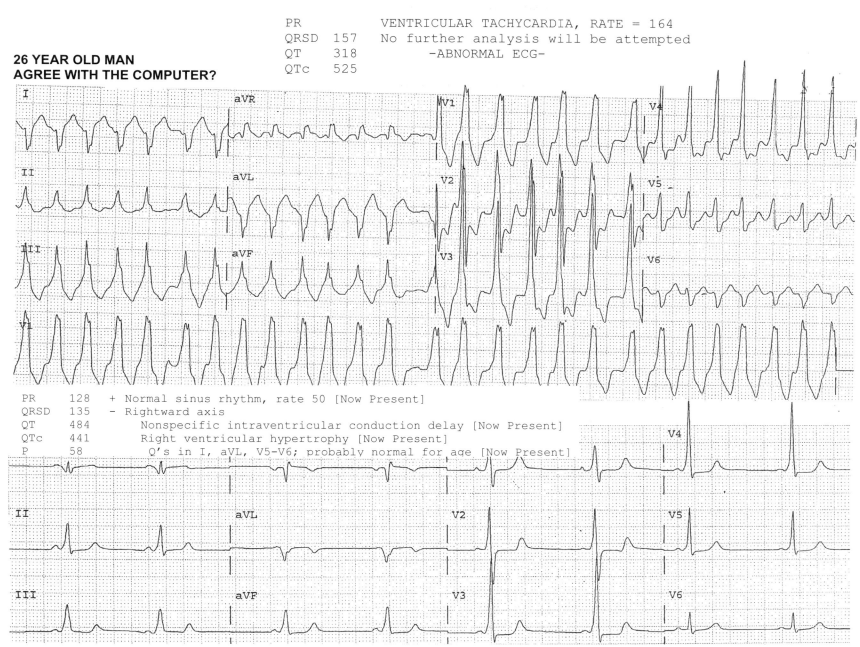

PR	128	+ Normal sinus rhythm, rate 50 [Now Present]
QRSD	135	- Rightward axis
QT	484	Nonspecific intraventricular conduction delay [Now Present]
QTc	441	Right ventricular hypertrophy [Now Present]
P	58	Q's in I, aVL, V5-V6; probably normal for age [Now Present]

The computer interpretation of the top tracing is based on the wide and bizarre QRS complexes, which could be consistent with ventricular tachycardia, but the evident irregularity denies this. This is another example of atrial fibrillation with conduction over an accessory pathway. In the bottom tracing, note the listing of ominous diagnoses that are provided by the computer. The preexcitation of the ventricles is responsible for all of the QRS abnormalities. Activation over an accessory pathway prevents our ability to validly interpret both the direction and duration of QRS forces.

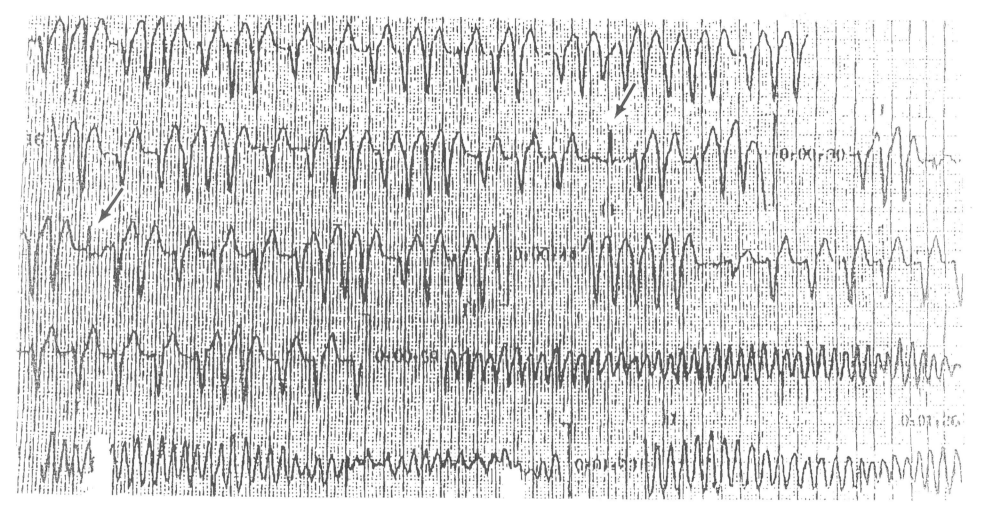

The source of this frightening tracing is not recalled, but, if "borrowed," the theft is perhaps justifiable. The gross irregularity and variable QRS morphology indicate that the rhythm is atrial fibrillation with dominant and rapid conduction over an accessory pathway. Single normally conducted beats are present (arrows) and the intermediate morphology complexes identify fusion beats. The burden of this tachycardia results in ventricular fibrillation!

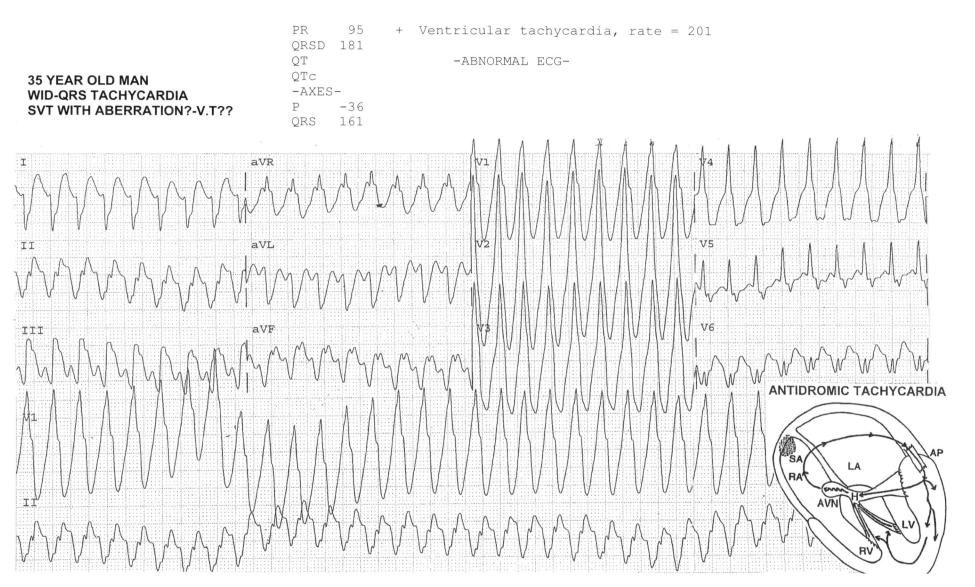

35 YEAR OLD MAN
WID-QRS TACHYCARDIA
SVT WITH ABERRATION?-V.T??

```
PR      95    +  Ventricular tachycardia, rate = 201
QRSD   181
QT                      -ABNORMAL ECG-
QTc
-AXES-
P      -36
QRS    161
```

ANTIDROMIC TACHYCARDIA

If a premature atrial impulse finds the normal AV bridge unavailable, and the accessory pathway responsive, it may establish a reentrant circuit with the accessory pathway the antegrade limb and A-V node the retrograde. This is depicted in the diagram and has been termed "antidromic tachycardia." Since the ventricles are abnormally activated, the QRS morphology may perfectly mimic ventricular tachycardia. The truth of the matter will become evident after rhythm conversion, with WPW complexes seen during sinus rhythm.

PR	100	+	Sinus tachycardia, rate 146
QRSD	95	.	Lateral region Q waves noted
QT	258	.	Nonspecific Inferior T wave abnormalities
QTc	402	.	Cannot exclude ischemia
-AXES-			-ABNORMAL ECG-
P	68		
QRS	78		
T	-36		

46 YEAR OLD MAN
SINGLE TRACING IN THE E.D.
DO YOU AGREE WITH THE COMPUTER?

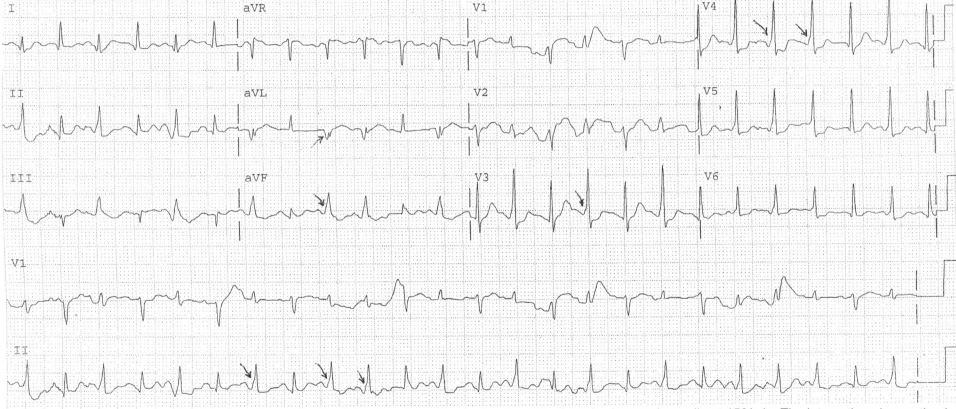

Let's disagree with the computer. The baseline artifact is distracting, but with careful attention, there is sinus tachycardia at 150/min. The interesting observation is that many of the atrial impulses are conducted over an accessory pathway, changing the initial part of the QRS complex, and producing delta waves (arrows). These are negative in leads I and AV L, indicating that the accessory pathway is *left lateral* in location. During part of the recording bigeminal WPW complexes are present.

PR	125	+ Sinus tachycardia, rate 120
QRSD	93	. Early transition
QT	316	. Consider left atrial enlargement
QTc	446	. Poor R-wave progression
-AXES-		. Diffuse ST-T abnormalities
P	45	. Consider ischemia
QRS	6	-ABNORMAL ECG-
T	237	

42 YEAR OLD WOMAN. DO YOU AGREE?
PLEASE SUGGEST AN ALTERNATIVE DIAGNOSIS.

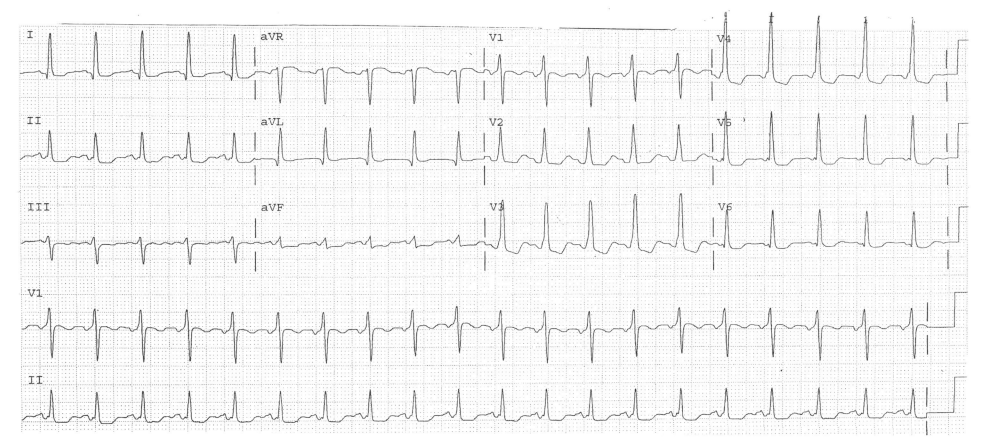

The computer identified the sinus rate, but struck out in everything else! The short P-R segment and evident delta waves in many leads indicates that an accessory pathway is present. Since there is an abnormal sequence of ventricular activation, it will be accompanied by abnormal repolarization. The ST-T changes with WPW, although diffuse and significant, do not allow the conclusion of "ischemia." Note that the delta wave in leads I and aVL are negative identifying a left lateral accessory pathway.

**44 YEAR OLD MAN-SCHEDULED
FOR T.M. TEST- WOULD YOU PROCEED?
WHY NOT?**

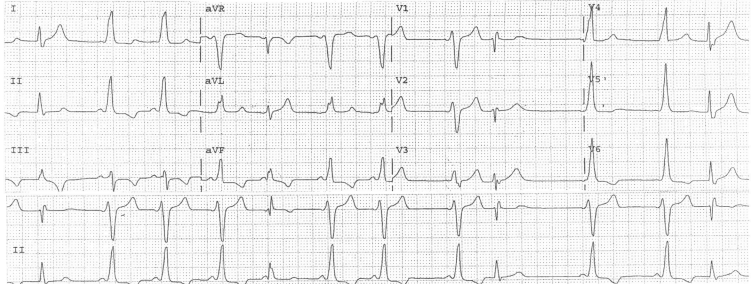

The sinus rhythm is irregular and the dominant QRS morphology occurs with a short P-R interval and a prominent delta wave on the upstroke --a rather typical WPW pattern. Significant repolarization abnormality accompanies the abnormal depolarization and this would make any EKG changes, with standard exercise testing, impossible to interpret. The narrow complexes are of interest. They are probably junctional in origin and do not share access to the accessory pathway. They are conducted over the normal A-V bridge and show incomplete RBBB and abnormal T wave vector in the frontal plane.

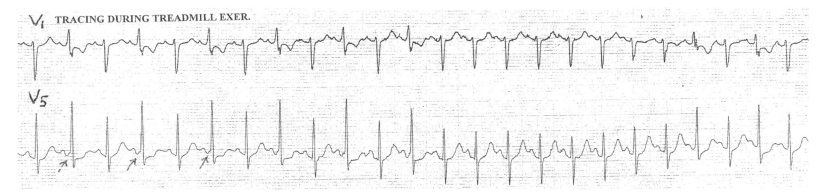

A case in point. This young man applied for pilot training, which was refused because his routine EKG showed "ischemia." A treadmill exercise test was performed with an interesting result. During exercise, many of the QRS complexes showed a short PR interval and delta waves (arrows) indicating the presence of an accessory pathway. The WPW complexes have significant ST segment depression, not present in the normally conducted beats. Happily, the conduction abnormality was recognized, or the incorrect diagnosis of ischemia" would have continued.

312

```
PR     117    +   Sinus tachycardia, rate 112
QRSD   115    .   Incomplete left bundle branch block
QT     346    .   Consider left atrial enlargement
QTc    472        -ABNORMAL ECG-
-AXES-
P       81
QRS      3
T      123
```

HIS HISTORY IS:?
1. **CHEST PAIN?**
2. **PULLED MY BACK AT WORK?**
3. **HEART RACING?**

35 YEAR OLD MAN
DO YOU AGREE WITH REVIEWER??

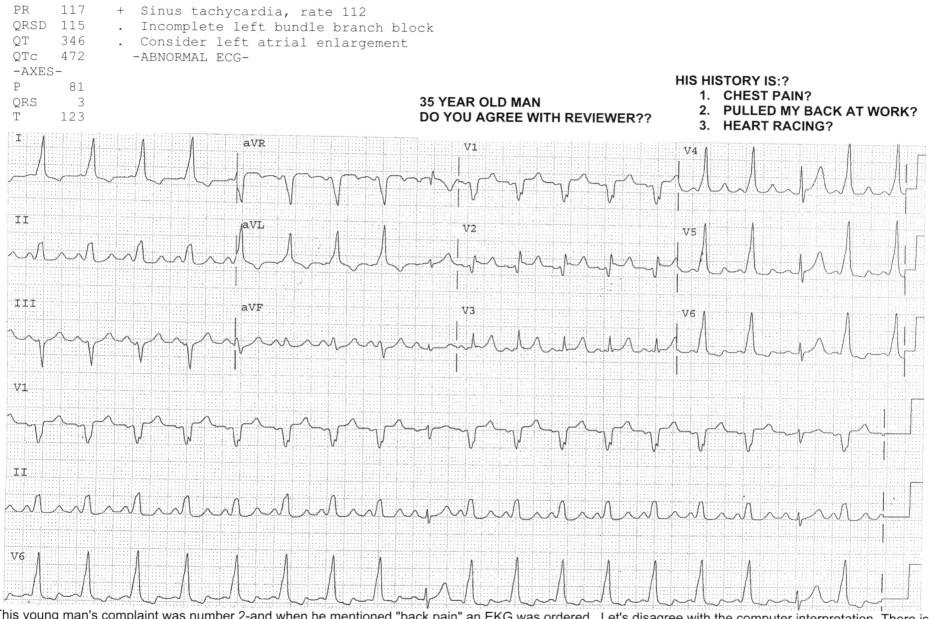

This young man's complaint was number 2-and when he mentioned "back pain" an EKG was ordered. Let's disagree with the computer interpretation. There is a conduction abnormality, but it's not left bundle branch block. The tracing shows sinus rhythm with a short P-R interval and a prominent delta "slur" on the QRS upstroke, consistent with accessory pathway activation of the ventricles. Note that two P waves are normally conducted. The dominant negative morphology in lead V1 indicates that the accessory pathway is probably located in the right ventricle.

```
PR      149    +  Normal sinus rhythm, rate 73
QRSD    166    .  Superior axis
QT      480    .  Right bundle branch block
QTc     529    .  Consider left anterior fascicular block
-AXES-         .  Lateral region ST-T abnormalities
P        53            -ABNORMAL ECG-
QRS     -88
T       102
```

77 YEAR OLD MAN
DO YOU AGREE?

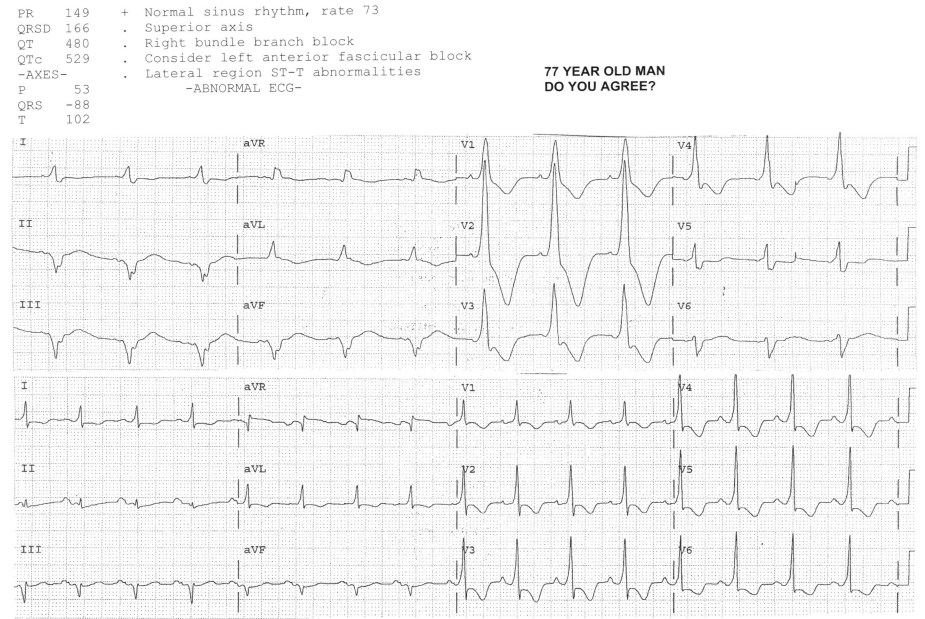

Although the QRS complex is broad and positive in lead V1, it is not due to right bundle branch block. Notice that the P-R interval is short and that delta waves are present-particularly in leads V3-V5. The bizarre QRS is due to *maximum* use of the accessory pathway-"complete preexcitation." (Perhaps this is why W-P and W mistakenly thought that the wide complexes were due to bundle branch block?). The bottom tracing was obtained a day earlier and shows less contribution over the accessory pathway and a more conventional degree of "preexcitation" and a more typical WPW <u>pattern</u>.

```
PR     160   +  Rhythm, rate 79
QRSD    83   .  Right Ventricular Hypertrophy
QT     362   .  Consider Pulmonary Emphysema
QTc    415      -ABNORMAL ECG-
```

64 YEAR OLD WOMAN
DO YOU AGREE?
HOW COULD YOU PROVE YOUR DX??

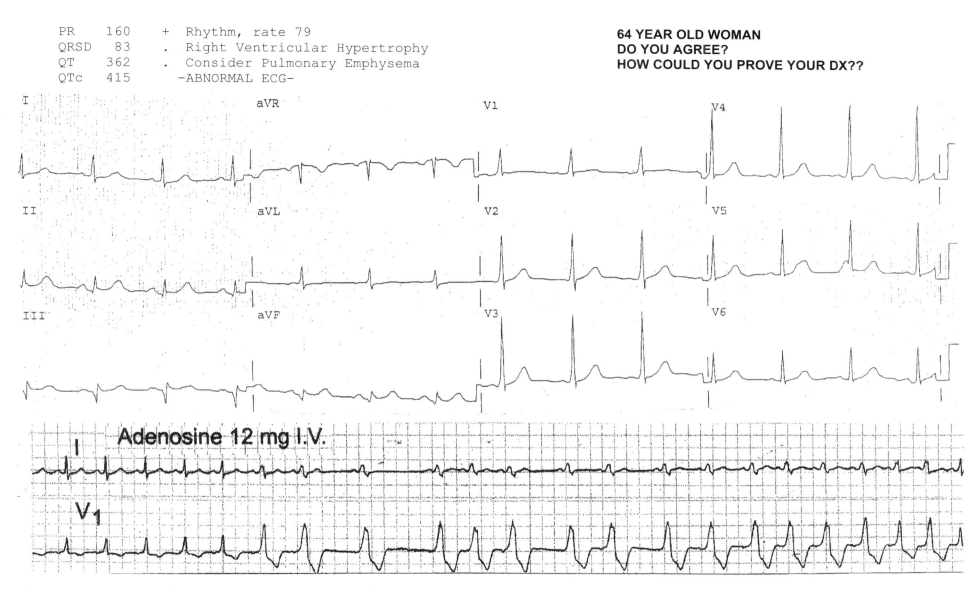

The computer interpretation may be correct, but the short PR interval in the precordial leads and the suggestion of a delta wave in leads V3-4 is evidence that there is a different problem. To clarify the situation, the AV nodal blocking drug adenosine was given. As it takes the effect, the sinus rate slows and AV nodal transmission decreases, and then ceases. The atrial stimuli are transmitted over the accessory pathway, since it is the only available route. QRS duration increases as complete AP activation occurs. The correct diagnosis is now proven.

(Tracing courtesy of Dr. J. Michael Criley)

315

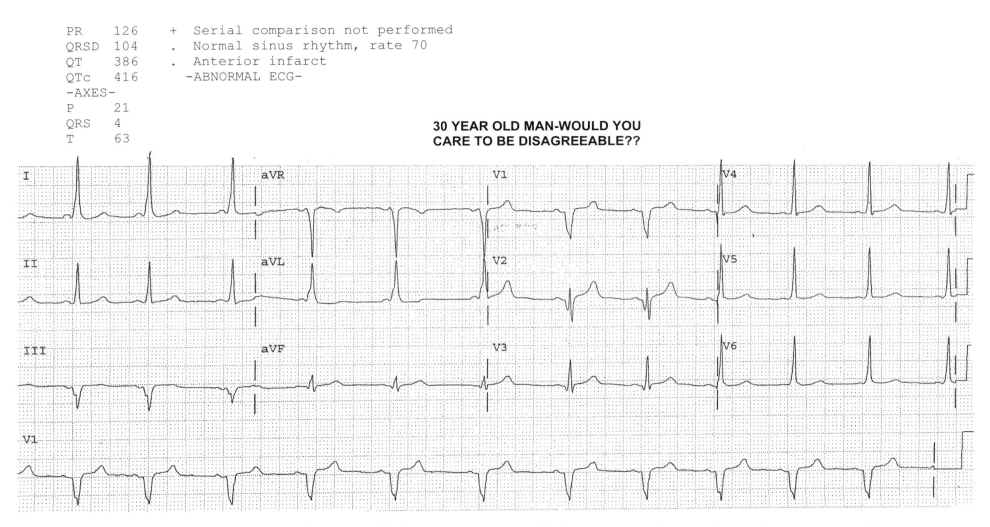

```
PR    126    +  Serial comparison not performed
QRSD  104    .  Normal sinus rhythm, rate 70
QT    386    .  Anterior infarct
QTc   416       -ABNORMAL ECG-
-AXES-
P      21
QRS     4
T      63
```

**30 YEAR OLD MAN-WOULD YOU
CARE TO BE DISAGREEABLE??**

The computer has misinterpreted the initial negative forces in V1-3 as due to an anterior MI. The morphology in most other leads shows a short PR interval and delta wave, indicating accessory pathway activation. The pathway is located in the right ventricle and the direction of the preexcited forces is to the left and posterior, resulting in the "pseudo Q waves" in leads V1-3. Obviously, it is undesirable to have WPW complexes, but it would be a greater calamity to carry the diagnosis provided by the computer!

Sinus tachycardia, rate 111 [Now Present]
Right axis deviation [Now Present]
RVH with ST-T abnormalities [Now Present]
Old Inferior infarct [Remains]
Lateral region infarct [Remains]   -ABNORMAL ECG-
[Now Absent] Probable Posterior region wall involvement
[Now Absent] Nonspecific Anterior T wave abnormalities

41 YEAR OLD WOMAN
DO YOU AGREE WITH THE COMPUTER?

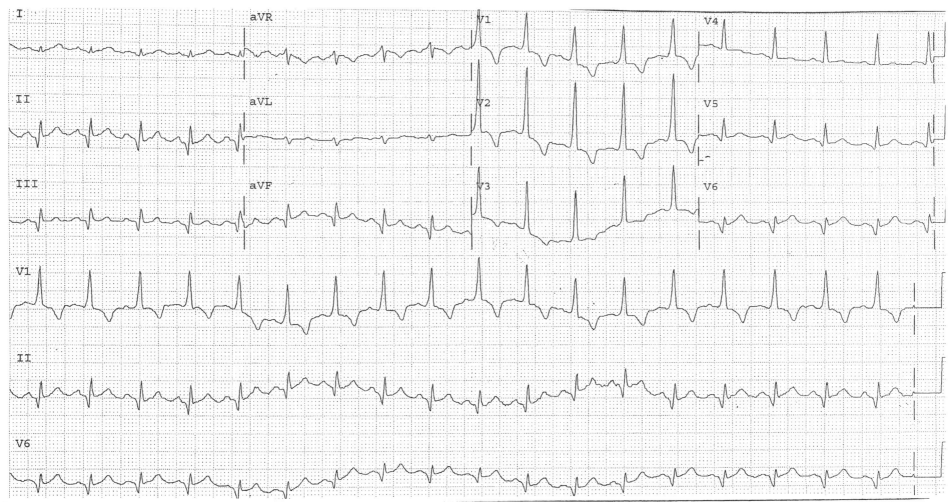

The computer incorrectly diagnoses the majority of tracings showing WPW; and here is a disappointing example. The left-sided accessory pathway has provided subtle delta waves in leads V1-3. They are recorded as negative deflections in the inferior and lateral leads, simulating an inferior and lateral M.I. The R wave in lead V1 is not due to RVH but to the anterior direction of the forces due to the accessory pathway.

317

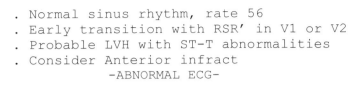

. Normal sinus rhythm, rate 56
. Early transition with RSR' in V1 or V2
. Probable LVH with ST-T abnormalities
. Consider Anterior infract
            -ABNORMAL ECG-

**64 YEAR OLD WOMAN
DO YOU AGREE WITH REVIEWER?**

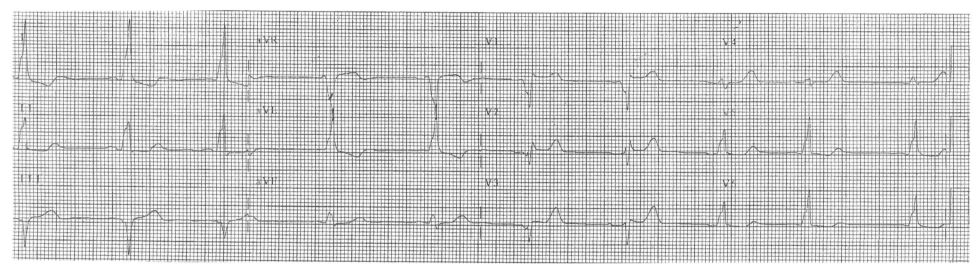

The reviewer has failed to identify this woman's WPW complexes. The abnormal sequence due to accessory pathway conduction results in <u>asynchronous</u> ventricular activation and removes the expected "cancellation" of opposing forces which are present during normal activation. This can result in an increase in the recorded QRS voltage, simulating left or right ventricular hypertrophy. There are no *validated* criteria to diagnose ventricular hypertrophy in the presence of an accessory pathway. The diagnosis of anterior infarction should be replaced, since the negative initial forces in V1-3 are really delta waves. The direction of these indicates that the accessory pathway is in the right ventricle.

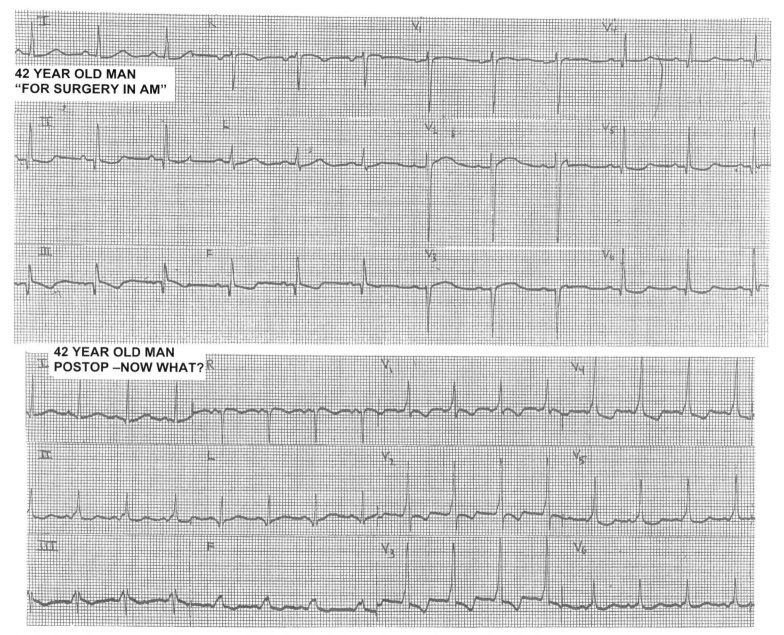

42 YEAR OLD MAN
"FOR SURGERY IN AM"

42 YEAR OLD MAN
POSTOP –NOW WHAT?

An interesting feature of accessory pathway activation is the ability to mask other abnormalities. In the top tracing, it is evident that this man has sustained inferior and anterolateral infarctions. Bypass surgery was performed and, postoperatively, his EKG showed WPW conduction which had not been previously identified. The reorientation of the initial forces due to the accessory pathway has removed the diagnostic Q waves of the prior MIs.

27 YEAR OLD MAN-1/13-OBSERVATIONS?

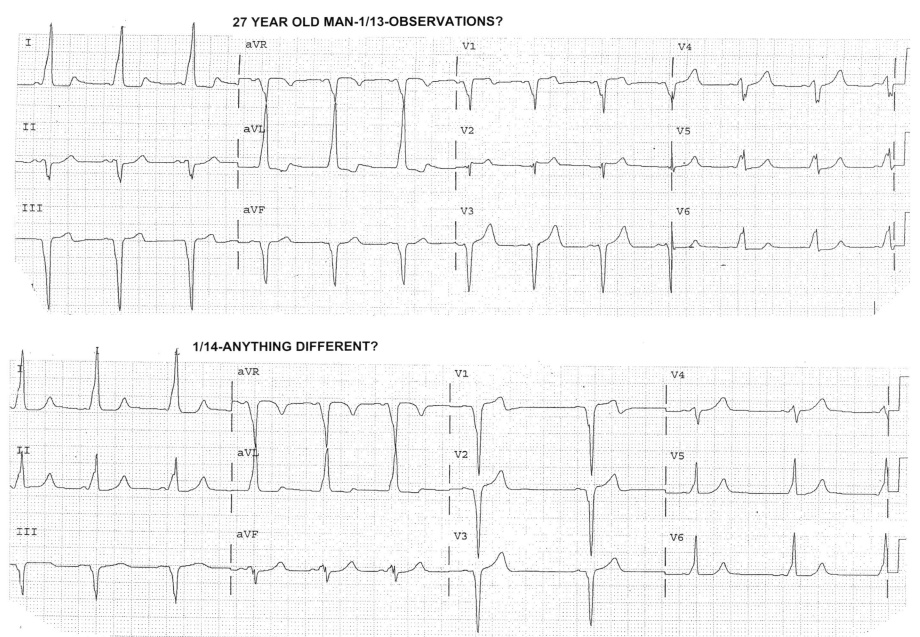

1/14-ANYTHING DIFFERENT?

In the top EKG, the short PR interval and delta wave in the QRS upstroke is obvious and typical of WPW with a right-sided pathway. The interesting change in QRS axis and morphology from the top tracing to the bottom may indicate the presence of two accessory pathways, or differing entry of the preexcited stimulus into the ventricle.

320

ELECTRONIC PACEMAKERS

The progress in electronic pacemaker therapy has been dramatic and the current generation of pacemakers represents an engineering triumph. The beginnings date to 1952 when Dr. Paul Zoll was able to successfully provide *external* pacing of the heart with a high-energy stimulus. In the 1960s, the pacing electrodes were applied directly to the left ventricle via a left thoracotomy, with effective cardiac stimulation at low energy levels. However the major surgery required in elderly sick patients resulted in a significant morbidity and mortality. The pioneering work of Dr. Seymour Furman led to the development of *transvenous* placement, requiring only minor surgery to expose a vein for the pacemaker procedure. When placed in the right ventricular apex, the pacer discharge results in a depolarization sequence that is directed superiorly and to the left (left axis deviation), with a later left ventricular activation simulating left bundle branch block.

The physician was offered an option in the pacing lead. It could be "bipolar" with electrodes closely spaced or "unipolar" with the active electorate at the tip and the metallic case of the generator the other electrode. Identification of the two varieties is usually simple. The pacing "spike" of a bipolar lead is small; the unipolar is much larger (sometimes gigantic!).

The indication for the original pacemakers was for patients with complete heart block. The early pacemakers discharged at a preset "fixed rate" providing a predictable stimulus. Although lifesaving, they had major disadvantages:

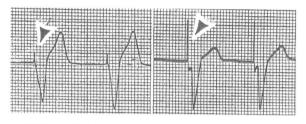

BIPOLAR LEAD   **UNIPOLAR LEAD**

1. The presence of competing rhythms was not recognized, and pacer discharge shortly following another ventricular depolarization could encounter the chamber's vulnerable period and possibly trigger serious ventricular arrhythmias.
2. If sinus impulses were present, there would be no synchronous relationship to pacemaker discharge, depriving the ventricle of the valuable, and often critically important, "atria kick."
3. If the AV bridge was intact, the ventricular stimulus could be conducted retrogradely to the atrium.
4. The preset rate of the pacer remained fixed, regardless of the level of the patient's activity.

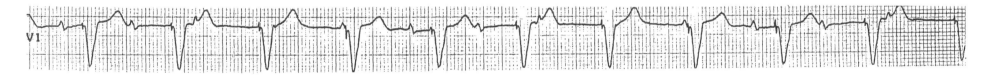

A 78-year-old woman with complete heart block was treated with a fixed-rate pacemaker. Although her heart rate is satisfactory, the dissociated P waves are not linked to the paced activity. They only inconsistently contribute to ventricular filling, which is a significant compromise to cardiac output.

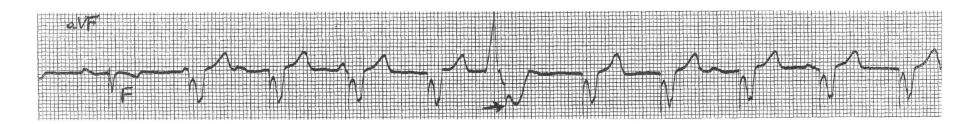

The 60-year-old man had type II A-V block with recurring "presyncope." An asynchronous pacemaker was inserted providing a predictable discharge at 74/min. In the first beat, discharge coincides with a conducted stimulus-a ventricular fusion complex (**F**) resulting. This is of no concern, but what is disturbing is that six beats later, a VPC occurs and the fixed-rate pacemaker fires during its repolarization phase. The pacer discharge is ineffective, but if it occurred in the "vulnerable period" of the VPC, it could initiate a serious or lethal ventricular arrhythmia.

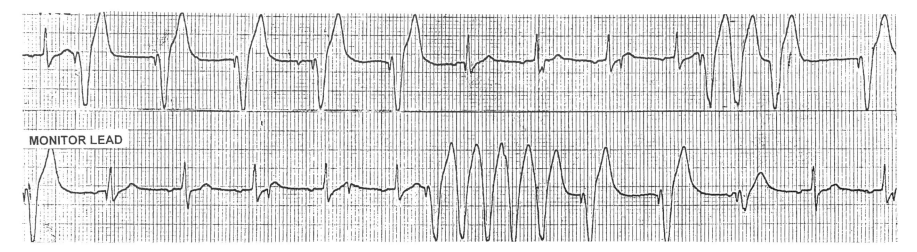

The 70-year-old woman had acute anterior infarction complicated by transient complete heart block. A temporary transvenous pacemaker was inserted, but because of poor positioning, it could not sense conducted QRS complexes. When the pacer discharge occurred in the vulnerable period of conducted beats, bursts of ventricular tachycardia resulted.

322

A major advance occurred with the ability of the electronic unit to "sense" the presence of competing rhythms (conducted beats or VPCs). The pacemaker, thus, functioned as an "escape" mechanism. If spontaneous ventricular activation occurred, the electronic circuitry sensed its presence and inhibited pacer discharge, but awakened to stimulate the heart if needed. The "demand" pacemaker, by switching off for a cycle whenever a natural beat occurred, overcame the first disadvantages of the fixed-rate pacemaker, but the other problems remained.

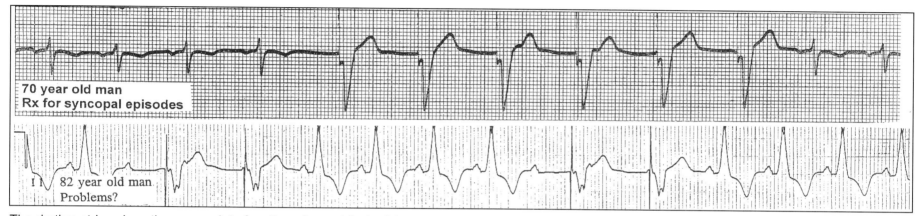

70 year old man
Rx for syncopal episodes

I 82 year old man
Problems?

The rhythm strips show the appropriate function of a ventricular "demand" pacemaker. In the 70-year-old man with "sick sinus syndrome," when P waves are present and conducted, the pacing electrode "senses" the QRS and does not discharge. If the sinus impulses default, the pacer awakens. When sinus rhythm resumes, the pacer returns to sleep. In the 82 year old man the problem is abnormal A-V conduction—type 2 A-V block. When the atrial impulse is not transmitted over the A-V bridge, the pacer assumes command until conduction returns. Both of these examples show an "escape interval" of 0.88sec. (pacer rate = 70/min). The sensing function of the demand pacemaker prevents the competitive rhythms seen with the fixed-rate variety.

The development of this variety of pacing led to the formulation of a useful three component pacemaker code system.

	CHAMBER PACED	CHAMBER SENSED	MODE OF RESPONSE
FIXED-RATE PACER	V	O	O
VENTRICULAR "DEMAND" PACER	V	V	I

The application of the code is apparent. If the ventricle is paced, but has no sensing ability, it will function as a "fixed-rate" unit. Code = _VOO_. If sensing is added, the pacemaker will respond to conducted beats or VPCs, and inhibit its discharge and "reset"--Code = _VVI._

The next major step in pacemaker therapy was the development of "dual chamber" pacing, requiring a stimulating electrode in both the right atrium and ventricle. This mode of "physiologic pacing" simulates sinus rhythm. The atrial and ventricular limbs have the ability to both pace and sense. This variety of pacing was particularly advantageous in patients without predictable P waves (e.g., "sick sinus syndrome"). Lacking a P wave, the atrial electrode discharges and after an "A-V delay," the ventricle is activated. The response mode can be either "inhbition" (I) of discharege in atrium or ventricle or "triggered" (T). Thus, if a P wave is sensed, the atrial discharge is inhibited, but the ventricle is paced (triggered). Sensing ventricular activity inhibits both atrium and ventricle.

The pacemaker codes now became:

	CHAMBER PACED	CHAMBER SENSED	MODE OF RESPONSE
FIXED-RATE PACER	V	O	O
VENTRICULAR "DEMAND" PACER	V	V	I
DUAL CHAMBER PACER	A + V = D	A +V =D	I + T =D

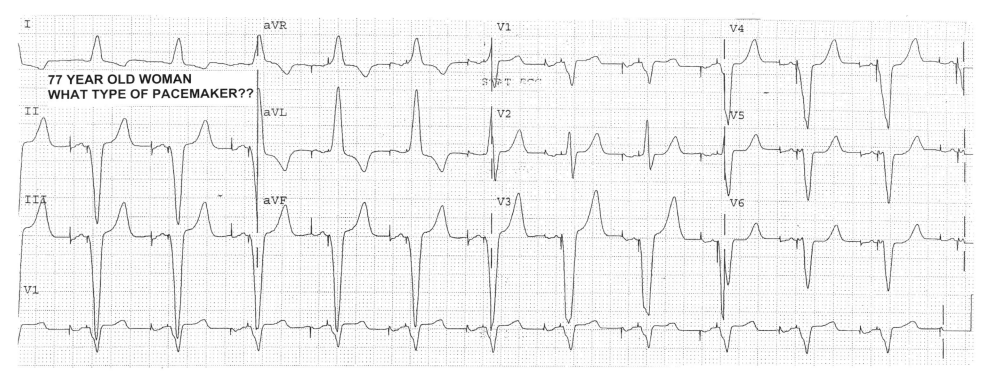

77 YEAR OLD WOMAN
WHAT TYPE OF PACEMAKER??

An example of DDD pacemaker function. The atrial electrode has not sensed atrial depolarization and it discharges. After an A-V delay of 0.18 sec the ventricular electrode is activated and ventricular depolarization occurs. The sequence of electrical stimulation of the cardiac chambers nicely simulates sinus rhythm.

Less frequently used pacing modes:

ATRIAL-TRIGGERED (VAT) PACEMAKER--this variety senses the sinus P waves and, after an appropriate A-V delay, delivers a ventricular stimulus. It maintains a normal A-V sequence of contraction, and has the advantage of keeping pace with the patient's varied activity--if the patient exercises, the atrial and therefore the ventricular rate accelerate "physiologically." The evident disadvantage is that there must be P waves available, and in patients with "sick sinus" this is unpredictable. Tracing **A** is an example.

ATRIAL (AAI) PACEMAKER--this variety paces the atrium and, like the VAT mode, also overcomes the handicap of losing one's "atrial kick." Obviously, it is not applicable in the presence of A-V block, since the AAI pacemaker paces and senses _only_ the atrium. An early and significant problem was the difficulty of securing the lead in the atrial appendage. This has been largely resolved with the use of electrode fixation devices. An example is shown in tracing **B.**

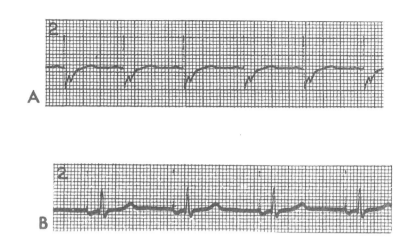

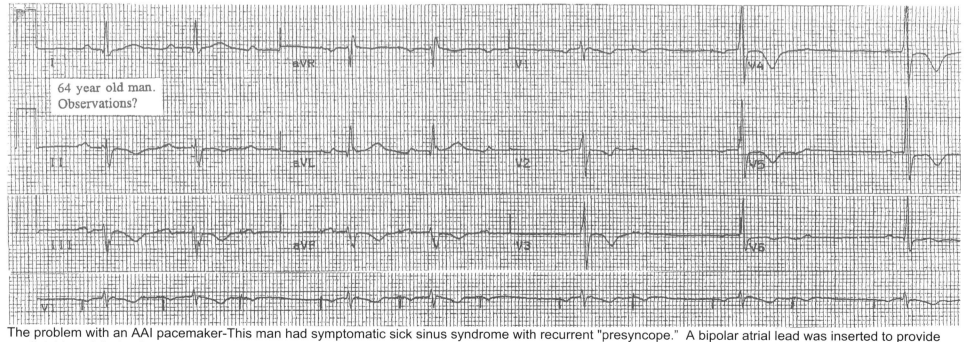

64 year old man. Observations?

The problem with an AAI pacemaker-This man had symptomatic sick sinus syndrome with recurrent "presyncope." A bipolar atrial lead was inserted to provide predictable atrial stimulation. The paced P waves are seen in lead V1 rhythm strip (pacer discharge is darkened for clarity). Unfortunately, although P waves are available, consistent A-V transmission is not! Note that the PR intervals prolong with repetitive 3:2 and 2:1 Wenckebach A-V block. The resulting long pauses returned his symptoms. The AAI pacemaker was replaced with a DDD unit.

325

With the realization that some patients required the pacemaker to increase its rate with an increase in activity, there was another development. A sensor, usually related to motion, was added to the generator and changed the pacemaker rate depending on activity. The pacemaker code now became:

	CHAMBER PACED	CHAMBER SENSED	MODE OF RESPONSE	RATE RESPONSIVE
FIXED-RATE PACER	V	O	O	
VENTRICULAR "DEMAND" PACER	V	V	I	R
DUAL CHAMBER PACER	A + V = D	A +V =D	I + T =D	R

The demand ventricular and dual chamber pacemaker may now function VVIR and DDDR, indicating that they will respond with increased rate if the sensor determines that there is a change in the patient's activity.

A later and valuable development was the ability to alter pacemaker functions with an external "programmer". A radio-frequency signal, like that of a TV "remote," can change many pacemaker parameters including: rate; upper rate limit; sensitivity; refractory period; stimulus strength; and A-V interval. It can also "interrogate" the pacemaker performance regarding threshold, resistance of the pacing lead, and residual battery strength.
The pacer code now has five possible components:

	CHAMBER PACED	CHAMBER SENSED	MODE OF RESPONSE	RATE RESPONSIVE	PROGRAMMABLE
FIXED-RATE PACER	V	O	O		
VENTRICULAR "DEMAND" PACER	V	V	I	R	P
DUAL CHAMBER PACER	A + V = D	A +V =D	I + T =D	R	P

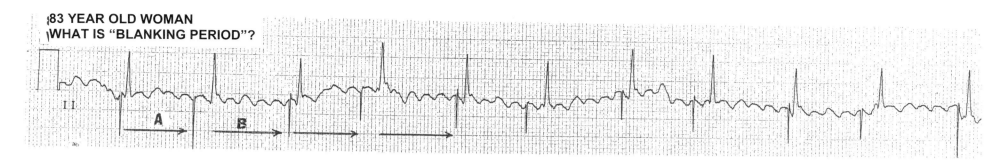

83 YEAR OLD WOMAN
WHAT IS "BLANKING PERIOD"?

A programmable function that has been added for "safety" is the pacemaker "blanking period." After its discharge, the pacemaker will not accept another stimulus if it occurs within this brief period of time. In this example, ignoring the obvious pacemaker's spikes for a moment, the patients own rhythm is atrial flutter with varying A-V conduction. Quite clearly, the QRS complexes are not due to the electronic pacemaker. The changing interval between pacemakers spikes shows that it is intermittently sensing the ventricular depolarization and "resetting." When the ventricular discharge occurs in the blanking period after pacer activation, it is not sensed and a shorter pacing interlude is seen (**A**). When the ventricular depolarization occurs after the blanking period, it is sensed and the pacer discharge is inhibited and reset.

12/10 –PACER CODE?   WHAT IS THE PURPOSE OF "MAGNET MODE"?

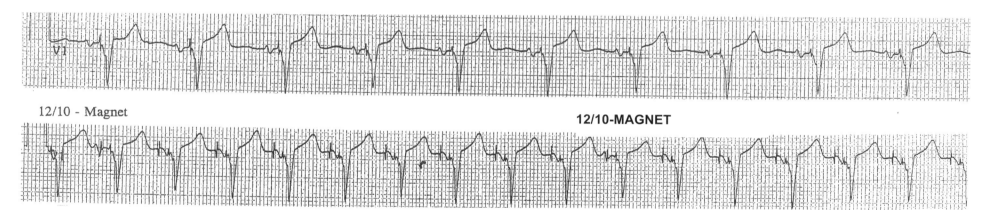

12/10 - Magnet   **12/10-MAGNET**

The upper tracing shows a consistent relationship of P waves and paced QRS complexes. This must be a dual chamber pacemaker. In order to insure that the atrial electrode will awaken if the P wave does not surface, a testing mechanism was devised. In the lower tracing, a magnetic field is provided over the pacemaker generator. It disarms the sensing function of both atrial and ventricular limbs. Atrial pacing appears and the ventricular lead is "triggered" to respond. To indicate that the "magnet mode" is present, the atrial rate is increased to 100/min and the A-V delay decreased. When the magnet is removed, normal DDD pacing will return.

PACEMAKER PROBLEMS

The recognition of appropriate function of single or dual chamber pacemakers is easy. When there is "peculiar" or abnormal behavior, analysis is more difficult. The tracings to follow are examples of unusual or incorrect pacemaker function. The pacemaker can only perform as it is instructed to do.   Problems occur either due to electrode placement, programming, or the wrong type of pacemakers selected for the patient's problem. Included are:

1. Undersensing
2. Oversensing
   -of other EKG events
   -of environmental signals
   - of muscle potentials

3. Lack of capture
   - displaced electrode
   - loss of electrode continuity
4. Retrograde conduction
5. Pacemaker-mediated tachycardia

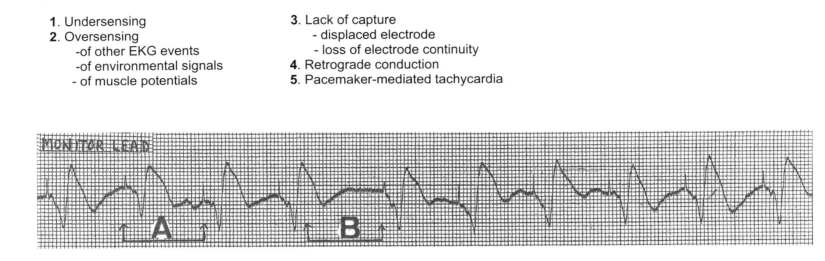

The sensing function of a demand pacemaker requires the recognition of a signal amplitude (voltage) that develops in a brief period of time. If voltage + time requirements are met, the event will be sensed and inhibit pacer discharge. The interval between the paced QRS complexes (A) is the preset pacer rate. When a pause occurs in the pacing cycle, "something" has been sensed. In this example, the tall, high frequency T wave has been sensed and delays the pacemaker discharge (B). This is an example of "over-sensing" and requires adjustment of the pacemaker.

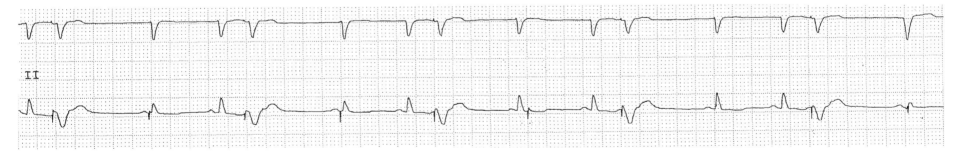

The 62-year-old woman had a ventricular demand pacemaker inserted because of intermittent A-V block. The sensitivity level was not properly established and the pacer is functioning as a fixed-rate unit. Proper programming will eliminate this "under-sensing" problem.

328

The computer can sense pacemaker activity (sometimes) but its response is limited. Its diagnoses will only be-- "Electronic Pacemaker--Rate = xx" or--"Electronic Pacemaker--Demand mode--Rate = xx". It often does not sense dual chamber pacing activity and does not recognize departures from normal function. The reviewer should not depend on the computer analysis. The examples below will emphasize this.

```
Electronic pacemaker, ventricular capture, rate = 65 [Now Present]
[Now Absent] Intraventricular conduction delay [? Atypical LBBB]
[Now Absent] Left atrial enlargement    -ABNORMAL ECG-
```

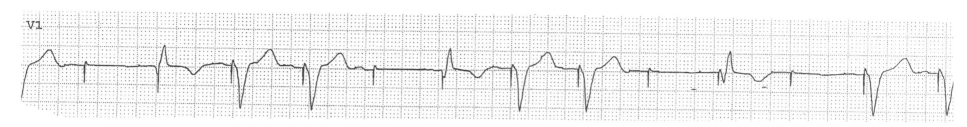

The computer ignores this pacemaker malfunction. The unit is functioning VOO; neither sensing nor consistently pacing. The computer does not recognize that there are pacer discharges without ventricular stimulation. This is a disaster and may be an indication of a fractured pacing lead.

```
Electronic pacemaker, demand mode, ventricular capture rate = 54
No further analysis attempted due to pacemaker rhythm          -ABNORMAL ECG-
```

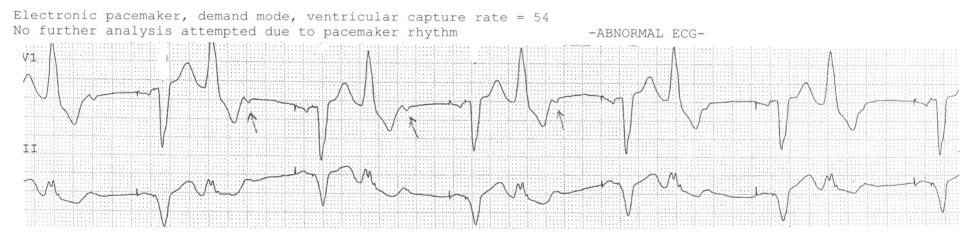

The computer diagnosis is correct, but clearly inadequate. Small pacer spikes identify the bipolar leads of a dual chamber electronic pacemaker. Unfortunately, each paced ventricular depolarization is married to a fixed-coupled VPC of L.V. origin. The VPC's conduct retrogradely to the atria with variable V-A conduction delay (arrows). For some reason, the atrial lead does not sense the retrograde impulses and the paced atrial discharge is not delayed. Although the electronic pacemaker function is appropriate, the premature ventricular discharge may not result I effective contraction. Thus, the <u>effective</u> ventricular rate may be only 35/min. A bad situation!

63 YEAR OLD MAN-OBSERVATIONS
PROPER LACER PERFORMANCE??

CHAMBER PACED	CHAMBER SENSED	MODE OF RESPONSE

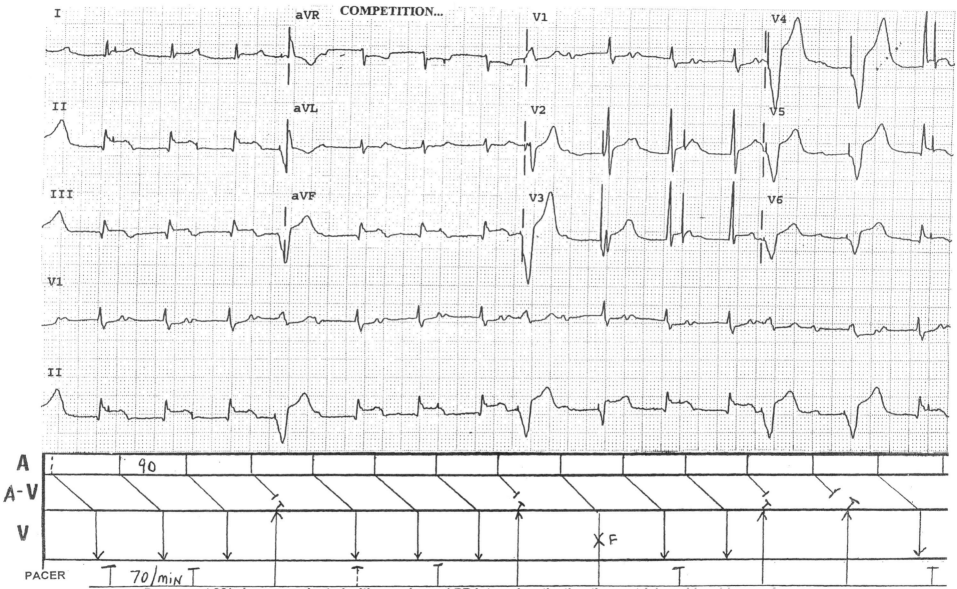

COMPETITION...

Regular sinus P waves at 90/min are conducted with a prolonged PR interval, activating the ventricles with evidence of acute inferior-posterior-lateral infarction. Clearly the pacemaker is this behaving! It is "nonsensical," and is functioning as a fixed-rate unit, and stimulating the heart only when its discharge is beyond the refractory period of the conducted sinus impulses. This is a worthless and potentially hazardous competition.

330

78 YEAR OLD MAN
PECULIAR PACER PERFORMANCE
WHAT IS HAPPENING?

CHAMBER PACED	CHAMBER SENSED	MODE OF RESPONSE

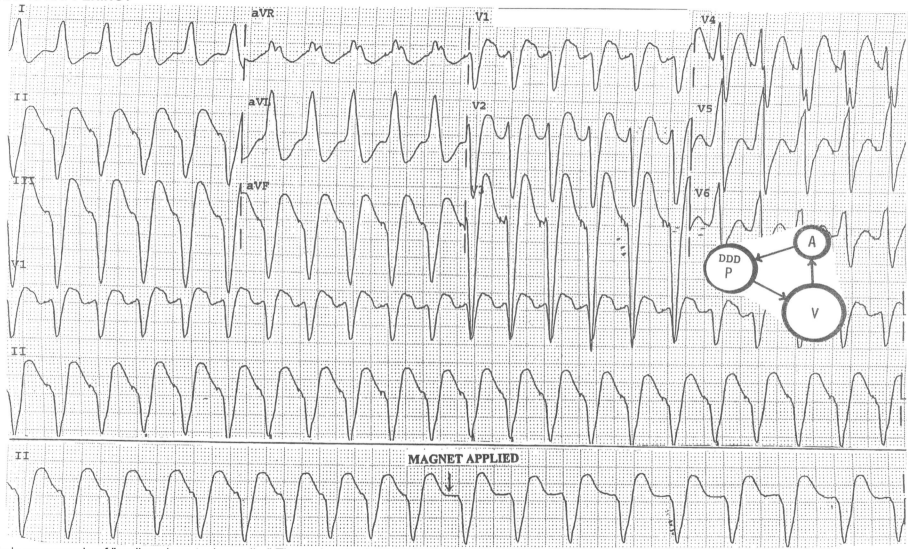

This is an example of "endless-loop tachycardia." The patient had a dual chamber pacemaker implanted several weeks before presenting to the E.D. with this rhythm. Dual chamber (A-V sequential) pacemakers are designed to simulate normal sinus rhythm; however; if the A-V bridge is intact, and the atrial refractory period is short, the ventricular stimulus may return to the atrium. The atrial discharge is sensed and the ventricular limb is triggered to fire again. The sequence then becomes repetitive: ventricle--to--atrium--to ventricle--to--atrium-etc.--and an "endless loop" tachycardia results. The magnet influence prevents atrial and ventricular *sensing* and interrupts the "pacemaker mediated tachycardia."

79 YEAR OLD WOMAN
WHAT IS "PVARP"??

CHAMBER PACED	CHAMBER SENSED	MODE OF RESPONSE

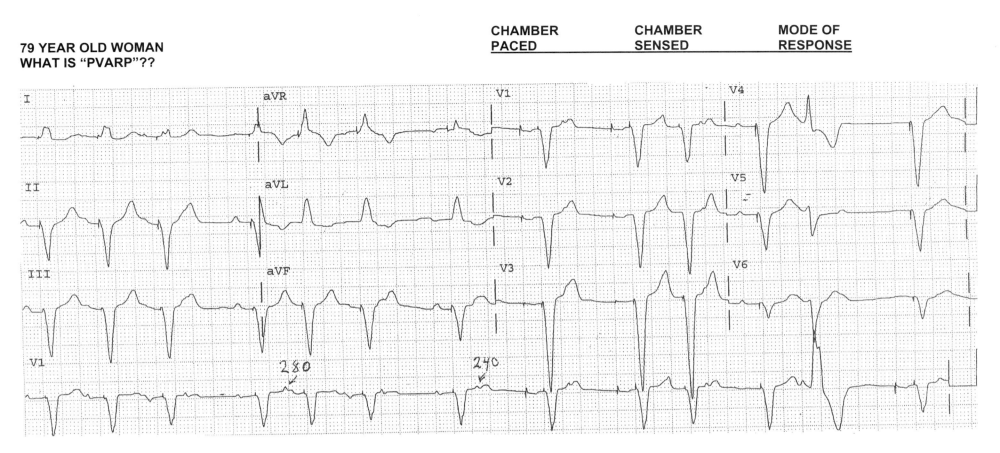

"PVARP" is an abbreviation for "post ventricular atrial refractory period," and is a programmable pacemaker function. In a dual chamber unit, the circuitry is designed to sense an atrial impulse and "tell" the ventricle to fire. Clearly, it would be undesirable to sense a "very early" APC--thus the PVARP. Note that an APC which is 240 msec, or sooner, after the preceding paced beat is ignored, while one slightly beyond the PVARP--280 msec. is sensed and results in ventricular pacing. The PVARP was added by the pacer engineers to prevent the problem of "endless loop tachycardia."

75 YEAR OLD MAN
HOW MANY OBSERVATIONS??

	CHAMBER PACED	CHAMBER SENSED	MODE OF RESPONSE

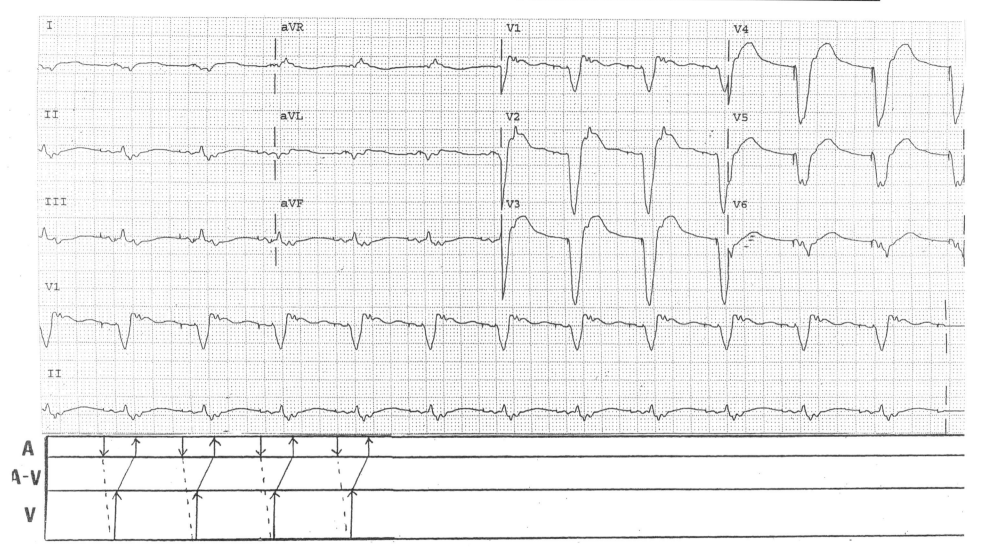

Clearly a dual-chamber electronic pacemaker is present. The disturbing thing is the retrograde transmission from the paced ventricular beats. Happily, the retrograde atrial impulse is not sensed by the pacemaker or an "endless-loop" tachycardia could result. The "post ventricular atrial refractory period" (PVARP) is sufficiently long that the retrograde P waves are ignored.

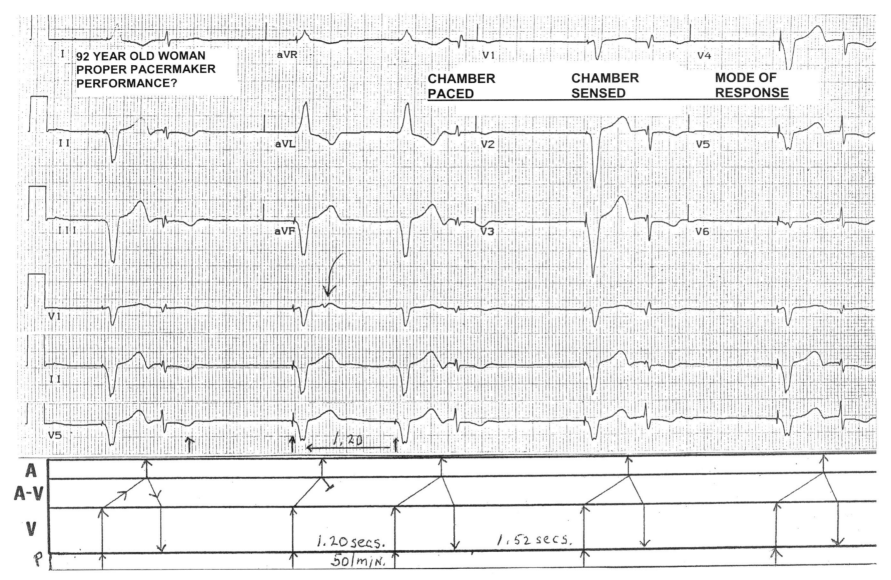

The pacer spikes are separated by 120msec, indicating a rather slow discharge rate of 50/minute. As diagrammed, the pacemaker is able to conduct retrogradely with a marked and variable delay. When the V-A conduction is long enough this stimulus "reciprocates," and returns to activate the ventricle in normal fashion. When the V-A delay is less (arrow), the returning reciprocal beat does not occur. The question of some concern is why, after the normal ventricular beat, does the pacemaker wait for 1.52sec. before awakening? A possible explanation is that the unit is "sensing something" such as the T wave of the normal beat, and has inhibited its discharge ("oversensing"). That could mean a potentially serious problem. The markedly low QRS voltage and the Q waves in limb and precordial leads in the conducted beats would suggest extensive myocardial disease-perhaps amyloidosis is elderly man?

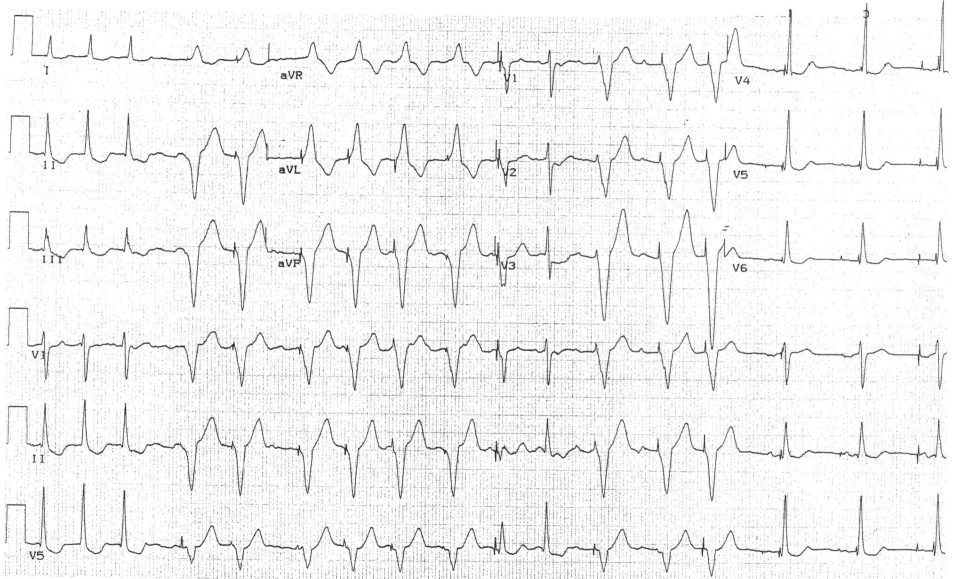

Dual chamber pacemakers, with both atrial and ventricular sensing and pacing, have a lurking, but predictable, complication. The atrial limb is instructed to sense atrial depolarization and trigger the ventricular lead to fire. If the patient develops atrial fibrillation, and if the intra-atrial signals are large enough, the pacer will frequently interpret the irregular atrial events as "P waves" and activate the ventricle, resulting in irregular ventricular paced beats. The pacemaker performance is appropriate, but obviously undesirable.

66 YEAR OLD WOMAN-12/6
WHAT IS HER PACEMAKER CODE?

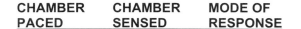

CHAMBER PACED	CHAMBER SENSED	MODE OF RESPONSE

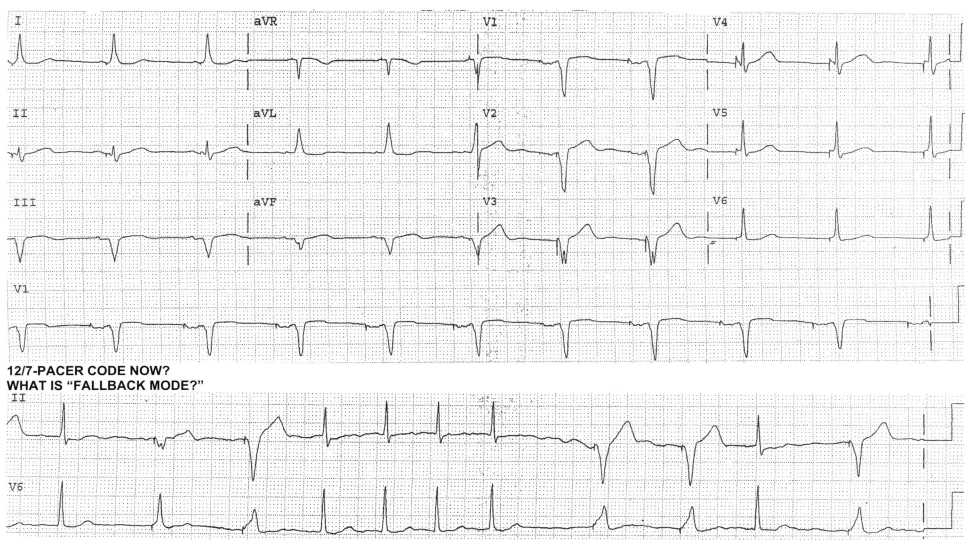

12/7-PACER CODE NOW?
WHAT IS "FALLBACK MODE?"

The upper tracing shows normal function of a bipolar DDD pacemaker. The paced atrial discharge is shared between normal A-V conduction and electrical activation of the ventricle (fusion complexes). However the next day, atrial fibrillation developed and the atrial lead began "tracking" the AF stimuli with rapid, irregular ventricular pacing resulting. An obvious treatment would be--turn off the atrial lead and stop atrial sensing. Some pacemakers do this automatically. If the atrial does not sense regular atrial stimuli, it turns off the atrial lead and "falls back" to VVI pacing, as shown in the lower tracing. A very desirable feature.

336

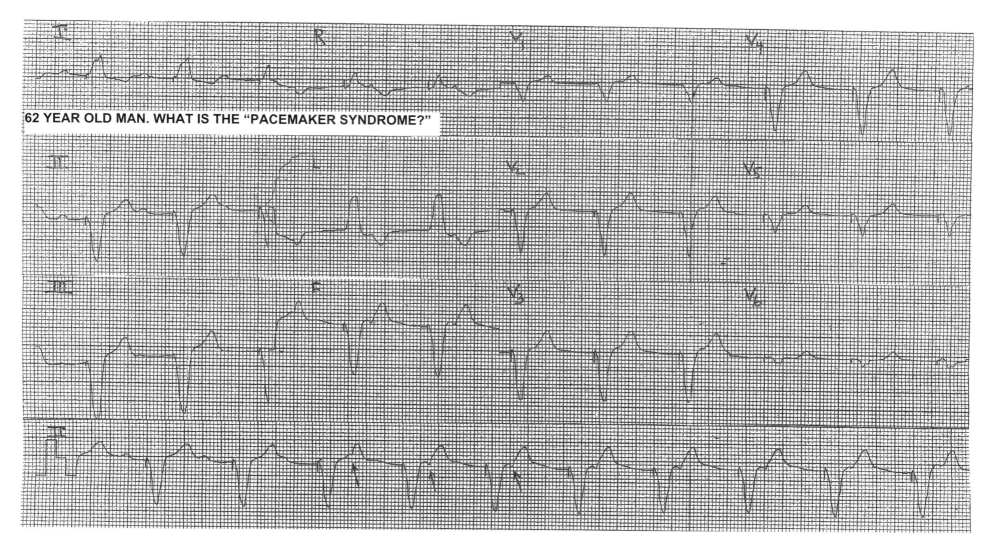

62 YEAR OLD MAN. WHAT IS THE "PACEMAKER SYNDROME?"

This man received a fixed-rate ventricular pacemaker for intermittent A-V block. An interesting, but troubling, paradox resulted. Although P waves are not conducted in anterograde direction, the ventricular pacemaker succeeds in retrograde transmission. After the third beat in the rhythm strip, there is 1:1 V-A conduction (arrows). Atrial contraction now occurs during ventricular systole, producing *retrograde* flow in both systemic and pulmonary venous circuits. This can lead to breathlessness and hypotension and may make the patient more symptomatic than before pacemaker insertion→ the "pacemaker syndrome."

73 YEAR OLD WOMAN
PACER PERFORMING PROPERLY?

CHAMBER PACED	CHAMBER SENSED	MODE OF RESPONSE

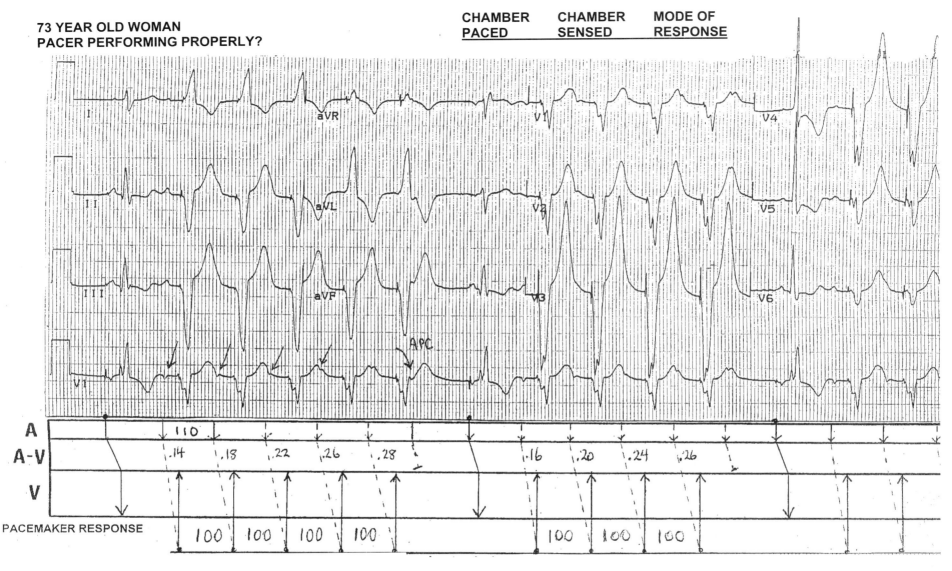

This dual chamber pacemaker is functioning properly-if you understand what is has been told to do! Stimuli are available to pace and sense both the atria and the ventricles. What you need to know is that the pacemaker has been told that, no matter what the atrial rate, the ventricular rate should not be faster than 100/min.-- _the upper rate limit_. The P waves evident in lead V1 (arrows) indicate an atrial rate of 110/min. but, since the ventricular activation cannot exceed 100/minute, the A-V delay gradually prolongs. The first pause is produced by an APC (reversed arrow) which is sufficiently early that is not sensed by the pacer. The second pause ends a series of prolonging A-V delays-a "pseudo Wenckebach phenomenon," The ladder diagram depicts this interesting phenomenon. Despite the irregularity in the pacemaker activity, it is only doing what it was told to do! This feature protects against pacemaker-mediated tachycardia and against SV tachycardia that would result in ventricular pacing at 1:1.

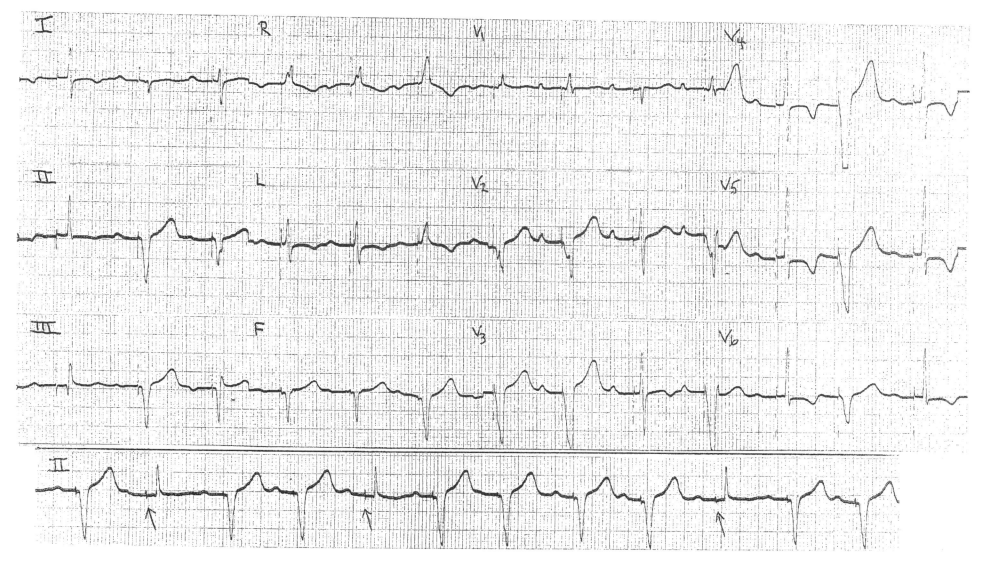

The pacemaker discharge is regular, activating the right ventricle at 75/min; however, note that there are P waves consistently related to the QRS complexes. This is a dual chamber pacemaker. The disturbing thing is that there are 3 pacing stimuli (arrows) that the do not succeed in ventricular activation. Happily, the sinus P waves are conducted, with a long PR interval and a normal QRS complex. The lack of predictable pacing is very threatening and requires an explanation. Investigation revealed that the pacing cable was fractured and could not consistently transmit the electrical stimulus to the distal electrode. It must be replaced!

70 YEAR OLD MAN
HOW MANY ABNORMALITIES?

CHAMBER PACED	CHAMBER SENSED	MODE OF RESPONSE

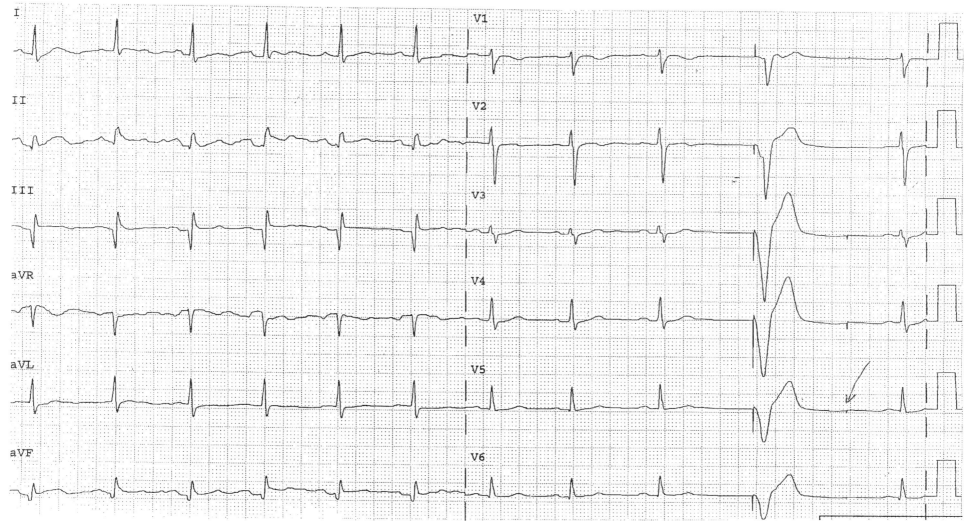

I V1
II V2
III V3
aVR V4
aVL V5
aVF V6

This man had an acute inferior myocardial infarction complicated by marked sinus node suppression. A VVI pacemaker was inserted, initially with appropriate sensing and "capture." This later tracing shows consistent sensing of the sinus-conducted QRS complexes, until suddenly the P wave fails to appear and the pacemaker "escapes" with a large spike. This is followed by a smaller spike, without ventricular activation. Investigation revealed that the ineffective output was due to a lead insulation defect, with intermittent "short circuit" of the electrical pulse. A returning sinus impulse saves the day.

Tracing courtesy of Dr. Ronald Vlietstra.

72 YEAR OLD MAN
RECOMMENDATIONS??

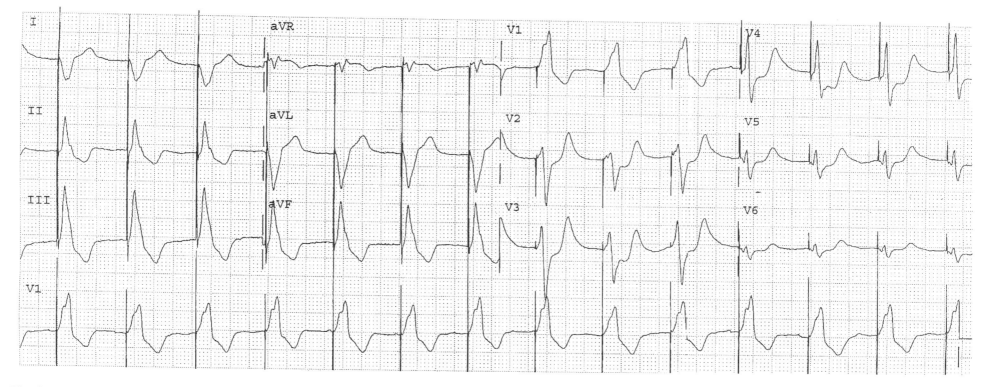

The huge spikes indicate that the pacemaker activity is being conducted via a unipolar lead. If it is stimulating the RV apex, the direction of electrical spread should be left-superior (left axis) with a sequence of the RV depolarization before the LV (simulating LBBB). The morphology of the QRS complexes in this man should raise a red flag! They show _right axis deviation_ and a V1 pattern of _right bundle branch block_. The evident concern is that the pacing electrode is stimulating the LV.

Possibilities include:
1. The electrode has perforated the ventricular septum and is pacing the left side of the septum.
2. The electrode has perforated the RV apex and is in the pericardial space over the LV.
3. The electrode entered the coronary sinus and is in a coronary vein over the lateral wall of the LV.
A chest x-ray and echocardiogram should help clarify the location of the pacing electrode.
The third possibility was the explanation in this case.
Emerging knowledge, in fact indicates that LV pacing produces more efficient LV ejection than RV pacing. Therefore, in patients with low cardiac output and heart failure, bi-ventricular pacing (so-called "cardiac resynchronization therapy"-CRT) has shown to be clinically very beneficial.

61 YEAR OLD WOMAN
WHY THE CHANGING PATTERN??

CHAMBER PACED	CHAMBER SENSED	MODE OF RESPONSE

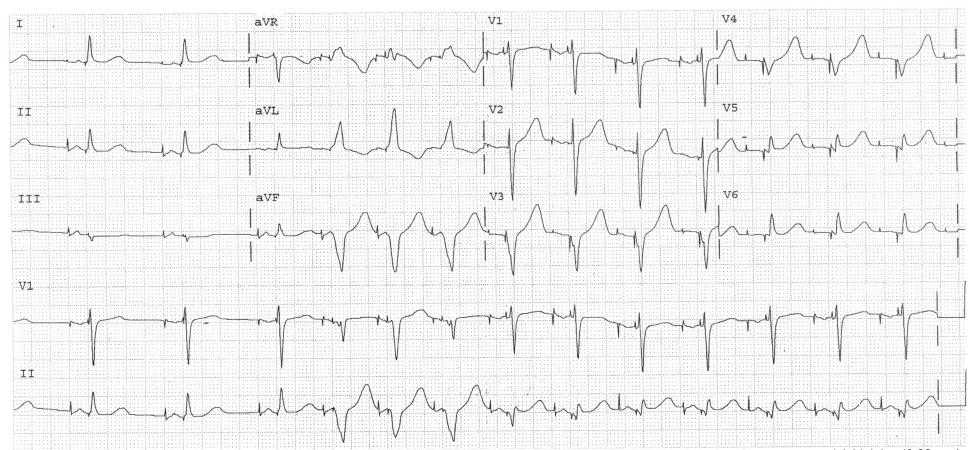

The twin spikes identify a dual chamber pacemaker. In the first complex, the initial stimulus activates the atria at 70/min, but the programmed A-V delay (0.20 sec) is sufficiently long that it permits the signal to cross the A-V bridge and activate the ventricles normally. The ventricular lead of the pacemaker fires, but does not participate in ventricular depolarization—a phenomenon called "pseudo-fusion." The next three complexes show appropriately dual chamber pacing. Note that the rate has increased to 100/min and the A-V delay has decreased to 0.12 sec. This is the response when a magnet is placed over the pacemaker generator. During the last seven beats, the atrial pacing rate "falls back" to 85/min; the initial A-V delay returns; and the QRS complexes are fusion beats, indicating that ventricular activation is due to both paced and conducted stimuli.

83 YEAR OLD MAN-IS THE PACER PERFORMING PROPERLY-WHY NOT?

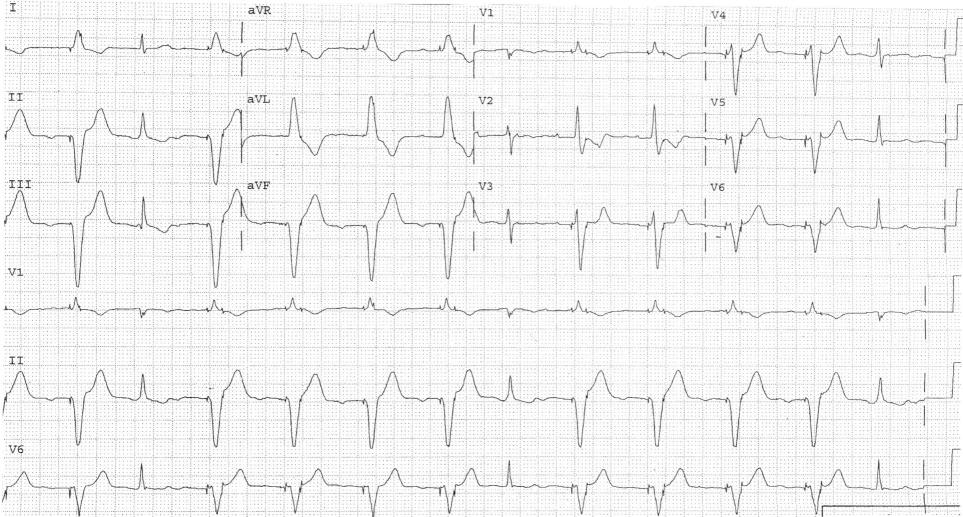

Although there are two pacing "spikes" note that the first is at the leading edge of, and is the cause of the QRS; and the second is hiding at its end. Something is awry! Explanation: the atrial electrode of a dual chamber pacer has dislodged and has slipped across the tricuspid valve and is now stimulating the ventricle. After a delay of 160 msec, the ventricular limb is activated, and arrives at the end of the QRS complexes, and is obviously ineffective. With the recognition of the problem, the atrial lead was repositioned and all's well that ends well. Since it is in the right ventricle, the atrial electrode can sense the three conducted beats, inhibit its discharge, and reset the timing clock.

```
PR          +   Atrial fib. w/rapid ventr. Response of 173 [Remains]    CHAMBER     CHAMBER     MODE OF
QRSD  224   .   Multiple ventricular premature complexes [Now Present]  PACED       SENSED      RESPONSE
QT    362   -   Right axis deviation [Now Present]
QTc   614   +   Nonspecific intraventricular conduction delay [Now Present]
            -   Early Transition
--AXES--    -   Lateral region infarct, possibly acute [Now Present]
P           -   Diffuse Nonspecific T abnormalities [Now Present]
QRS   94    -   [Now Present] Consider right ventricular hypertrophy    71 YEAR OLD MAN
T     -1                  - ABNORMAL ECG -                              COMPUTER A LITTLE OFF BASE??
```

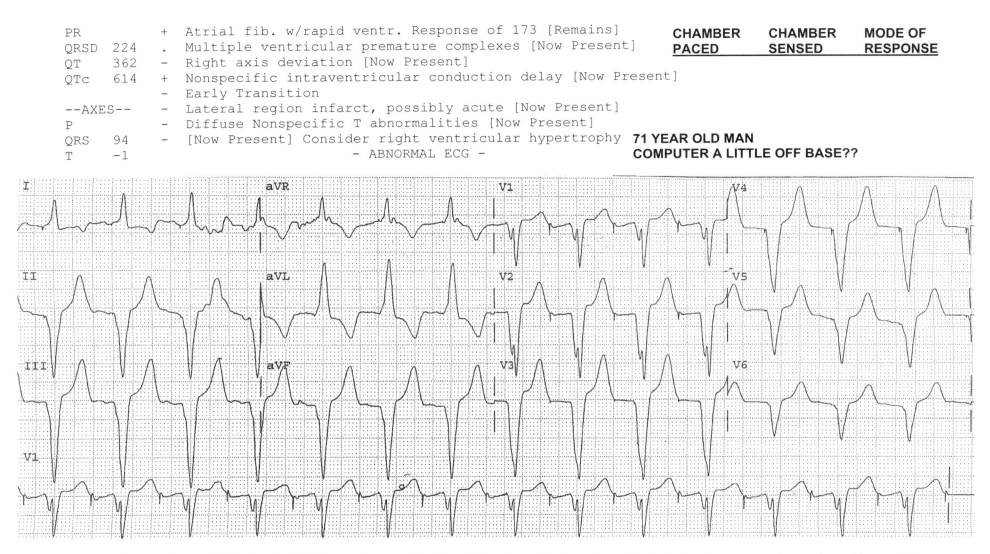

The computer really struck out with this tracing! It does not appreciate the atrial and ventricular spikes of a dual chamber pacemaker and provides multiple diagnoses--all of which are wrong. Since the discharge of the pacemaker alters the sequence of both depolarization and repolarization, diagnoses of myocardial infarction, atrial abnormality, ventricular hypertrophy, and ST-T changes can no longer be made.

```
PR     203    +   Electronic pacemaker, ventricular capture. Rate = 117
QRSD    94    -   No further analysis attempted due to pacemaker rhythm
QT     348    -   [Now Absent] QT interval long for rate
QTc    437    -   [Now Absent] Diffuse ST-T abnormalities
--AXES--
P       20                            - ABNORMAL ECG -
QRS     15
T
```

CHAMBER PACED	CHAMBER SENSED	MODE OF RESPONSE

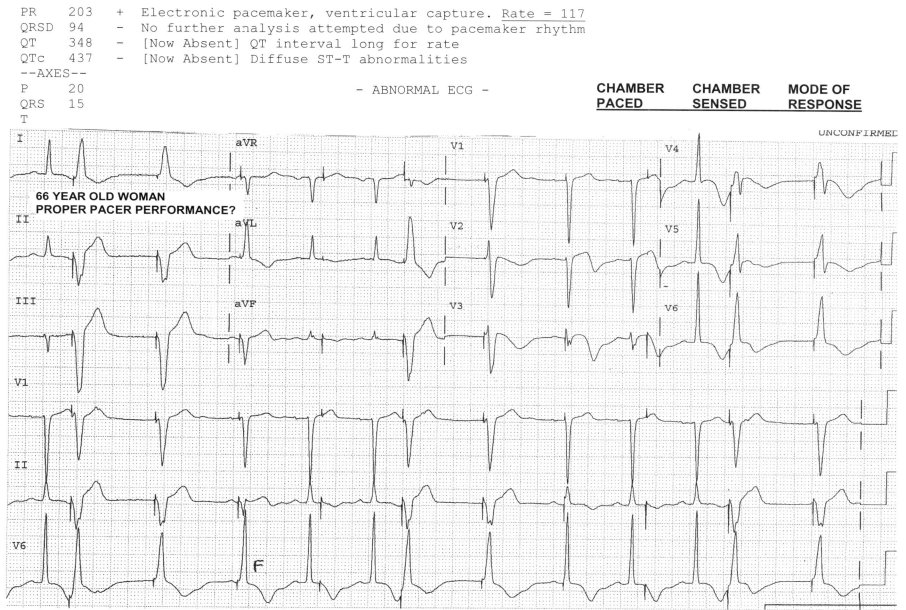

66 YEAR OLD WOMAN
PROPER PACER PERFORMANCE?

UNCONFIRMED

The computer has recognized the presence of a single chamber ventricular pacemaker, but had trouble counting the pacer spikes and determining the discharge rate. A glance at the pacing interval indicates that the rate is +/- 63/min and not 117. In addition, the computer ignores the fact that the pacemaker is not sensing and is behaving as a fixed-rate unit. As the pacer discharge meanders through the sinus conducted rhythm, it is able to "capture" if it is beyond the refractory interlude established by the sinus beats. The coincidence of the sinus impulse and electronic pacemaker results in a fusion complex (**F**).
Conclusion: the pacemaker sensitivity needs to be adjusted, and the computer needs to be instructed!

```
PR      168   (DIS15)  .    No analysis attempted for this ECG due to defective data
QRSD    139   (QMA04)  $    Lead (s) I, II, III, V1, V2, V3, V4, V5, V6 were not used for morphology analysis
QT      373   (ST)          [Now Absent] Sinus tachycardia, rate 104
QTc     414   (LBBB)   - *  [Now Absent] Left bundle branch block
              (LAE)    - *  [Now Absent] Left atrial enlargement
--AXES--      (AMIA)   - *  [Now Absent] Consider Acute Anterior infarct
P        84                        - Defective ECG -
QRS       2
T       120
```

CHAMBER PACED	CHAMBER SENSED	MODE OF RESPONSE

70 YEAR OLD MAN
SUGGESTIONS FOR THE COMPUTER?

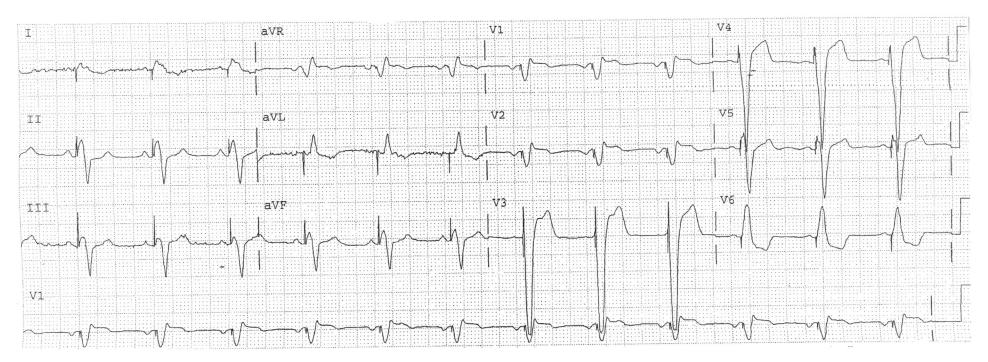

For reasons unclear, the computer was unable to recognize the obvious pacer "spikes" and regards the tracing as "defective," rather than the appropriate function of a dual chamber pacemaker.

```
PR              (VTACH) + VENTRICULAR TACHYCARDIA, rate = 169.
QRSD    192     No further analysis will be attempted
QT              [Now Present]
QTc             (QMA04) $ Lead(s) aVR, aVL, aVF, V1, V2 were not used

--AXES--
P                              - ABNORMAL ECG -
QRS      68                                           73 YEAR OLD MAN
T                                                     COMPUTER'S HAD A BAD NIGHT!
```

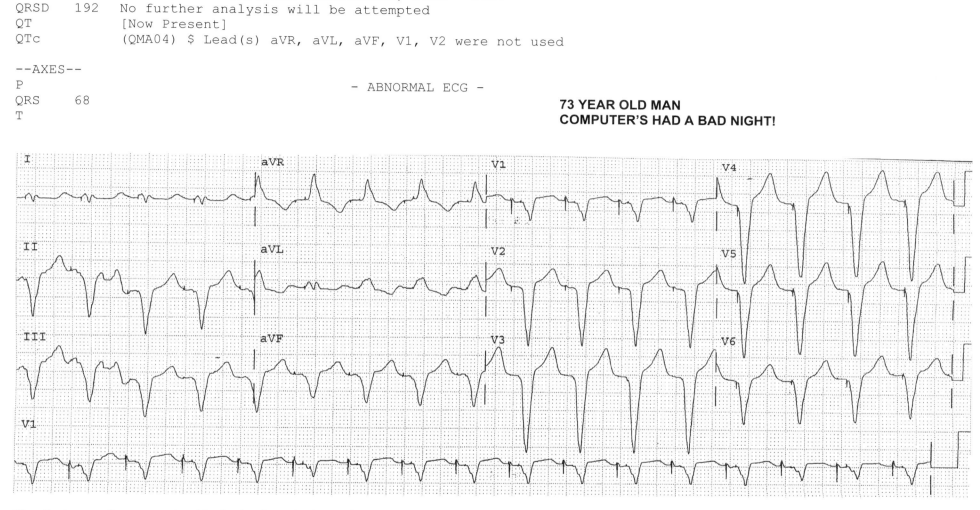

The discharge of a pacemaker bipolar lead results in small spikes that are sometimes difficult to see. Presumably, that is the reason that the computer does not recognize the pacemaker activity. It attributes the wide QRS paced beats as due to "ventricular tachycardia" and, for unclear reasons, thinks that the rate is 169/min. The dual chamber pacing function identifies a DDD pacemaker. The rate of 100/min and the short A-V delay indicates that this is the "magnet mode" of the unit.

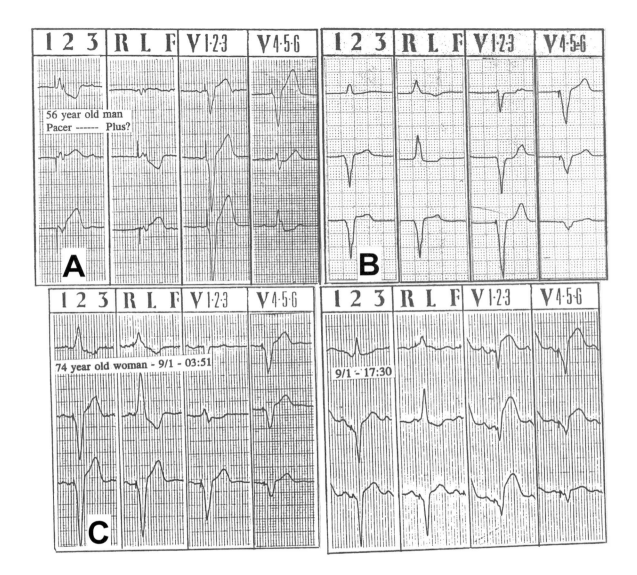

Since a right ventricular pacemaker activates the heart with the sequence of depolarization of RV before LV, the paced QRS morphology resembles LBBB. The criteria for the diagnosis of acute myocardial infarction in the presence of an electronic pacemaker are the same as those defined for acute MI with LBBB.

1. *ST segment elevation 1 mm or more concordant with the QRS complex.* In patient **A**, note that the QRS in lead II, although small, shows concordant ST elevation indicating an acute inferior M.I.

2. *ST segment depression 1 mm or more in leads V1 or V2 or V3.* This is present in V1 and V 2 in patient **B** and is consistent with acute posterior infarction.

3. *ST segment elevation > 5 mm discordant with the QRS complex.* In contrast to tracing **C** at 03:51, the later tracing at 17:30 shows marked ST elevation in leads V1-V4, due to an acute anterior MI.

Sgarboss, et al Am. J. Cariol. 1996: 77:423.

TECHNICAL ERRORS AND ARTIFACTS

The reviewer must stay alert to recording errors in the EKG, as well as distracting and disconcerting mistakes in the computer interpretation. Obviously, our dedicated, talented, and trained EKG technicians would never willfully present an incorrectly recorded tracing for interpretation. The majority of errors occur with untrained personnel obtaining EKGs in the emergency department, or on the wards, at night or on weekends.

The possibility for technician errors are numerous. Reflect on this: if there are four extremity and a single precordial lead, the number of different lead combinations is--1 x 2 x 3 x 4 x 5 = 120-only one of which is correct! With the current precordial display of six electrodes, the possibility of error exceeds 3 million.

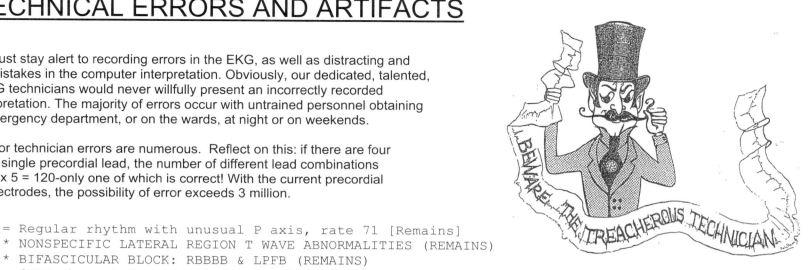

```
PR      152     = Regular rhythm with unusual P axis, rate 71 [Remains]
QRSD    124     * NONSPECIFIC LATERAL REGION T WAVE ABNORMALITIES (REMAINS)
QT      400     * BIFASCICULAR BLOCK: RBBBB & LPFB (REMAINS)
QTc     435     - [NOW Absent] Consider left atrial enlargement
--AXES--
P       121
QRS     100
T       113
```

                                                        - ABNORMAL ECG -

76 YEAR OLD WOMAN ANY CHANGES IN DX NEEDED?

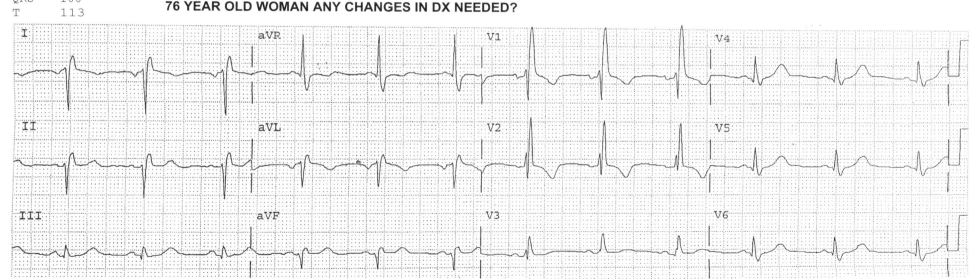

Probably the most frequent recording error is the interchange of rt. and lt. arm electrodes, which is present in this tracing. Since this reverses the polarity of lead I, the normally upright P wave becomes negative, and the QRS complex becomes inverted. The QRS recorded as lead II is really lead III, lead aVR is aVL, and the only correct frontal plane lead is aVF. Note that the precordial leads show typical RBBB. Lead I now shows an "upside-down" RBBB pattern. A worthwhile alert is to compare the QRS morphology in lead I and V6. Since their electrical axes are similar, there should be a reasonable similarity in the two leads.

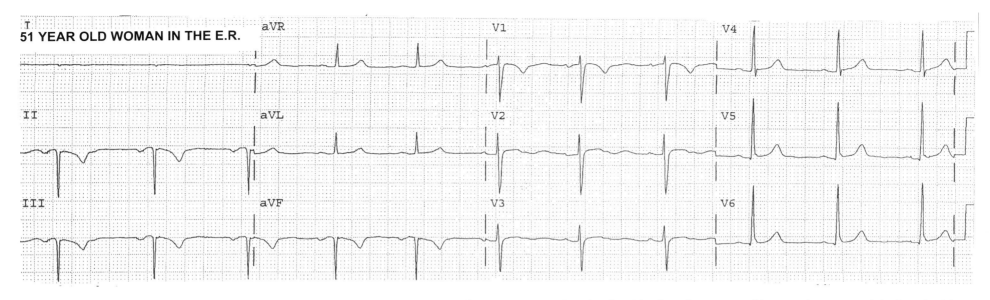

51 YEAR OLD WOMAN IN THE E.R.

If the electrodes of a bipolar lead are placed on both ankles, the potential difference recorded in that lead is virtually zero, and it records as a straight-line. In this example, the right and left arm electrodes have been so placed (i.e., the arm leads are on the legs, and vice versa). This makes the frontal plane leads invalid and warrants a repeat tracing (and a gentle reprimand!). In the repeat tracing, notice that the ST segment elevation and PR segment depression are consistent with the patient's problem of pericarditis.

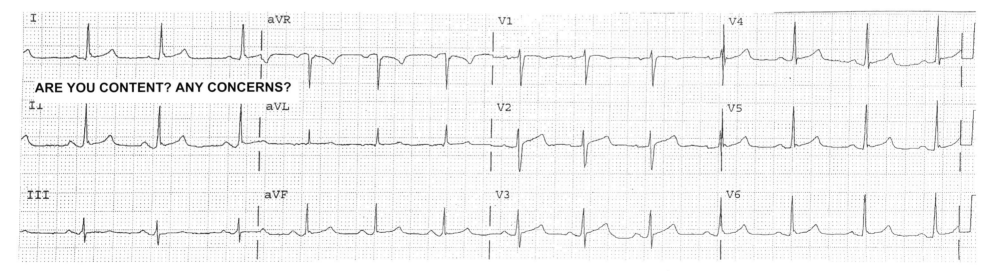

ARE YOU CONTENT? ANY CONCERNS?

81 YEAR OLD WOMAN -12/19 06:31
YOUR OBSERVATIONS?
A MAJOR PROBLEM IS?

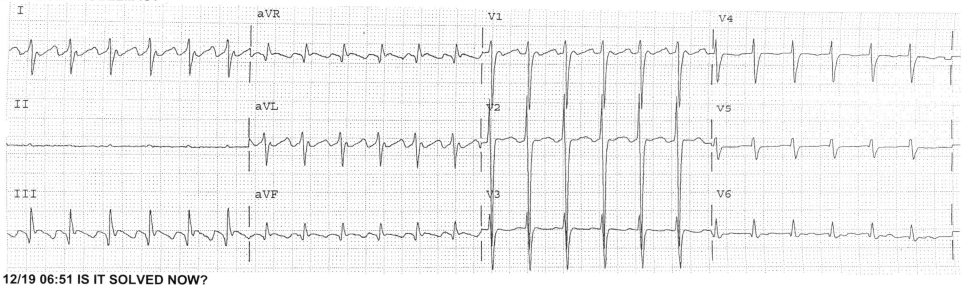

12/19 06:51 IS IT SOLVED NOW?

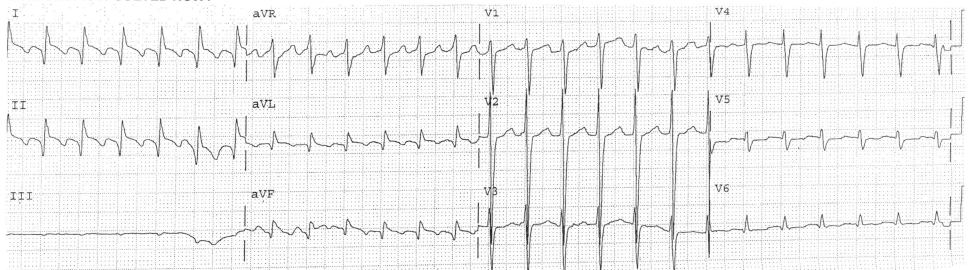

In the top tracing, the rhythm is atrial flutter at 300/min with 2:1 AV conduction, and with precordial lead evidence of LVH. The "major problem" is a sleepy technician! The flat QRS complex in lead II is evidence that somnolent Sam has placed the right arm electrode on the ankle. The lead is now registering the potential across the ankle bones, where little exists! The QRS complexes in frontal plane leads should be regarded as uninterpreable. 20 minutes later the tracing was repeated: this time with the left arm electrode on the ankle and lead III becomes the lead without voltage. Another tracing that is uninterpretable!

351

```
PR      178     = Normal sinus rhythm, rate 77 [Remains]
QRSD     81     * Prominent anterior forces (? RVH or post. MI) [Now Present]
QT      358     * Consider Anterior infarct [Now Present]  - Borderline ECG -
QTc     405
```

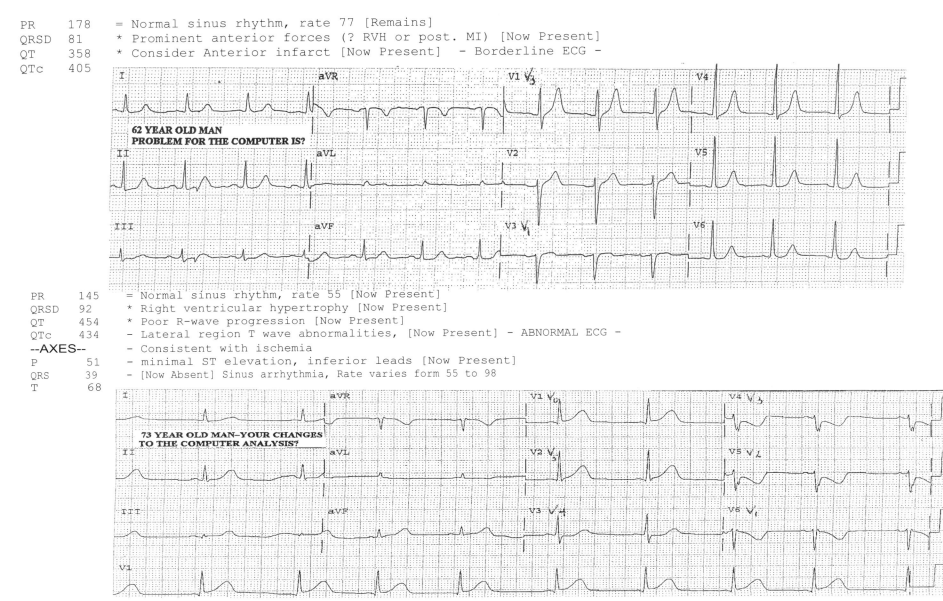

62 YEAR OLD MAN PROBLEM FOR THE COMPUTER IS?

```
PR      145     = Normal sinus rhythm, rate 55 [Now Present]
QRSD     92     * Right ventricular hypertrophy [Now Present]
QT      454     * Poor R-wave progression [Now Present]
QTc     434     - Lateral region T wave abnormalities, [Now Present] - ABNORMAL ECG -
--AXES--        - Consistent with ischemia
P        51     - minimal ST elevation, inferior leads [Now Present]
QRS      39     - [Now Absent] Sinus arrhythmia, Rate varies form 55 to 98
T        68
```

73 YEAR OLD MAN–YOUR CHANGES TO THE COMPUTER ANALYSIS?

Lest we are sometimes too hard on the computer, let's acknowledge that if the wrong information is provided, a wrong analysis will result. A frequent technician error is to rearrange the precordial leads. In the top tracing, the electrodes for leads V1 and V3 are switched and a large R wave is recorded in V1, prompting an incorrect diagnosis by the computer. When the precordial leads are corrected, the EKG is normal. In the bottom tracing, _all_ of the precordial leads are rearranged and the corrected leads are indicated. The tracing is abnormal, with slight ST segment elevation in leads II, III, and aVF; ST segment depression in V1-V3; and ST elevation in V5 and V6 consistent with an acute inferior-posterior and lateral myocardial infarction.

352

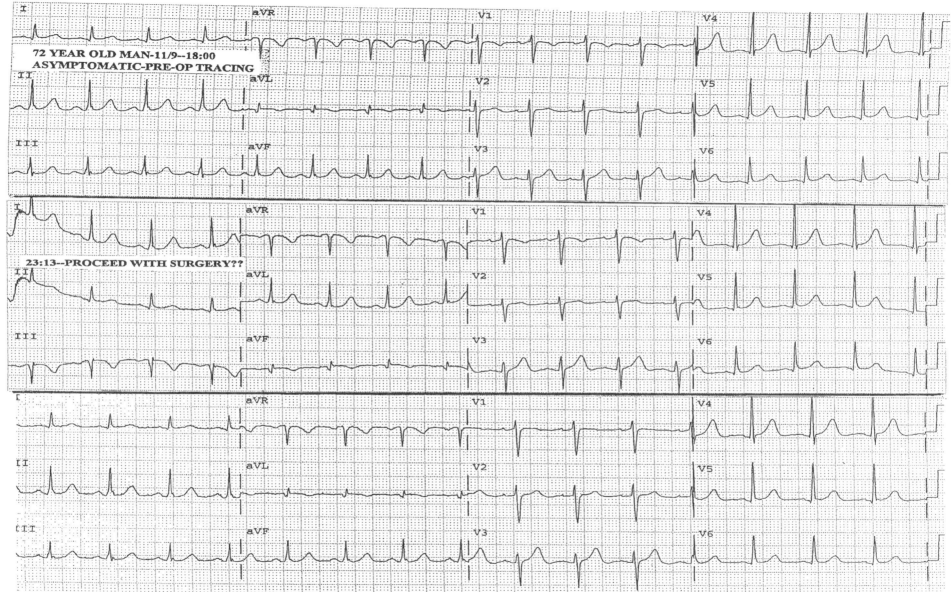

72 YEAR OLD MAN-11/9--18:00
ASYMPTOMATIC-PRE-OP TRACING

23:13--PROCEED WITH SURGERY??

An interesting and disturbing thing resulted from this technician error. The top tracing was obtained prior to scheduled surgery and is normal. Later the same evening, a nurse, who was not aware that the preoperative EKG had already been obtained, repeated the tracing. Understandably, it was interpreted as showing an inferior M.I. and surgery was canceled. The bottom tracing, the following morning, is identical to the first EKG. Why is the second tracing so different and so abnormal? The error was due to an interchange of the left arm and left leg electrodes. The major alterations in the QRS and T waves in leads III and aVF that resulted simulate an inferior infarction. This is a lead switch that is difficult to recognize unless prior tracings are available, and happily, is infrequently encountered.

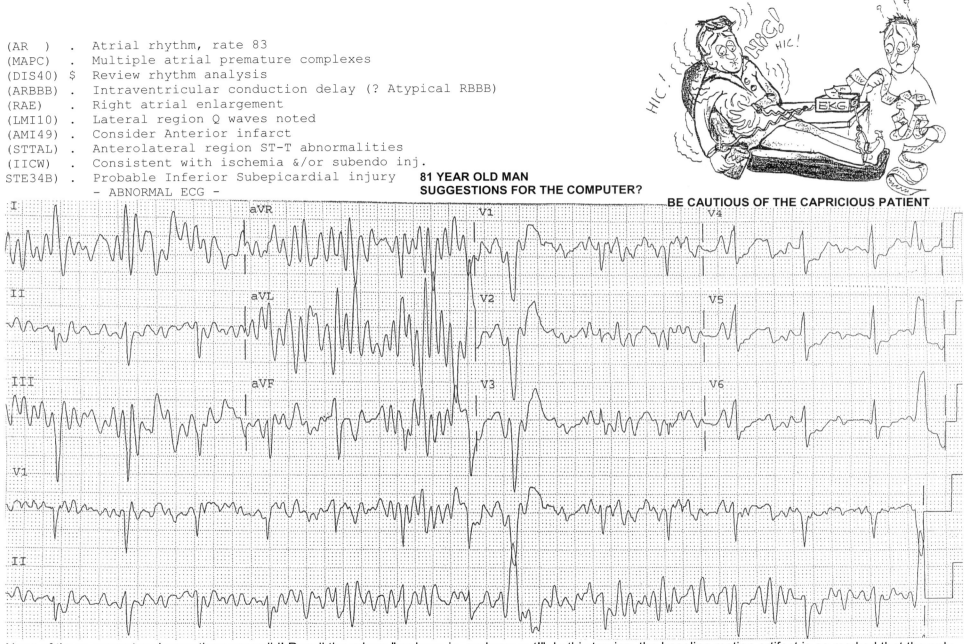

(AR　)　.　Atrial rhythm, rate 83
(MAPC)　.　Multiple atrial premature complexes
(DIS40)　$　Review rhythm analysis
(ARBBB)　.　Intraventricular conduction delay (? Atypical RBBB)
(RAE)　.　Right atrial enlargement
(LMI10)　.　Lateral region Q waves noted
(AMI49)　.　Consider Anterior infarct
(STTAL)　.　Anterolateral region ST-T abnormalities
(IICW)　.　Consistent with ischemia &/or subendo inj.
STE34B)　.　Probable Inferior Subepicardial injury
　　　　　- ABNORMAL ECG -

81 YEAR OLD MAN
SUGGESTIONS FOR THE COMPUTER?

BE CAUTIOUS OF THE CAPRICIOUS PATIENT

None of these computer observations are valid! Recall the adage "garbage in, garbage out!" In this tracing, the baseline motion artifact is so marked that the only possible conclusion is: "EKG is unsuitable for interpretation-please repeat." It is prudent to instruct the patient that moving, wiggling, coughing, hiccupping, and seizing during the EKG recording is **FORBIDDEN**!

```
PR      201    = Normal sinus rhythm, rate 75 [Remains]
QRSD     95    = Indeterminate QRS axis
QT      390    + Inferior injury (Acute infarct) [Now Present]
QTc     436     *Nonspecific lateral region T abnormalities [Now Present]
                   - ABNORMAL ECG -
```

75 YEAR OLD WOMAN
DO YOU AGREE?

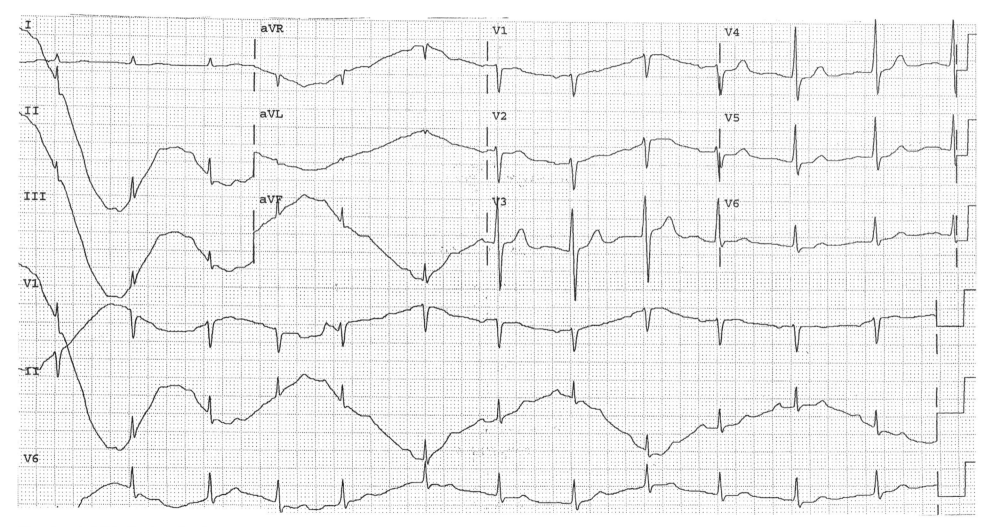

The abrupt shift in the baseline is due to the patient's movement. It results in an apparent ST segment elevation in leads II, IIII, and aVF. The computer diagnosis of acute inferior M.I. is not warranted. The tracing should be repeated before a final judgment can be made.

87 YEAR OLD MAN
"PLEASE TAKE THE EKG WHILE I'M SITTING IN MY CHAIR!"

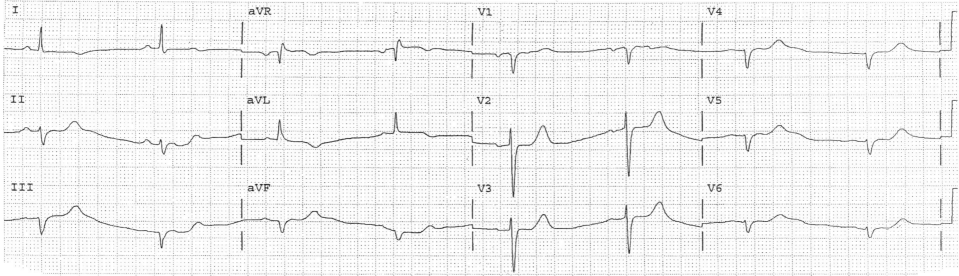

"OH ALL RIGHT – I'LL LIE DOWN"

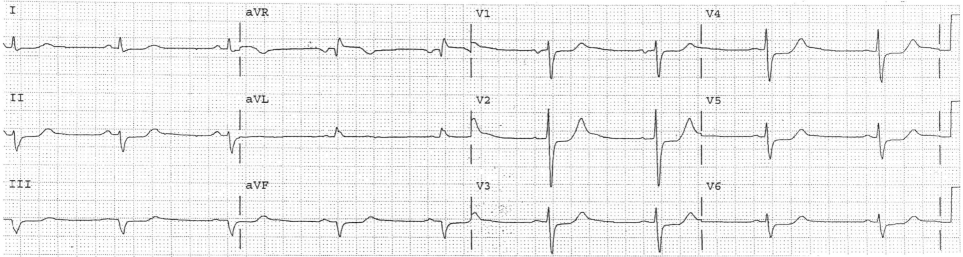

The EKG technician should always alert the clinician if the tracing was not obtained with the patient recumbent. When recorded lying on the side, and particularly when sitting, the change in cardiac position can alter the recording significantly. In the top tracing, the rhythm is sinus bradycardia at 45/min. The left axis deviation of (-) 60° is probably due to a prior inferior infarction. The negative T waves in leads I and aVL are abnormal and the QS pattern in leads V4-V6 is consistent with a lateral M.I of uncertain age. When the tracing was repeated in recumbency, the frontal plane T waves are upright in I and aVL and the pattern of lateral infarction is no longer present.

80 YEAR OLD WOMAN-RHYTHM?
THE FLB's REPRESENT:
   1.   **PERNICIOUS PVC's?**
   2.   **SIMPLY SINGULTUS?**

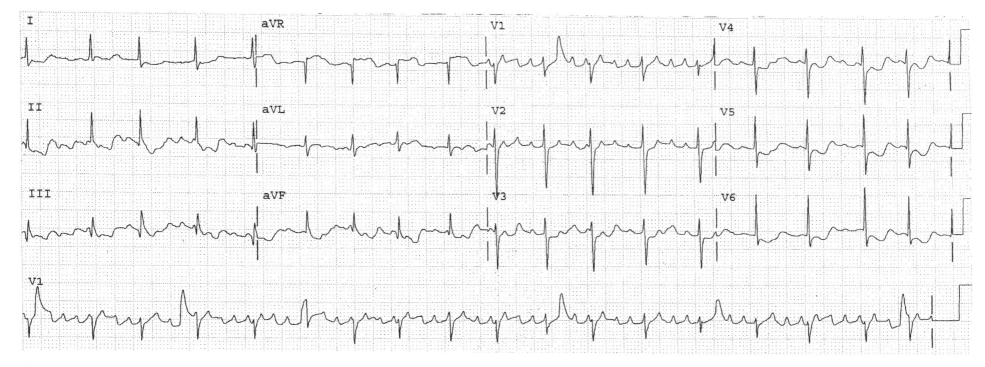

The underlying rhythm is atrial flutter with variable A-V conduction. The startling "funny looking beats" are due to the forceful chest motion of "hiccups" (more precisely, in medical parlance, known as "singultus").

```
PR    131   (TACHO) . Tachycardia of undetermined origin, rate 134
QRSD   86   (PC  )  . Premature complexes
QT    276   (CLAE)  . Consider left atrial enlargement
QTc   412   (SDJ )  . Junctional ST depression

--AXES--
P     IND              - ABNORMAL ECG -
QRS    36
T      72
```

55-YEAR OLD MAN OBSERVATIONS?

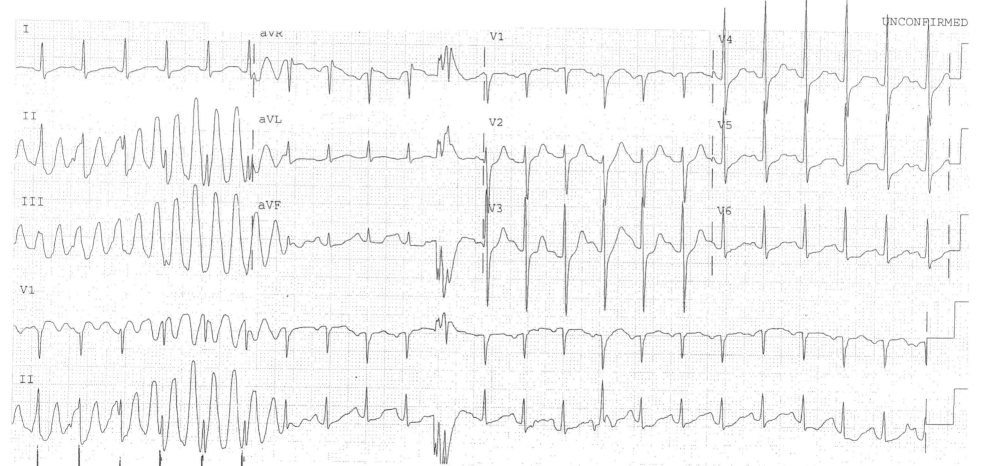

Despite having simultaneous leads available, the computer does a poor job of recognizing gross artifact. Lead I is free of the baseline motion artifact seen in leads II and III—therefore that "moving part" is the left leg. Sometimes patients inadvertently try to fool us!

80 YEAR OLD WOMAN 8/26
EVIDENCE OF ANTERIOR M.I.??

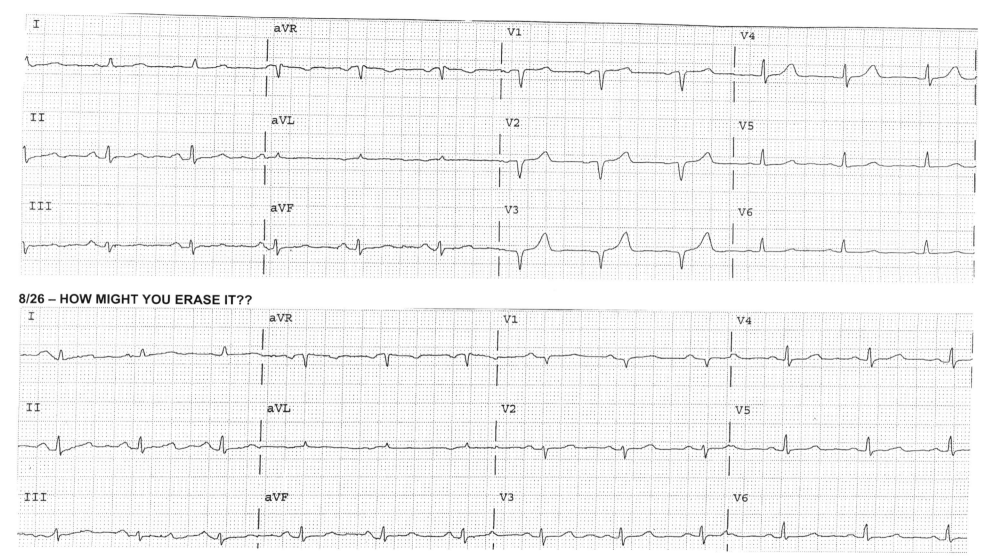

8/26 – HOW MIGHT YOU ERASE IT??

The upper tracing shows low QRS voltage in both frontal and horizontal planes. Absence of r waves in V1-3 is consistent with anterior MI. Could this be artifactual? If the decreased voltage is due to hyperinflation pulmonary disease, the heart would be trailing the low-lying diaphragm. Thus, the appropriate precordial electrode position would be "too high" for the cardiac position. The lower tracing was recorded three interspaces below the normal position and eliminates the concern about anterior infarction. This exploration is called "precordial mapping," and is a simple and inexpensive procedure in the patient with C.O.P.D.

In bygone days, the "machine" problems were in the electrocardiograph itself. There was a need for careful maintenance to insure proper standardization, recording stylus pressure and heat, and frequency response. Today, the problem for the clinician is the computer! Computer interpretation of EKGs became available in the early 1970s and was greeted with enthusiasm and anticipation. Unfortunately, the computer's ability to provide an accurate interpretation or provide comparative analysis has been sorely lacking.

The requirement for "oversight" by a reviewer remains more important than ever.

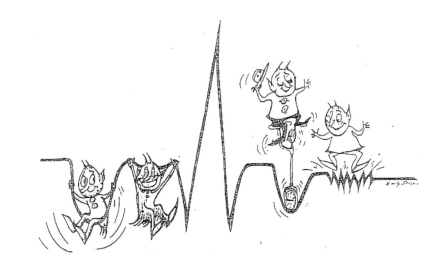

BE MINDFUL OF THE MISCHIEVIOUS MACHINE

```
PR              3rd degree AV block. Ventricular rate = 44
QRSD   96
QT     424
QTc    363
--AXES--
P       54                      - ABNORMAL ECG -
QRS     36
T       46
```

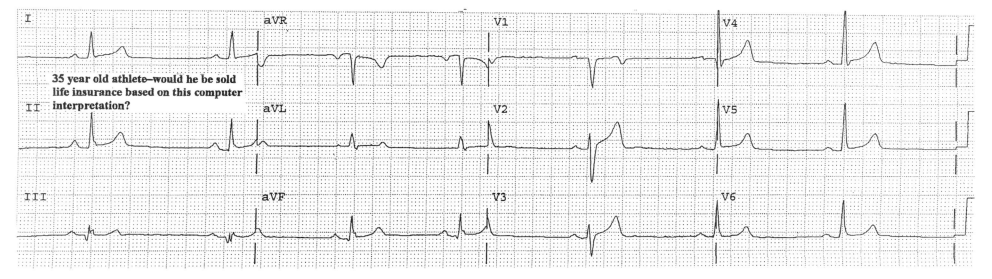

I   aVR   V1   V4

35 year old athlete--would he be sold life insurance based on this computer interpretation?

II   aVL   V2   V5

III   aVF   V3   V6

An example in point--this man's EKG and is normal and the computer interpretation defies understanding.

74 YEAR OLD MAN –
DO YOU AGREE WITH THE COMPUTER?

SERIAL COMPARISON NOT PERFORMED
REGULAR RHYTHM, UNDETERMINED ORIGIN, RATE 75
MULTIPLE VENTRICULAR PREMATURE COMPLEXES
LEFT AXIS DEVIATION
INFERIOR INFART
                         ABNORMAL ECG

The underlying rhythm is sinus and the conducted impulses are normal. Despite the computer's recognition that the wide complexes are ventricular, it misinterprets them as the conducted impulses, and misdiagnosis them as showing left axis deviation and inferior MI.

```
PR     198   * Normal sinus rhythm
QRSD   109   + Low voltage in frontal leads [Now Present]
QT     346   + Nonspecific Inferior T abnormalities [Now Present]
QTc    430

--AXES--
P       5.                          - ABNORMAL ECG -
QRS    54
T      -8            66 YEAR OLD MAN
                     DO YOU AGREE?
```

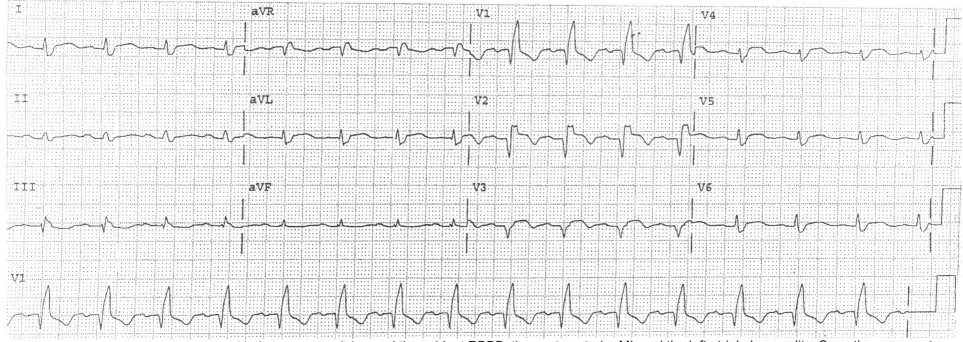

There should be major disagreement with the computer. It ignored the evident RBBB, the acute anterior MI, and the left atrial abnormality. Sometimes computer interpretations are not particularly helpful.

Sinus rhythm, rate 96 [Remains]
Borderline first degree AV block [Remains]
Bifasicular block: RBBB & LAFB [Now Present]
LVH by voltage [Now Present]
                 -   ABNORMAL ECG -

**54 YEAR OLD MAN
DO YOU AGREE WITH THE
COMPUTER?**

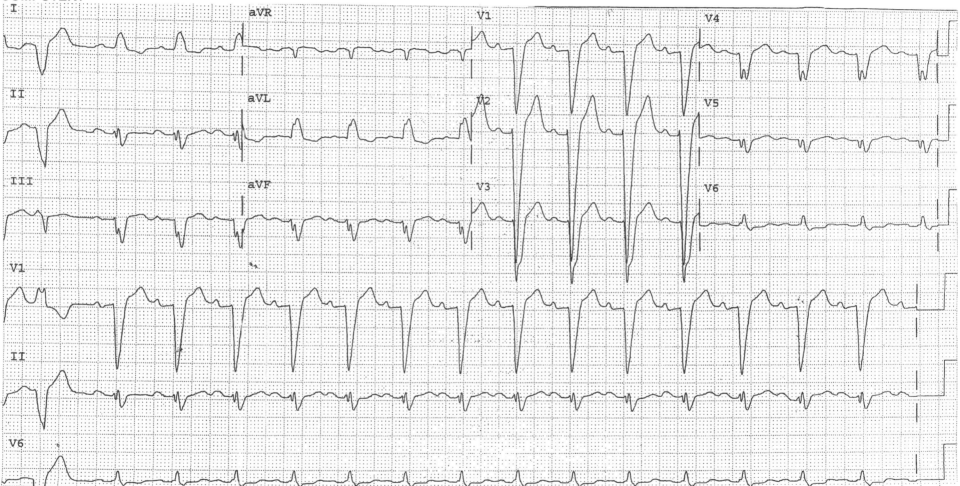

All complexes, except the first, are due to sinus rhythm conducted with first-degree A-V block and LBBB. The computer has mistaken the first beat, which is clearly a ventricular ectopic complex, as the morphology to interpret, and arrives at the bizarre diagnosis of RBBB plus LAFB.

PATTERNS AND EPONYMS

"We see only what we look for, we recognize only what we know."
Dr. Benjamin Felson

66 YEAR OLD MAN
HOW MANY FEATURES OF COPD?
WHAT IS "SCHAMROTH'S SIGN"?

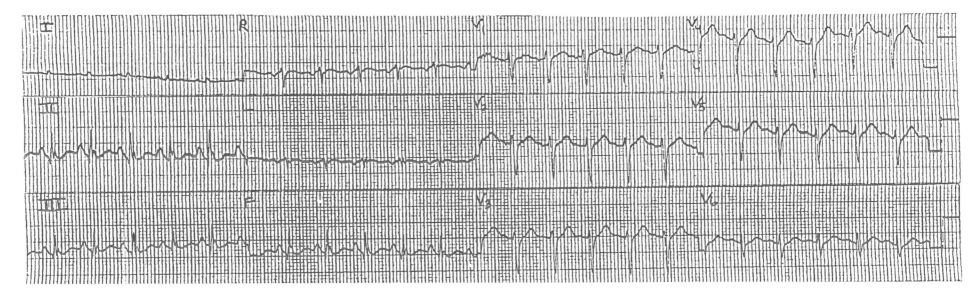

Dr. Leo Schamroth provided a valuable EKG sign which is available at a glance. The clue is: when the P-QRS-T are all <u>reasonably</u> isoelectric in lead I, the patient has advanced COPD. The correlation with this pattern and the patient's pulmonary disease is excellent. Hyperinflation results in low-lying diaphragms. The heart shares in the lower position, and the frontal plane vectors are directed inferiorly. In addition, the appropriate location of the precordial leads is now "too high" for the cardiac position and there is a monotonous rS pattern in all the chest leads. Usually, evidence of right atrial abnormality is present.

79 YEAR OLD MAN – LOW VOLTAGE
IN LEAD V6 MAY BE DUE TO?

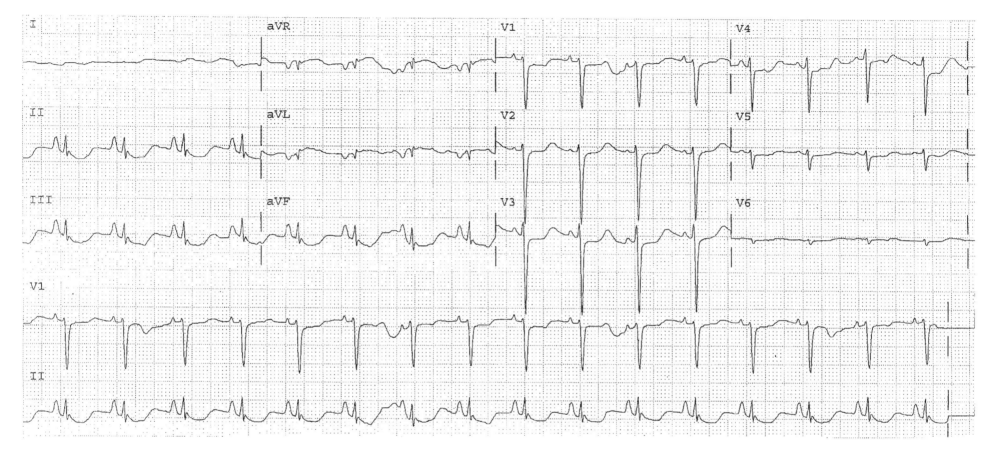

Another example of the "Schamroth sign." The lead I pattern is accompanied by impressive P waves indicating right atrial abnormality. The Q-T-U interval is prolonged, probably due to hypokalemia. The precordial leads are unusual. Prominent rS complexes are present in V1-V3 because these lead locations have a "proximity effect" to the heart. Leads V4-V5 are further removed from the heart and their voltage is less. Lead V6 has the insulating effect of the hyperinflated left lung and displays a diminutive QRS complex. All in all-far advanced obstructive pulmonary disease

WHAT IS A "PRECORDIAL MAP"?

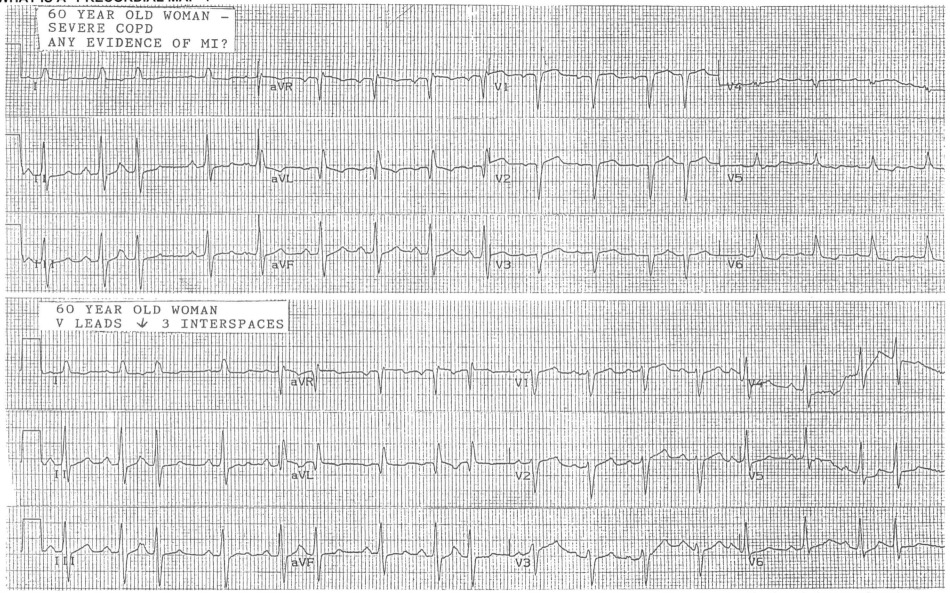

60 YEAR OLD WOMAN —
SEVERE COPD
ANY EVIDENCE OF MI?

60 YEAR OLD WOMAN
V LEADS ↓ 3 INTERSPACES

One of the potential traps in the patient with COPD is due to the low-lying cardiac position. The precordial leads, although correctly placed, do not reflect the location of the heart. As in this woman, the result is an EKG lacking R waves in V1-V4, simulating an anterior myocardial infarction. A simple and inexpensive expedient is to record the horizontal plane leads lower than normal. A "precordial map" is a series of tracings recorded 1-2 & 3 interspaces below the normal. When performed in this patient, the tracing obtained 3 interspaces "low" shows no evidence of MI. Although she still has serious pulmonary disease, she hasn't had a heart attack!

85 YEAR OLD MAN
HOW MANY OBSERVATIONS?
THE FLBs REPRESENT?

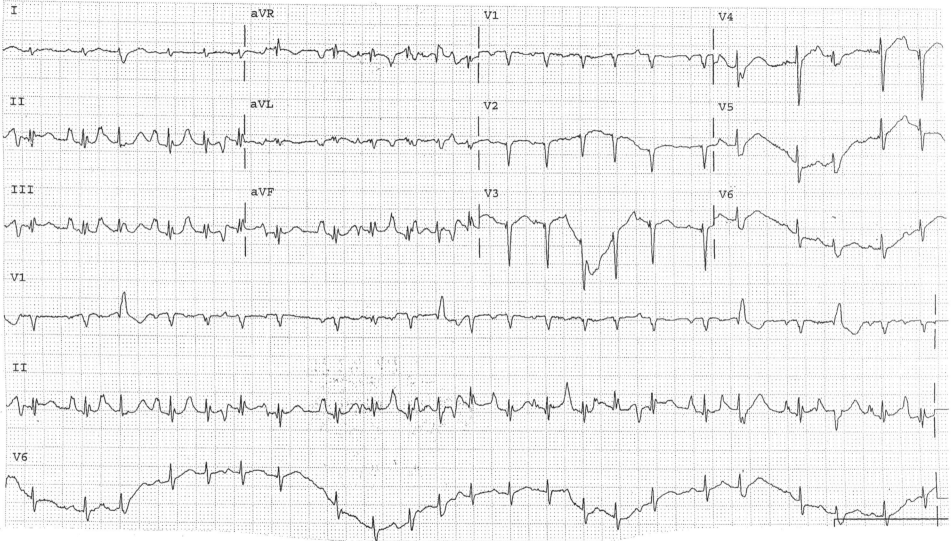

Observations include the following:

1. The rhythm is irregular and the P waves are multiform--a good example of multifocal atrial tachycardia.

2. Lead I shows isoelectric P-QRS-T ("Schamroth's sign") indicating advanced COPD.
   The dyspnea pattern at the bottom is evident.

3. Some of multiple P waves suggest right atrial abnormality.

4. The "funny looking beats" (FLBs) result when four of the APCs are aberrantly conducted with typical RBBB morphology.

367

WHAT IS THE "McGINN-WHITE PATTERN?

57 YEAR OLD MAN 9/25 PREOP EKG

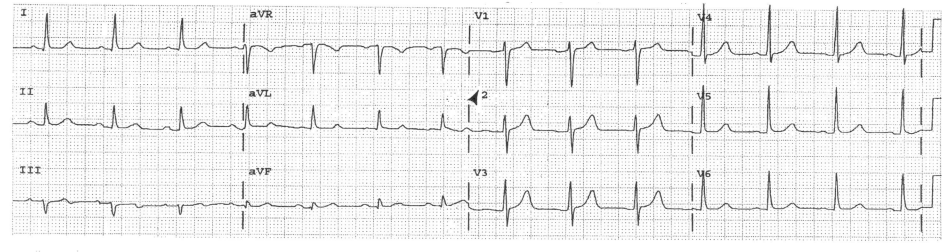

9/26-CONCERNS INCLUDE?

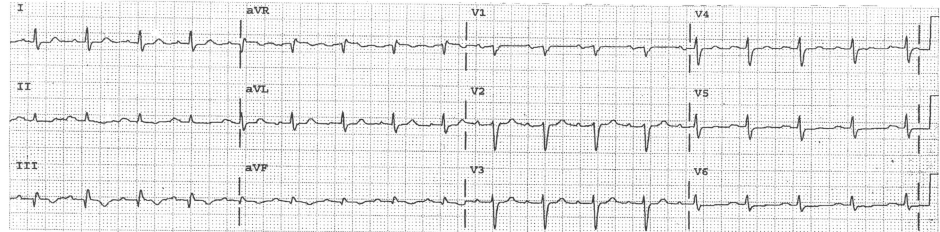

In 1935, with only the frontal plane leads available, Drs. McGinn and White described an important EKG pattern. They observed in patients with an S wave in lead I, Q wave in lead III and T wave inversion in that lead, a correlation with acute pulmonary emboli. The common abbreviation is "S I, Q III, T III pattern." Although the explanation for the changes is disputed, the pattern serves as a valuable alert to acute cor pulmonale, particularly pulmonary embolization. The top tracing, before projected surgery, is normal. Late the next day, he was found hypotensive and the bottom tracing shows major differences. The initial reaction might be inferior wall MI, but the lack of ST segment changes would be against that diagnosis. Massive pulmonary embolization was proven by angiography.

368

32 YEAR OL MAN
DIFFERENTIAL DIAGNOSIS?

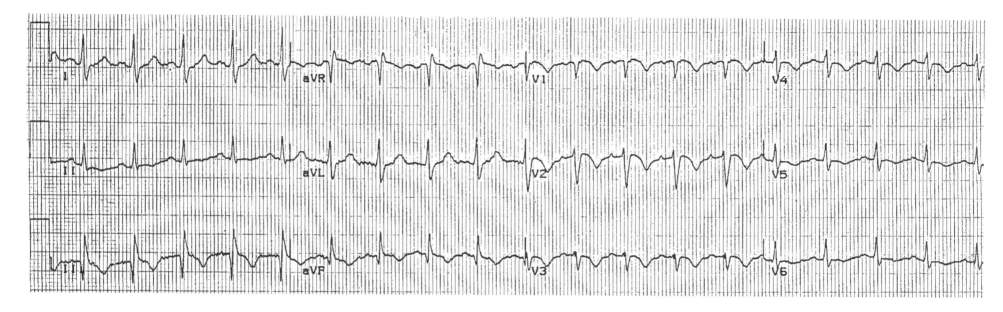

With the development of the precordial leads, there was an addition to the limb lead pattern of Drs. McGinn and White. Often, the frontal plane features of acute cor pulmonale are accompanied by prominent T wave inversions in the precordial leads. These are thought to represent "ischemia" of the right ventricle. This young man was injured in an auto accident and was confined for years to a wheelchair. He presented with marked leg edema, increasing dyspnea, and oppressive chest discomfort. His EKG shows a classic pattern of acute cor pulmonale-S I-Q III-T III with T wave inversion in V1-V5. Major pulmonary emboli were documented. At first glance, the frontal plane changes could be consistent with inferior MI, and the precordial lead T wave abnormality could reflect "anterior ischemia." An important aphorism is: *in the same EKG, when the limb leads suggest inferior MI and the precordial leads anterior MI, think pulmonary embolization.*

Important patterns to distinguish are those that are due to acute pericarditis and acute myocardial infarction. Since the pericardium itself has no electrical activity, pericarditis, with EKG changes, must be due to myocarditis of variable wall depth. The injury process is diffuse and not zonal as is that due to MI. Thus, there will be ST segment elevation in both frontal and horizontal planes, without reciprocal depression, except in lead aVR. In addition, in pericarditis there is an injury vector involving the atria. This is manifested by PR segment depression in most leads, but with PR segment elevation in lead aVR.
The upper tracing shows all the features of acute peri-myocarditis.

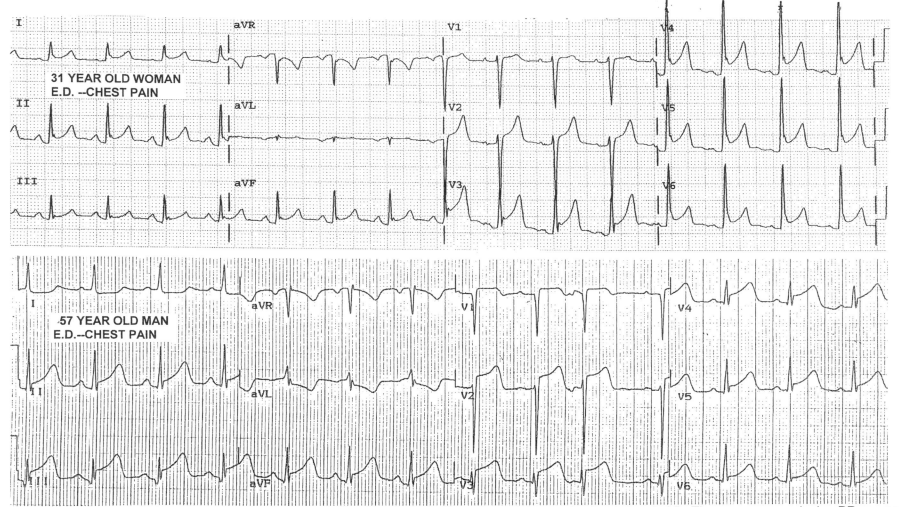

In contrast, this EKG shows ST segment elevation in the majority of leads, but with reciprocal depression leads I and aVL. There are no convincing PR segment depressions. This tracing indicates an extensive acute myocardial infarction.

**39 YEAR OLD MAN – WHOSE NAME IS
ATTACHED TO THIS PATTERN?
WHAT IS THE SIGNIFICANCE?**

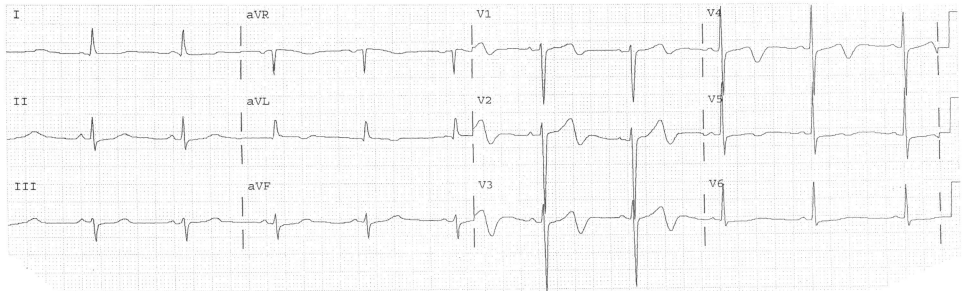

The major EKG abnormality is the striking ST-T change in leads V1-V4. The ST segment is not elevated in these leads, and it rises in a concave fashion to the apex of the T wave, and then drops sharply into the deep trough. This pattern has been termed "Wellens' warning." Dr. Wellens and his colleagues reported that when patients presented with chest pain and this EKG pattern, cornary arteriography revealed a proximal and high-grade lesion in the left anterior descending coronary artery. If untreated, these patients had a significant incidence of extensive anterior infarction within a few weeks to months.

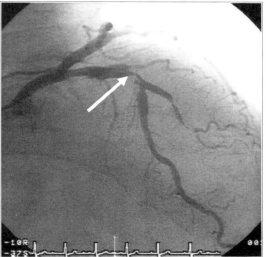

This 39-year-old man presented with increasingly frequent and lasting angina pectoris. After myocardial infarction was excluded, coronary arteriograms were performed. The illustration shows a highly obstructive lesion in the L.A.D., proximal to the first septal perforating branch. The other coronary vessels were normal.

Angioplasty was performed with good results.

WHAT IS A "SWINGING HEART"?

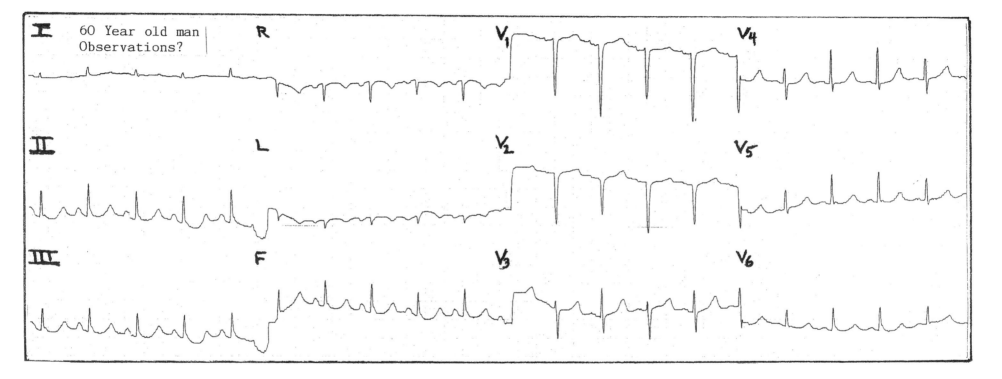

The most important observation in this EKG is the alternating amplitude of the QRS complexes, well seen in leads V1-V3. "Electrical alternans" is virtually diagnostic of pericardial effusion with tamponade. The cause has been clarified by echocardiography. Pericardial fluid accumulations with cardiac compression results in a pendular motion of the heart--a "swinging heart." This man had lung cancer with pericardial metastases.

49 YEAR OLD MAN
LOW QRS VOLTAGE – WHY?
CLUE: NORMAL [NA] X 3 = BW

Low QRS voltage is present when the limb lead amplitude is 5 mm or less, <u>and</u> the precordial 10 mm or less. It can be due to a loss of "signal" from the cardiac generator, or to some form of "insulator" present. The math quiz posed for this tracing provides an answer: Na = 145 X 3 = 435--which is this man's weight. The cardiac voltage on the inside is insulated from the outside by adipose tissue!

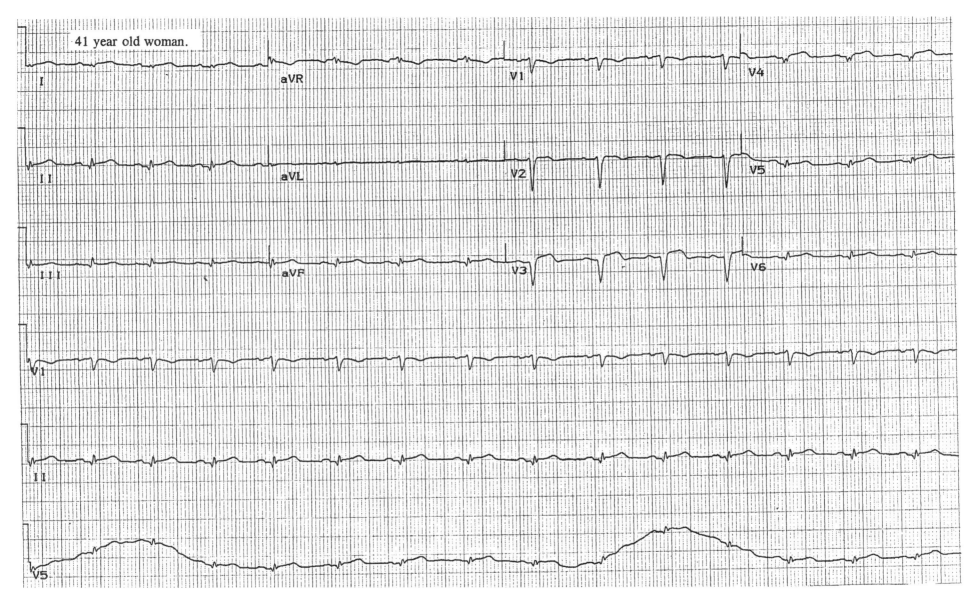

41 year old woman.

Low QRS voltage in this woman was due to her multiple myocardial infarctions--inferior and anterolateral. She presented with profound heart failure and required intubation. The rhythm strip of lead V5 shows a respiratory excursion due to the ventilator at 12/min. She died during this hospitalization.

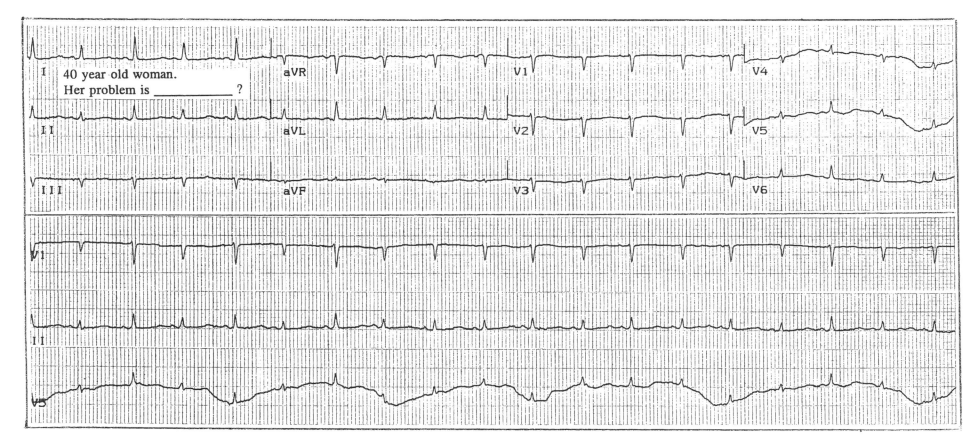

I — 40 year old woman. Her problem is _____ ?

aVR — V1 — V4

II — aVL — V2 — V5

III — aVF — V3 — V6

V1

II

V5

This unfortunate woman had metastatic breast cancer and had a malignant pericardial effusion. In addition to the low QRS voltage, note the electrical alternation in the rhythm strip of lead V1, indicating pericardial tamponade. Her dyspnea is reflected in the respiratory undulations in lead V5. Pericardiocentesis produced 2000 ml of bloody fluid, which was teeming with cancer cells.

63 YEAR OLD MAN -9/18 07:43
WHAT IS "KILLIP'S RULE"?

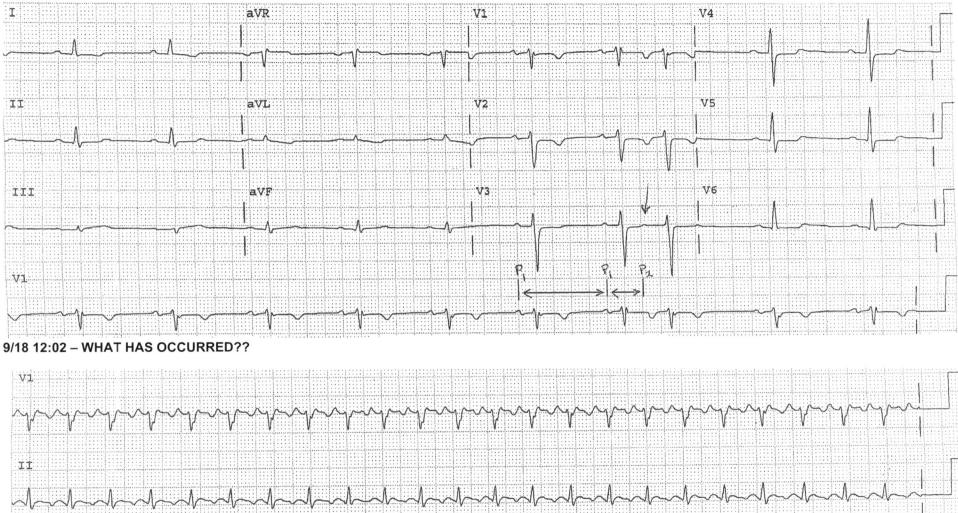

9/18 12:02 – WHAT HAS OCCURRED??

Years ago, Dr. Thomas Killip pointed out that when APCs are sufficiently premature, they are likely to precipitate a supraventricular tachycardia--either atrial flutter or fibrillation. This has become known as "Killip's rule" which states: when the timing of the atrial premature is less than 50% of the basic P-P cycle, an atrial arrhythmia can be anticipated. In this example the sinus cycle (P1-P1) is 1 sec; and the APC arrives with a coupling interval of 0.40 sec (P1-P2). The bottom tracing shows that Killip's prophecy was correct. The patient has developed atrial flutter with 2:1 conduction.

72 YEAR OLD WOMAN
THE "GUSTO CIRTERIA" INCLUDES?

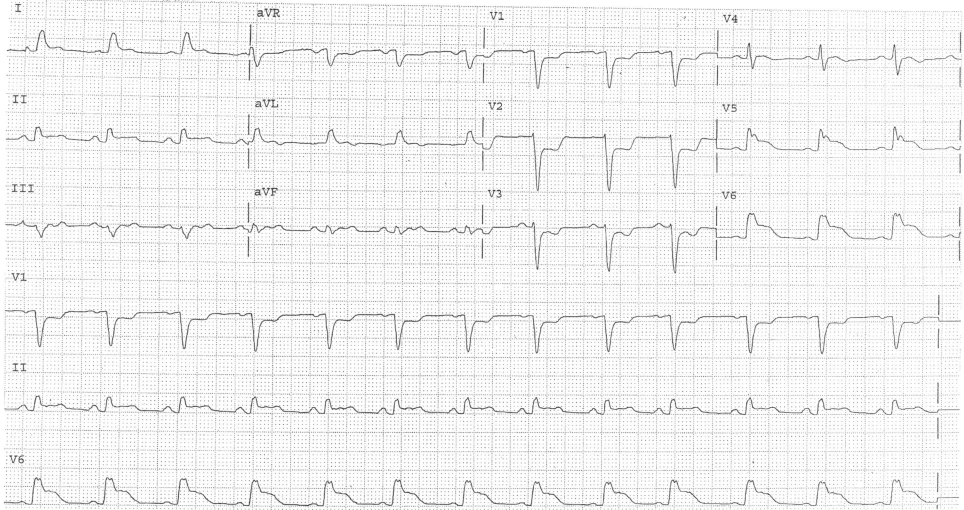

They "GUSTO" study was an international investigation, designed to determine the efficacy of thrombolytic drugs in the treatment of acute myocardial infarction. A subsequent substudy provided criteria for the recognition of acute MI in the presence of left bundle branch block.

Criterion #1 = ST segment elevation of 1 mm or more concordant with the QRS complexes (i.e. the ST segment is elevated in a lead in which the QRS is positive). This is present in leads I, II, aVF, V5 and V6.

Criterion #2 = ST segment depression in V1 or V2 or V3 of 1 mm or more. This is present in all 3 leads.

Criterion #3 = ST segment elevation discordant with the QRS of 5 mm or more (i.e., the QRS is negative in a lead in which there is ST segment elevation of 5 mm or more.) This is not present in this tracing.

The frontal and horizontal plane directions of the "injury vector" suggests that the acute infarction involves the posterolateral wall.

28 YEAR OLD WOMAN
WHAT IS THE "SI, SII, SIII PATTERN"?

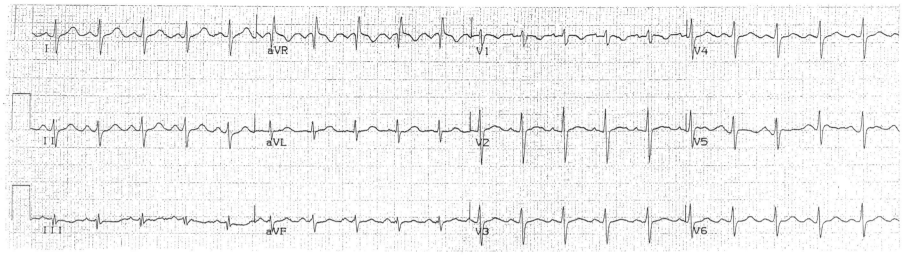

56 YEAR OLD MAN
PULMONARY FIBROSIS

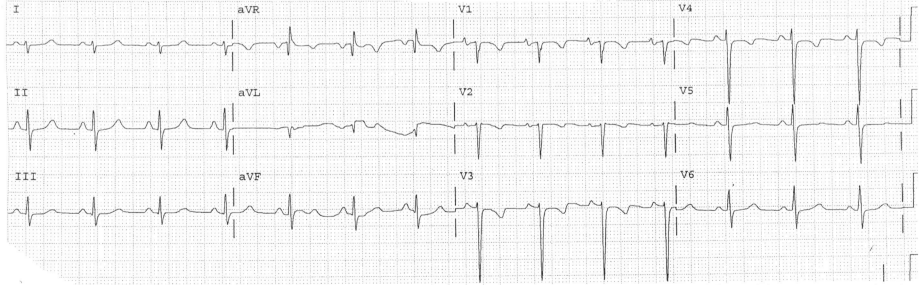

A reminder: in childhood and young adult life, the right ventricle is electrically the dominant chamber. As life continues, the left ventricle assumes control and remains "in charge" for the remainder of one's life. There is normally a period of transition when the R.V. and L.V. are competing. The result is a "tug-of-war" which renders the frontal and horizontal plane leads equiphasic. Today, this is called an indeterminate axis. In earlier days, when only the three bipolar limb leads were available, the description used was "S1, S2, S3 pattern." It is normal in the 28-year-old woman, but is abnormal in the 56-year-old man. His progressive pulmonary disease has resurfaced his latent R.V., which is again competing with the dominant L.V. This pattern is one of the indicators of developing R.V.H.

WHAT ARE "OSBORN WAVES"?

THIS MAN'S PROBLEM IS?
CLUE=HEAT-WAVE PARADOX

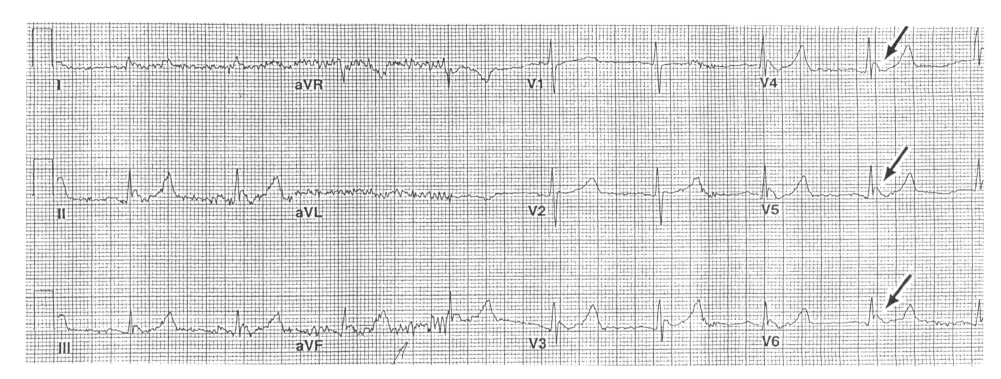

This EKG pattern was first described in 1953 by Dr. J. J. Osborn. Osborn was a cardiac surgeon investigating the application of induced hypothermia, to increase the time that the heart could be stopped for the correction of defects. He noted that as body temperature decreased, the EKG developed a late contribution to the QRS complex. This has become known as an "Osborn wave." The EKG shown was from an alcoholic man, who, during a heat wave "passed out" under a window air-conditioner. He was comatose when found by friends and had a temperature of 86°. Note the sinus bradycardia, the shiver artifact, and the "Osborn waves" (arrows), particularly in leads V4-6. A picturesque term that has been applied is "hypothermic humps." The obvious conclusion is--sometimes cold hands did not indicate a warm heart!   Tracing courtesy of Dr. Howard Burchell.

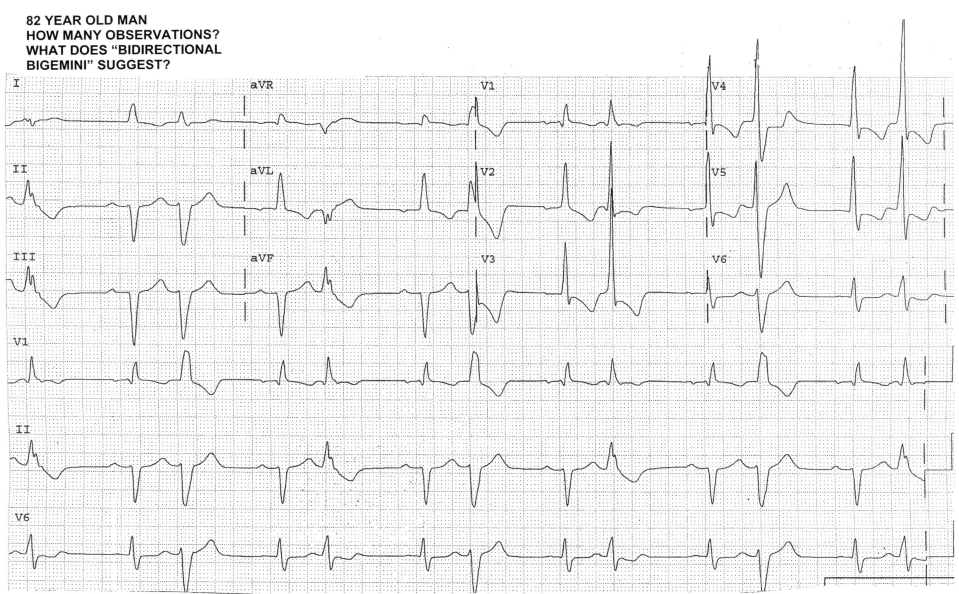

The sinus impulses are conducted with RBBB, and are coupled to VPCs-ventricular bigemini. The frontal plane "pre-blocked axis" is (-) 60°. The left axis is due to inferior MI, and the large initial R waves in V2-3 to a posterior infarction. Note that the polarity of the VPCs alternates in the rhythm strip of lead II. This is been termed "bidirectional bigemini," and is very suggestive of digitalis toxicity.

49 YEAR OLD MAN-POSSIBILITIES?
WHAT IS "BRUGADA'S SYNDROME"?

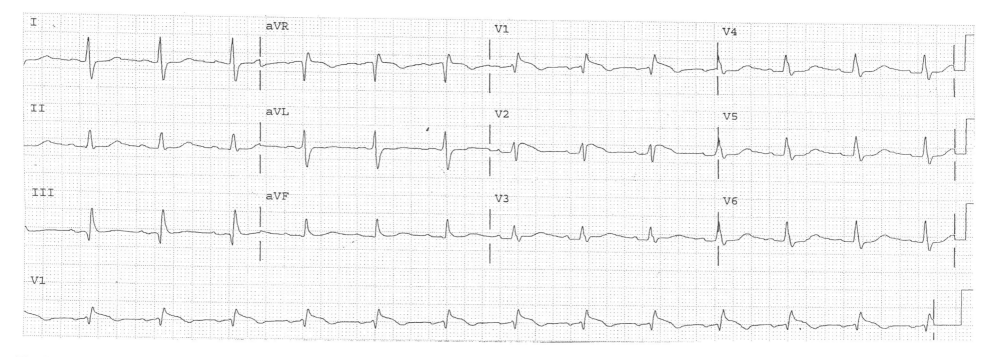

The Brugada brothers reported patients with an abnormal pattern of repolarization which was associated with a threatening clinical course. The EKG showed RBBB, normal QT interval, and persistent ST segment elevation in precordial leads V1-V3. It was not explained by ischemia, electrolyte abnormality, or structural heart disease. Patients presented with recurrent episodes of aborted sudden death, due to a rapid polymorphic ventricular tachycardia. Since the early report of the "Brugada syndrome," many cases have been encountered, particularly in Asiatic countries. It appears to be the result of a genetic abnormality. The most effective treatment has been an implantable defibrillator, rather then antiarrhythmic drugs.

Some Final Thoughts and a Quiz

It is a natural inclination to want to shrug off the tedium, the time and the effort of interpreting the electrocardiogram to the ever vigilant eye of the computer. It appears doubly desirable when you, the overseer, can still be paid while the computer does most of the work. The hope, however, that a computer's interpretation can be substituted for that of a well-trained human is beguiling but misplaced.

In these pages we have presented examples of the inadequacy of the computer's efforts, and we believe it is irresponsible to ignore such evidence as that collected in these pages. The computer occasionally misses an acute myocardial infarction, usually misses an electrolyte imbalance, sometimes overlooks the presence of a functioning artificial pacemaker, almost invariably fails to suspect pulmonary embolism and is quite incapable of recognizing most of the not-so-simple arrhythmias. Surely it is time to blow the whistle on an expensive, time-consuming, sometimes risky exercise?

Even the most enthusiastic supporters of the computed interpretation agree that all interpretations must be checked and, if necessary, corrected by a competent human eye. This being so, the computer's effort is not only unreliable but also redundant. The skilled interpreter can dictate an original interpretation in less time than it takes to correct the computer's errors; thus the capable and conscientious reader has no use or need for the computer's assistance, while the less competent reader may be lulled into faulty security.

The following tracings have been selected not only to represent important clinical diagnoses but also to illustrate the computer's inadequacy as an interpreter.

1

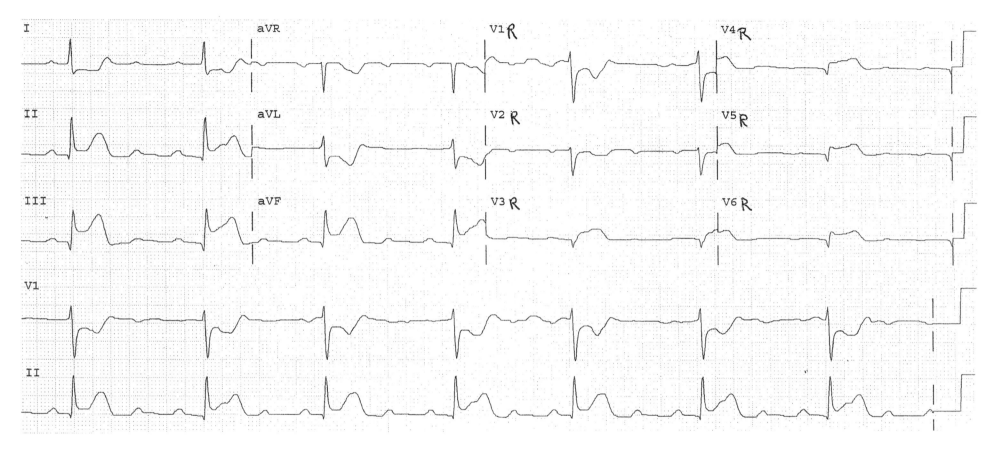

1

Computer: 53 yrs Female

```
PR              + Atrial flutter or fib with 3rd deg. AV block. (Atrial rate = 479, Ventricular rate 44)
                  [Now Present]
QRSD  92        + possible Acute Inferior infarct [Now Present]
QT    484       + Acute Anterolateral region infarct with reciprocal ST depression [Now Present]
QTc   414       - [Now Absent] Sinus tachycardia, rate 102
                - [Now Absent] Consider left atrial enlargement
--AXES--        - [Now Absent] Abn. R wave progression (?ASMI or lead loc'n)
P                                     - ABNORMAL ECG -
QRS   83
T     97
```

Comment: The computer has an exaggerated impression of the atrial rate which is, in fact, 130/min with sometimes 3:1 and sometimes 4:1 A-V conduction, giving a resulting ventricular rate of about 44/min. The P waves appear to be normally directed" and so we will assume a sinus tachycardia with 3:1 and 4:1 A-V conduction. The computer is not programmed to recognize, let alone interpret, <u>right chest leads</u>. The ST segment elevations in leads V3R-V6R identify a right ventricular infarction accompanying the inferior M.I. Given that these are not the standard precordial leads, the computer interpretation of "anterolateral region infarction" is incorrect.

2

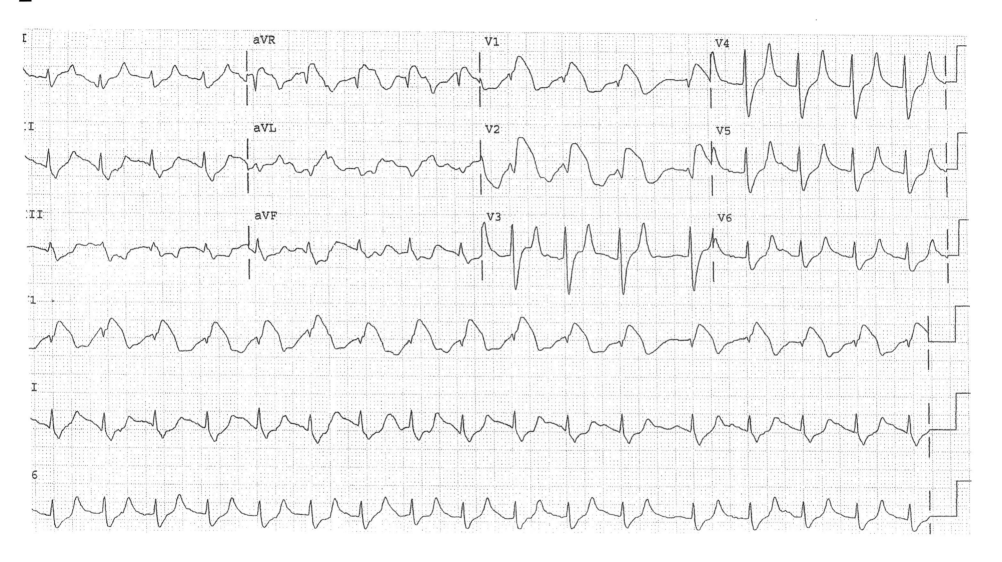

2

Computer: 35 yrs Male

```
PR     146    . Atrial tachycardia, rate 105
QRSD   148    . Right axis deviation
QT     366    . Nonspecific intraventricular conduction delay
QTc    484    . QT interval long for rate
              . ST-T abnormalities
--AXES--      . Anterolateral region Subepicardial injury
P      190                            - ABNORMAL ECG -
QRS    211
T       -2
```

Comment: This patient, aged 35 years, was taken to the lab and cathed only to find normal coronaries. It is difficult to take exception to any of the computer's assumptions and the only one that is emphatically wrong is the declaration of subepicardial injury; this is a dangerous assumption because it results in delayed appropriate treatment, combined with risky, inappropriate interventions.

The diagnosis here is severe **hyperkalemia-serum** potassium was 8.1 mEq/L. High levels of potassium are sometimes accompanied by marked ST elevations which expose the unfortunate patient to inappropriate and risky interventions.

A subtle clue that may help the clinician avoid this potentially fatal error is the detail of the upright T waves:

Whereas in most situations the upstroke of the upright T wave is more gradual than the downstroke, in' hyperkalemia the upstroke may be delayed so that the T waves are narrow-based with upstroke and downstroke forming symmetrical sides (as in the T waves in V3-6 in this tracing).

3

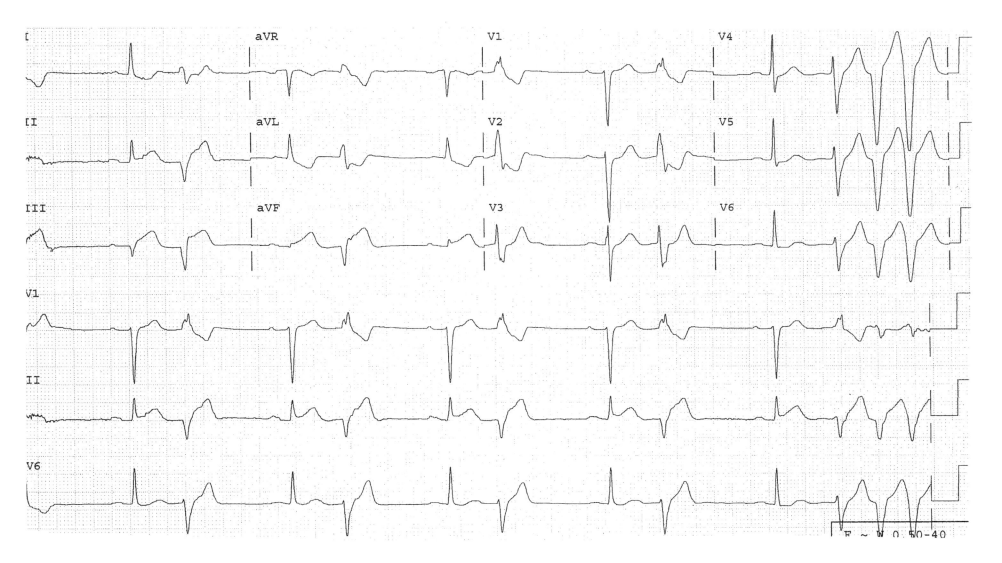

3

Computer: Male

```
PR      227     . Ventricular Bigeminy, Mean V-rate = 93
QRSD     81     . First degree AV block
QT      355     . Lateral region ST-T abnormalities
QTc     441


--AXES--                          - ABNORMAL ECG -
P        40
QRS       9
T       100
```

Comment: There is indeed ventricular bigeminy, slight prolongation of the PR interval (first degree A V block) a little ST depression in the left precordial leads and abnormally low T wave in V6.

But the most important diagnosis here is the early, acute inferior myocardial infarction with the ST-Ts elevated in leads 2, 3 and a VF and reciprocal depression in leads 1 and a VL. Note that these elevations and depressions of acute injury are recognizable in the ectopic as well in the sinus beats.

The terminal burst of three ectopic ventricular beats just squeezes under the qualifying wire for ventricular tachycardia, but we will never know if it continued!

4

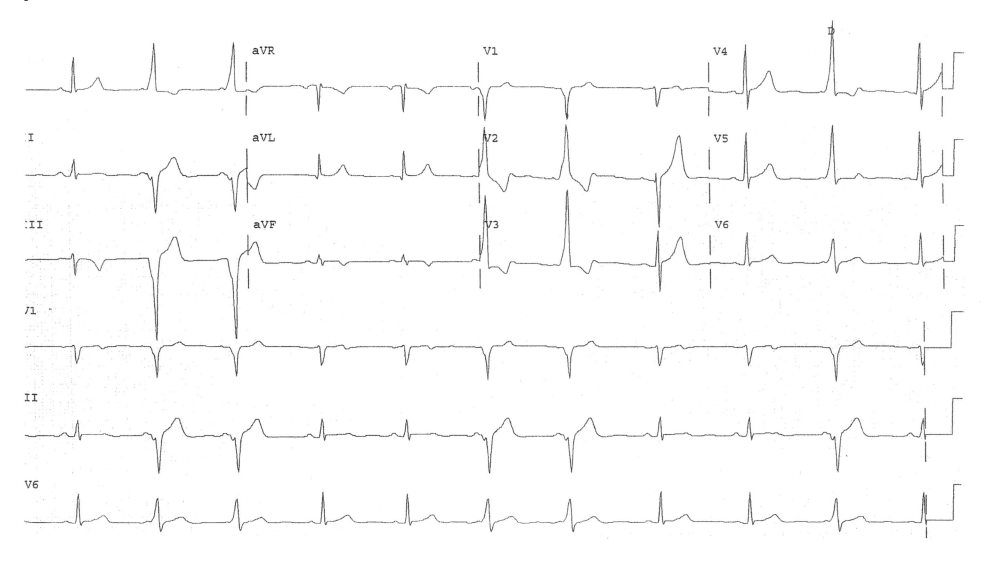

4

Computer: 51 yrs   Male   Other race

```
PR      167    = Sinus rhythm, rate 61 [Remains]
QRSD     80    + Ventricular premature complex [Now Present]
QT      361    = Consider Anteroseptal region infarct [Remains]
QTc     363    + Inferior T wave abnormalities, [Now Present]
               . Possible ischemia
--AXES--       -[Now Absent] Anterior infarct, possibly acute
P        46                              - ABNORMAL ECG -
QRS      16
T       -15
```

Comment: It is true that the preexcited complexes begin a little early, but they are not ventricular prematures as the computer would have them; and there is no sign of an anteroseptal infarct But there is, of course, **intermittent preexcitation** (WPW "syndrome").

It is worth keeping in mind the three entities that the WPW can somewhat simulate: ventricular hypertrophy, myocardial infarction and bundle-branch block. And the resulting diagnostic precaution: whenever you are *hesitantly* making any of those three diagnoses, ask yourself if you have overlooked a WPW.

5

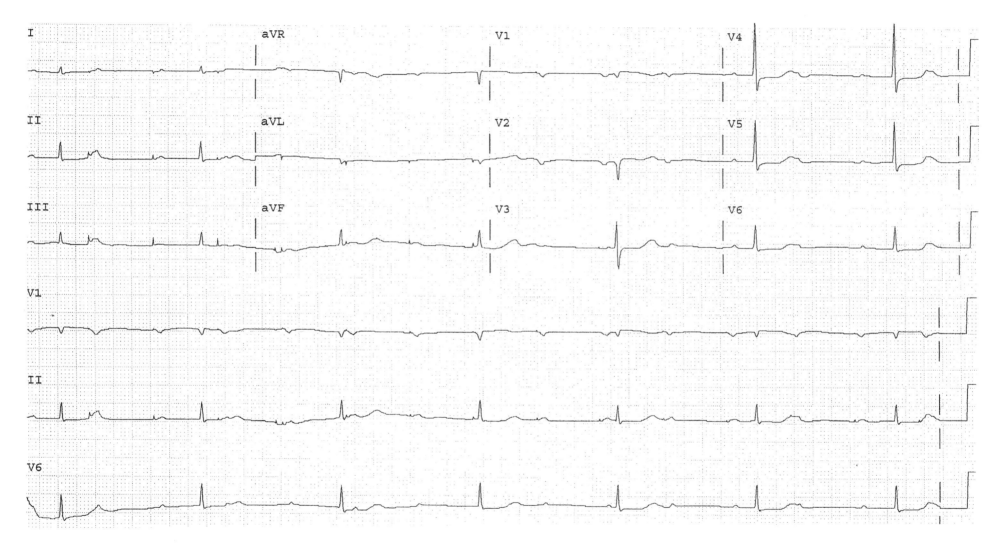

5

Computer: 87 yrs   Female   White

```
PR      160    + Electronic pacemaker, ventricular capture. Rate = 111 [Now Present]
QRSD     76
QT      342
QTc     469


--AXES--
P        12                                    - ABNORMAL ECG -
QRS      81
T       261
```

Comment: The computer recognizes an **electronic pacemaker** and abandons ship! The computer claims ventricular capture, of which there is no evidence and there is no rate approaching lll/min. The pacemaker is firing and controlling the atria at 86/min while the abandoned ventricles, thanks to **complete** A V block and now under the control of the A V junction, are enjoying a relaxed rate just under 40/min.

    The QRS complexes show unusually low voltage in most limb leads and somewhat increased amplitude in V4 and V5, while the ST segments are abnormally horizontal and a trifle depressed in several leads with a hint of elevation and no sign of an r wave in VI and V2-are we perhaps dealing with an **anteroseptal** infarct of uncertain date?

6

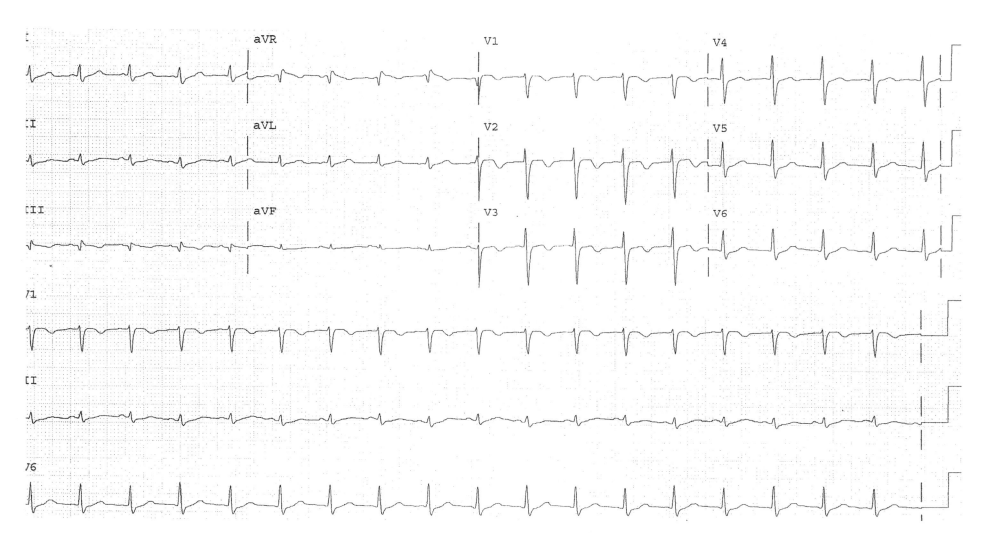

6

Computer: 50 yrs   Female Hispanic

    PR   112   + Sinus tachycardia, Rate = 110 [Now Present]
    QRSD   89   + Low voltage in frontal leads [Now Present]
    QT   322   = Nonspecific Anterior T wave abnormalities [Remains]
    QTc   435

    --AXES--
    P   49   - ABNORMAL ECG -
    QRS   70
    T   9

Comment: This is a diagnosis that is often missed by both computer and human eye-acute **cor pulmonale,** usually resulting from pulmonary embolism. It is often recognizable-as seen here--from the simultaneous inversion of T-waves in standard lead 3 and the right-sided precordial leads, VI-3, a combine that seems not to enjoy the recognition it deserves.

This patient also manifests the well known **S1Q3T3** combination commonly seen in pulmonary embolism.

7

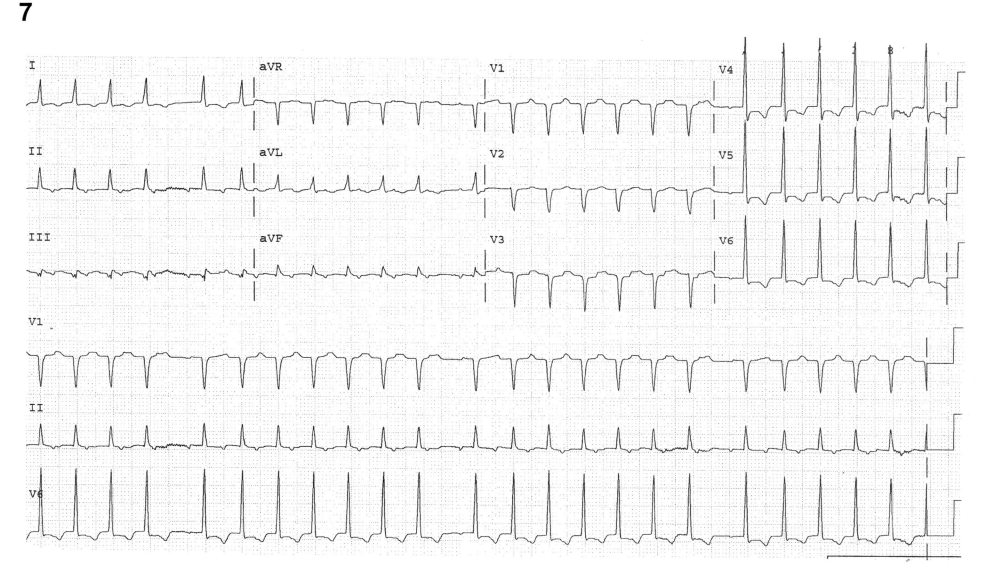

7

Computer: 85 yrs   Black

```
PR                . Supraventricular tachycardia, rate = 153
QRSD     86       * Aflutter/A Fib
QT       277      . Consider Anterior infarct
QTc      442      . Diffuse ST-T abnormalities

--AXES--
P                                         - ABNORMAL ECG -
QRS      32
T        179
```

Comment: The computer calls the supraventricular **tachycardia** but fails to recognize it as **atrial** and ccmment on the A V **Wenckebach periods** with **8:7 A-V ratios.**

Leads V4-6 present a QRS-T pattern that strongly suggests **left ventricular hypertrophy.**

The diagnosis of anteroseptal infarction is suggested by the computer because the right-sided chest leads are of QS configuration. But if you look at the more leftward leads (V4-6) you see that there are no normal little q waves, presumably thanks to the LVH; and this more readily and simply explains the absence of r waves in V1-3.

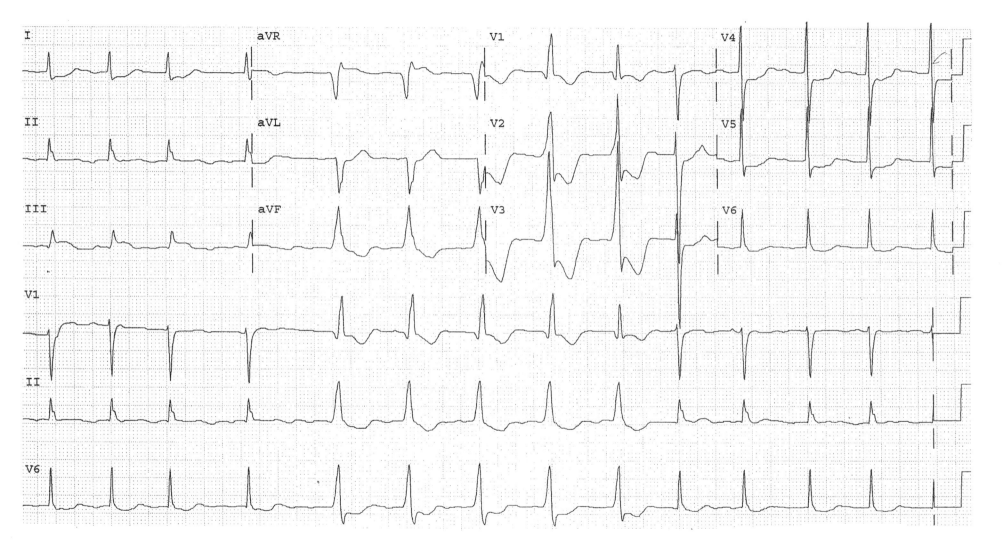

8

Computer: 69 yrs   Male White

```
PR      129    + Right axis deviation [Now Present]
QRSD    150    = Nonspecific intraventricular conduction delay [Remains]
QT      399
QTc     457


--AXES--
P       150                           - ABNORMAL ECG -
QRS     104
T       -76
```

Comment: This is a record that tempts one to make several misdiagnoses. First there is atrial fibrillation with ventricular response rate of about 85/min interrupted by a five-beat run of **accelerated left** idioventricular **rhythm.** Confirmation that this is indeed a rhythm of ventricular origin is seen in the fifth and last of these beats which, from its changed configuration especially in VI, is presumably a **fusion** beat.

The **acute inferior infarction,** recognizable from the ST elevation in lead 3, is confirmed by the reciprocal ST depression in the conducted beats in leads 1, aVL, and V2 to V6. The increased QRS amplitude of the conducted beats in the precordial leads implies significant **left ventricular hypertrophy.**

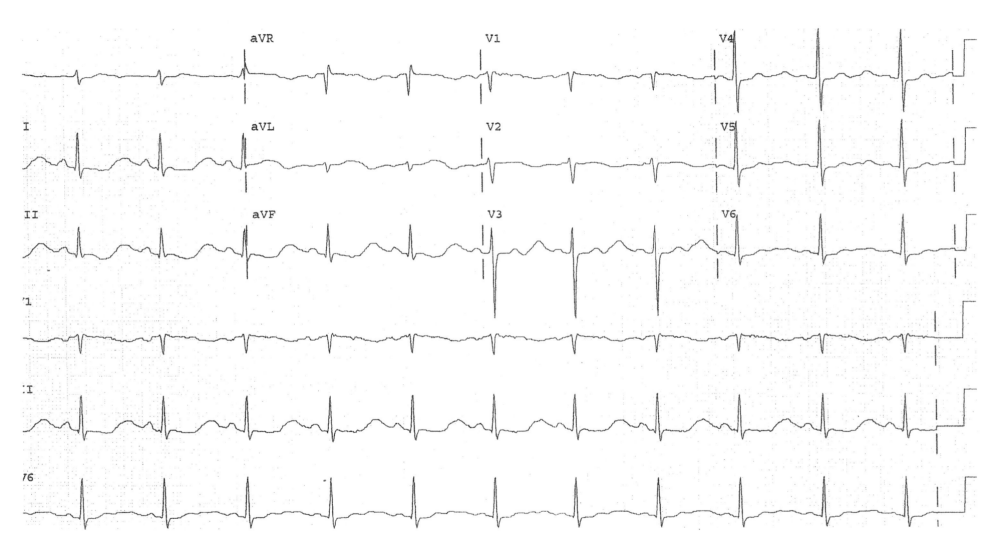

9

Computer: 73 yrs   Female White

```
PR     185   = Normal sinus rhythm, rate 67 [Remains]
QRSD    94   +  Vertical axis, unusual for age [Now Present]
QT     451   . RSR' in Vl or V2
QTc    476   = Consider left atrial enlargement [Remains)
             + QT interval long for rate [Now Present)
             + Diffuse T wave abnormalities, [Now Present)
               . .  Possible ischemia

--AXES--
P       82                        - ABNORMAL ECG -
QRS     86
T      -79
```

Comment: There are several inaccuracies in the computer's effort: There is no significant R prime in VI or V2; the QT interval, said to be prolonged, can be seen most clearly in V3 and is obviously not prolonged; we are asked to "consider" left atrial enlargement, but we certainly cannot make that diagnosis; the QT interval is said to be prolonged but is not.

But the one and only important, potentially disastrous error, is its failure to recognize the typical pattern of **hypokalemia.** Note the typical roller coaster (down-up) pattern of the T-U amalgam in leads II, III, and aVF; and U wave towering over the T wave in leads V3 and V4. The patient's potassium was 2.3 mEq/L.

The QT interval is often thought to be prolonged in hypokalemia because the end of the T wave in many/most leads is unrecognizable (because of the "T-U amalgam" referred to above) and so the U wave is incorporated in the Q-T measurement. In this tracing the best leads for recognizing where the T waves end are V3 and V 4, and in these leads it is evident that the QT is well within its normal range.

10

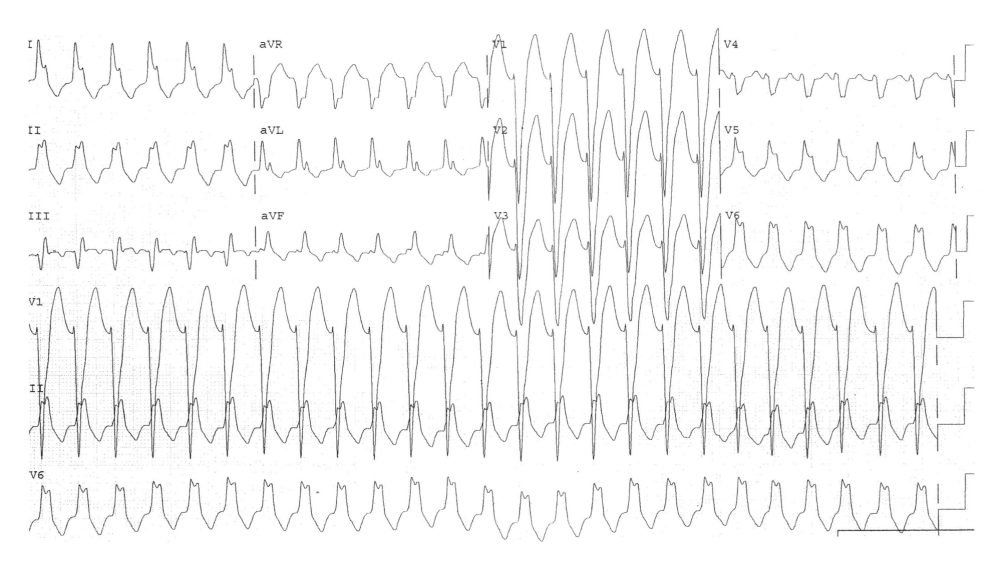

10

Computer: 54 yrs   Male White

```
PR              (VTACH) + VENTRICULAR TACHYCARDIA, rate = 152.- - - - - - V-rate > 150, QRSD > 150 ms
QRSD  161               No further analysis will be attempted [Now Present]

QT    335       (LBBB ) - [Now Absent] Left bundle branch block
QTc   533

--AXES--
P                                        - ABNORMAL ECG -
QRS    31
T     219
```

Comment: Although one cannot claim absolute certainty in the diagnosis, without doubt the probability is overwhelming-this tachycardia has all the hallmarks of **supraventricular tachycardia** with **LBBB.**

First we see that the patient previously ("now absent") had LBBB. Second, his QRS in lead VI has one of the most characteristic features of LBBB, namely a slick downstroke reaching the nadir in less than 0.06 s well within the first half of the 0.16 s wide complex. And third, all the other V leads sport QRS complexes that are certainly consistent with LBBB. Thus, the reasonable diagnosis to make is an SVT with LBBB and not ventricular tachycardia.

11

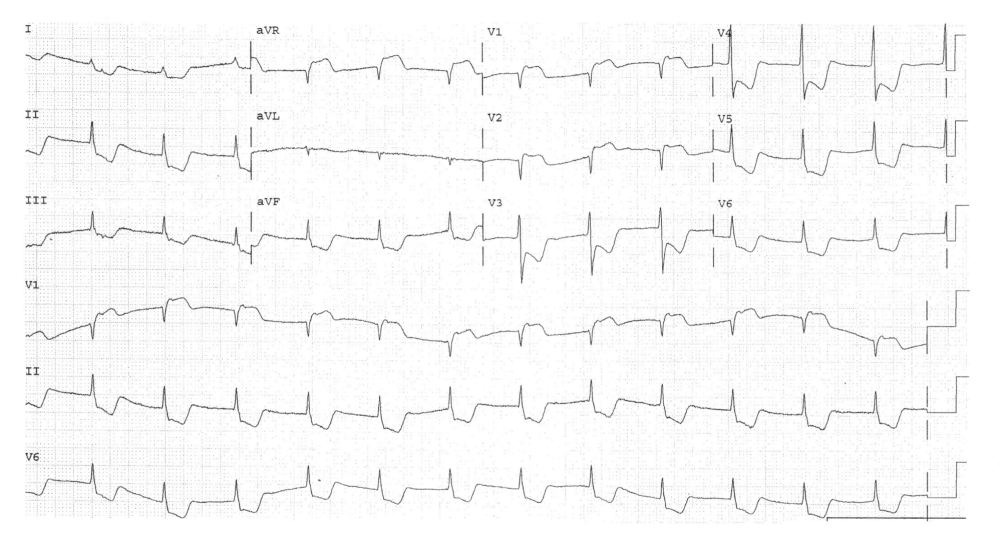

11

Computer: 68 yrs   Female

```
PR     202   + Diffuse St-T abnormalities, [Now Present]
QRSD    73   . . Also c/w ischemia &/or subendo, injury
QT     397   - [Now Absent] sinus bradycardia, rate 49
QTc    449

--AXES--
P      214                          - ABNORMAL ECG -
QRS     74
T      232
```

Comment: The computer suggests a borderline PR interval of 0.202 s, but as far as we can see there are no P waves and therefore no PR intervals (it is just possible that the last little positive part of the QRS in leads VI and V2 and tiny negative part in leads 2, 3 and a VF are the tail ends of retrograde P waves); in any case, the rhythm is clearly A V junctional at a rate of about 78/min-accelerated A V **junctional rhythm.**

   QS complexes with ST elevations in VI and V2 accompanied by reciprocal ST depressions in other leads are clear evidence of an **acute anteroseptal infarction.**

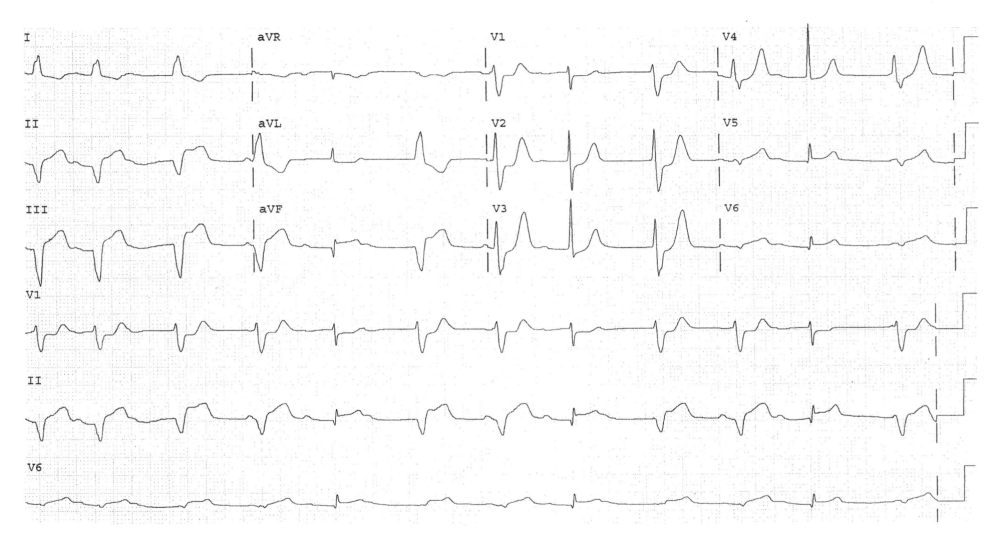

12

Computer: 29 yrs   Male Hispanic

        PR   236   + Sinus arrhythmia, Rate from 74 to 118 [Now Present]
        QRSD   71   + First degree AV block [Now Present]
        QT   335   + Probable Acute Inf. MI w /reciprocal ST dep [Now Present]
        QTc   403

        --AXES--
        P   56   - ABNORMAL ECG -
        QRS   6
        T   41

Comment: The computer's scant effort is indeed correct-the main diagnosis is an acute inferolateral myocardial infarction. But much additional diagnostic detail is omitted.

   The strip begins with an irregular accelerated idioventricular rhythm (AIVR at a rate about 68/min), dissociated from the sinus (rate about 90/min) which captures the ventricles in the 5th beat revealing the inferior infarct (though already recognizable in the ST - T pattern of the AIVR beats); this capture beat is conducted with a prolonged PR interval of 0.33 s (first degree A V block). The sequence of two AIVR beats followed by a conducted sinus beat is then repeated twice before the strip ends with a final independent beat.

13

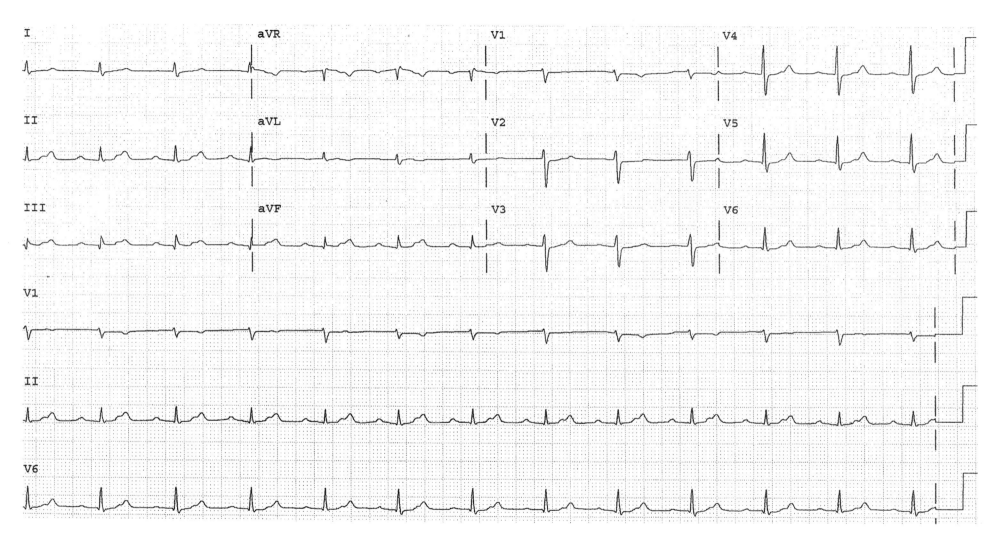

13

Computer: 72 yrs   Female White

```
PR    199   = Normal sinus rhythm, rate 80 [Remains]
QRSD   81   = Low voltage in frontal leads [Remains]
QT    366   + Nonspecific Anterolateral region T abnormalities [Now Present]
QTc   422    *Since previous tracing - no significant change

--AXES--
P      73                        - ABNORMAL ECG -
QRS    29
T      77
```

Comment: The important oversight here is an **atrial tachycardia** at 160/min with **2:1** A V **block,** not recognized by the computer, but easily spotted with the naked eye.

Index

A

Abdomen, acute, 45
Aberration, 109, 111,114, 115, 116, 134, 178, 237
Abnormality, left atrial, 82
Accelerated junctional rhythm, 131
   ventricular rhythm, 263
Accessory pathway, 46, 110, 221, 253, 296-320
   concealed, 225
Activation, WPW, 47
Acute pancreatitis, 277
  pericarditis, 286-87
  perimyocarditis, 370
Adenosine, 110, 205, 209, 215, 299, 315
Adipose insulation, 373
Alternation, electrical, 222-25, 301, 312, 372, 375
  repolarization, 239
Amyloid, 35,108
Angina, Prinzmetal's, 35, 44
Anorexia nervosa, 164
Antidromic tachycardia, 254, 309
Antihistamine, 275
Aortic valve stenosis, 85
Arrhythmia, sinus, 179
Artifact, motion, 89, 354, 358
Ashman phenomenon, 114, 115, 237
Atropine, 23
Athletes, ECG of, 270
Atrial fibrillation, 197- 99
Atrial flutter, 155, 200-06
Atrial kick, 321
Atrial tachycardia, 190
  multifocal, 196
  with block, 191
Atrial-tracking, 339
A-V block, 25

type I, 138
type II, 139
Axis, deviation, 6, 10, 50-57, 102
  left, 52
  right, 94
  indeterminate, 9
  mean, 16

B

Bachman's bundle, 80
Bezold-Jarisch reflex, 22, 23
Bigemini, 65
  atrial, 92, 112
  escape-capture, 22
  ventricular, 232-33, 380
Blanking period, 327
Block, A-V, 64,137- 59
  2:1, 79
  complete, 140, 148
  Type I, 149
  Type II, 146
  Wenckebach, 145, 203
  bifascicular, 72,-77
  bundle-branch, 49, 58-79
  bilateral, 153
  bifascicular, 33, 49, 50, 100, 102, 113
Bradycardia, 129
  sinus, 21
Brugada syndrome, 381
Bundle of His, 49
  of Kent, 296, 300

C

Cannon A wave, 239, 240
Capture beat, 119, 126, 239
Carcinoma, bronchogenic, 167, 372